ETHNOPHARMACOLOGY
Recent Advances

ETHNOPHARMACOLOGY
Recent Advances

Editors

Prof (Dr). P. Pushpangadan

Ph. D., FBRS, FES, FNSE, FNESA, FNAASc, FNASc.

Director General

Amity Institute for Herbal and Biotech Products Development

Trivandurm

Dr. V. George

Ph.D, FNSE, FABMS

Deputy Director and Head, Department of Phytochemistry and Phytopharmacology, Tropical Botanic Garden and Research Institute, Palode, Thiruvananthapuram

Dr. K.K. Janardhanan

Ph.D, FPSI, FNSE

Professor, Department of Microbiology, Amala Cancer Research Centre, Thrissur

2008

DAYA PUBLISHING HOUSE

Delhi - 110 035

ISBN10 81-7035-564-8
ISBN13 978-81-7035-564-9

Published by : **Daya Publishing House**
1123/74, Deva Ram Park
Tri Nagar, Delhi - 110 035
Phone: (011) 27383999
Fax: (011) 23260116
e-mail : dayabooks@vsnl.com
website : www.dayabooks.com

Showroom : 4760-61/23, Ansari Road, Darya Ganj,
New Delhi - 110 002
Phone: 23245578, 23244987

Laser Typesetting : **Classic Computer Services**
Delhi - 110 035

Printed at : **Chawla Offset Printers**
Delhi - 110 052

PRINTED IN INDIA

Acknowledgement

The present volume is a compilation of selected lectures presented in the 4th National Conference of the National Society of Ethnopharmacology and the International Conference on Ethnopharmacology and Alternative Medicine organized jointly by Amala Cancer Research Centre, Thrissur, Kerala, India and the National Society of Ethnopharmacology. This conference was meticulously planned and organized by the faculty and students of Amala Cancer Research Centre. We, therefore, express our sincere thanks to Rev.Fr. George Pius, Managing Director, Amala Hospital and Research Centre, and Amala Institute of Medical Sciences for his help, support and encouragements. We are also grateful to Rev. Fr. Gabriel, Founder Director, Amala Hospital and Research Centre for his blessings and Rev.Fr.Francies Kurissery, Rev.Fr.Sales, Rev.Fr.Deljo Puthoor for their support and Dr. Ramadasan Kuttan, Research Director, Amala Cancer Research Centre for his cooperation. We have great pleasure to acknowledge the whole hearted involvement of Dr. T.A. Ajith and B. Nitha, C.R. Meera, Thulasi G. Pillai, Mathew John, V.R. Vineesh, P.V. Fijesh and other research students in the successful conduct of the conference.

We acknowledge the support and co-operation of all the contributors of the articles in this volume. We specially thank them for the timely delivery of the articles. The assistance rendered by Sri. J. Anil John, Technical Officer, TBGRI, Palode, Thiruvananthapuram, for compilation and editing is gratefully acknowledged.

We sincerely thank M/s. Daya Publishing House, New Delhi for the neat and timely production of this volume.

Editors

Preface

Ever since Efron *et al.* introduced the term Ethnopharmacology in 1967, this new branch of Science has grown into a vibrant and dynamic scientific discipline during the past four decades. Ethnopharmacology as defined by Bruhn and Holmstedt (1981) is 'the interdisciplinary scientific exploration of biologically active agents traditionally employed or observed by man'. All ancient cultures and civilizations developed and fostered their own therapeutic systems, making use of the locally available bioresources and inorganic materials, through empirical observations and inference. They also attempted to provide rational explanations and interpretations to the prophylactic and curative properties of the drugs employed by them. Over the millennia, the accumulated knowledge were codified and edited into excellent treatises which has come down to us as the authoritative texts of the classical systems of medicine such as Ayurveda, Siddha, Unani, Amchi and the Chinese, Egyptian and Greek systems of medicine. Parallel to these classical systems of medicine which were mainly accessible to the urban elite and the nobility, the common village and tribal folks maintained a living, vibrant and down to earth healing art, transmitted to succeeding generations through the oral tradition.

Traditional medicines, both classical and oral, possess the advantage of having time tested remedies whose efficacy has been established by empirical observations. Ethnopharmacological research is chiefly targeted on traditionally used formulations and their ingredients. Ethnomedical knowledge which is normally community based, location specific or sometimes family based or individualized is a valuable resource base for ethnopharmacological investigations. Having realized the intrinsic value of traditional knowledge on plants used for food and medicine by various cultures, there has been a growing interest in the scientific community engaged in bioprospecting for drug development to gain access to this valuable knowledge base. This was further quickened by the fact that several laboratories from around the world reported a higher positive hit rate in their screening programmes, when they selected the target plants on the basis of their use in traditional medicine. As a result the positive hit rate of 0.001 normally obtained in most of the laboratories on random screening was substantially raised to a thousand fold on traditional knowledge based screening. This has considerably reduced the cost of screening resulting in saving of resources and manpower.

Having realized the immense value of traditional knowledge on plants used for food and medicine, several nations have brought in legislation for protection of such knowledge base, especially in the current IPR regime, conferring ownership rights to communities, societies and nations with a view to safeguard the interest of the custodians of traditional knowledge.

The great progress and impact that ethnopharmacological research has brought to mankind can be gauged by the number of novel bioactive molecules discovered from traditionally used medicinal and animal products. A few noteworthy examples are the discovery of artemisinin from *Artemisia annua*, quinine from *Cinchona* bark, vincristine and vinblastine from *Catharanthus roseus*, morphine from *Papaver somniferum* etc. Ethnopharmacologic research thus aims at scientific validation of traditional knowledge and development of new useful products through science and technology intervention.

The National Society of Ethnopharmacology established in a meeting of like minded people held in 1986 at Regional Research Laboratory, Jammu, has been in the forefront for promoting ethnopharmacological research in academic institutions and in research laboratories. Today several universities and research institutions are conducting M. Phil. and Ph. D. programmes in ethnopharmacology. The Society has organised four National Seminars and one International Seminar during the past 20 years. The Society has over 100 life members besides ordinary and student members. The Society has conferred Fellowships on 15 distinguished Scientists in recognition of their significant contribution for the advancement of ethnopharmacology. The book 'Glimpses of Ethnopharmacology' published by the Society was widely acclaimed by the Reviewers and the Scientific Communities. The present Volume is the second in the series. We hope this compilation will be welcomed by all those who are interested in the study and research in ethnopharmacology.

Editors

Contents

List of Contributors

Ahmed, Firoj
Pharmacy Discipline, Life Science School, Khulna University, Khulna – 9208, Bangladesh

Ajith, T.A.
Department of Biochemistry, Amala Institute of Medical Sciences, Amala Nagar, Thrissur, Kerala, India – 680 555

Balaram, Prabha
Division of Cancer Research, Regional Cancer Centre, Thiruvananthapuram – 695 011, Kerala, India
E-mail: prabhabalaram@yahoo.co.in; Phone: 0471-2522203

Bayry, Jagadeesh
INSERM U681, Université Pierre et Marie Curie, (UPMC – Paris 6), Institut des Cordeliers, Paris, France

Correa, Hernan
Vanderbilt University Medical School (Department of Pathology), Nashville, TN

Craver, Randall
LSUHSC and Children's Hospital of New Orleans (Department of Pathology)

Das, A.K.
Pharmacy Discipline, Life Science School, Khulna University, Khulna – 9208, Bangladesh

Das, Dipak K.
Cardiovascular Research Center, University of Connecticut School of Medicine, Farmington, Connecticut, 6030 1110, USA
E-mail: ddas@neuron.uchc.edu

Das, Samarjit
Cardiovascular Research Center, University of Connecticut School of Medicine, Farmington, Connecticut, 6030 1110, USA

Delignat, Sandrine
INSERM U681, Université Pierre et Marie Curie, (UPMC – Paris 6), Institut des Cordeliers, Paris, France

Elluru, Sriramulu
NSERM U681, Université Pierre et Marie Curie, (UPMC – Paris 6), Institut des Cordeliers, Paris, France Universite de Technologie, Compeiegne, France

Evangeline McKinnon
LSUHSC and The Children's Research Institute (Department of Pediatric Research), 200 Henry Clay Avenue, New Orleans 70118

Gardner, Renee Vanessa
Louisiana State University Health Sciences Center and Children's Hospital of New Orleans (LSUHSC; Department of Pediatrics), 200 Henry Clay Avenue, New Orleans, Louisiana 70118, USA

George, V.
Phytochemistry and Phytopharmacology Division, Tropical Botanic Garden and Research Institute, Pacha-Palode, Thiruvananthapuram, Kerala, India
E-mail: georgedrv@yahoo.co.in

Govindarajan, R.
National Botanical Research Institute, Lucknow, U.P.

Hari Kumar. K.B.
Amala Cancer Research Centre, Amala Nagar, Thrissur – 680 555, Kerala, India
Tel-91-487-2304190; Fax-91-48-2304030

Houghton, Peter J.
Department of Pharmacy, Pharmacognosy Research Laboratories, King's College London, Franklin-Wilkins Building, 150 Stamford Street, London SE1 9NH, UK

Janardhanan, K.K.
Department of Microbiology, Amala Cancer Research Centre, Amala Nagar, Thrissur, Kerala, India – 680 555
E-mail: kkjanardhanan@yahoo.com

John, J. Anil
Phytochemistry and Phytopharmacology Division, Tropical Botanic Garden and Research Institute, Pacha-Palode, Thiruvananthapuram, Kerala, India

Karunagaran, D.
Indian Institute of Technology Madras, Chennai – 600036
E-mail: karuna@iitm.ac.in

Kaveri, Srini V.
INSERM U681, Université Pierre et Marie Curie, (UPMC – Paris 6), Institut des Cordeliers, Paris, France

Kazatchkine, Michel D.
INSERM U681, Université Pierre et Marie Curie, (UPMC – Paris 6), Institut des Cordeliers, Paris, France

Kumar, V.
School of Natural Product Studies, Department of Pharmaceutical Technology, Jadavpur University, Kolkata – 700 032, India

Kuttan, Girija
Amala Cancer Research Centre, Amala Nagar, Thrissur – 680 555, Kerala, India
Tel-91-487-2304190; Fax-91-48-2304030

Kuttan, Ramadasan
Amala Cancer Research Centre, Amala Nagar, Thrissur – 680 555, Kerala, India
Tel-91-487-2304190; Fax-91-48-2304030

Latha, P.G.
Tropical Botanic Garden and Research Institute, Trivandrum – 695 562, Kerala

Maheshwari, Radha K.
Birla Institute of Technology and Science, Pilani 333031, India
E-mail: rmaheshwari@usuhs.mil

Mehrotra, Shanta
Pharmacognosy and Ethnopharmacology Division, National Botanical Research Institute, Lucknow – 226001, India

Mukherjee, Pulok K.
School of Natural Product Studies, Department of Pharmaceutical Technology, Jadavpur University, Kolkata – 700 032, India
E-mail: pknatprod@yahoo.co.in

Nair, C.K.K.
Department of Radiation Biology, Amala Cancer Research Centre, Thrissur – 680 555, Kerala, India
E-mail: ckknair@yahoo.com

Oommen, Suby
Rajiv Gandhi Centre for Biotechnology, Thiruvananthapuram, Kerala – 695 014

Paliwal, G.S.
NRO: NAEB, Ministry of Environment & Forests, B–1/9, Janakpuri, New Delhi – 110 058

Paliwal, Poonam
Department of Botany, I.P. College, Bulandshahr (U.P.)
E-mail: paliwalgk1@rediffmail.com

Preethi, K.C.
Amala Cancer Research Centre, Amala Nagar, Thrissur – 680 555, Kerala, India
Tel-91-487-2304190; Fax-91-48-2304030

Prost, Fabienne
INSERM U681, Université Pierre et Marie Curie, (UPMC – Paris 6), Institut des Cordeliers, Paris, France

Pushpangadan, P.
Amity Institute for Herbal and Biotech Products Development, TC 10/910 (1), VRA-173, Mannamoola, Peroorkada, Trivandrum – 695 005, Kerala, India

Rajasekharan, S.
Division of Ethnomedicine and Ethnopharmacology, Tropical Botanic Garden and Research Institute, Palode, Thiruvananthapuram – 695 562
E-mail: ethmed_tbgri@yahoo.co.in

Rajendran, K.
Department of Pharmacognosy, Manipal College of Pharmaceutical Sciences, Manipal – 576 104, Karnataka, India

Rao, Ch. V.
Ethnopharmacology Division, National Botanical Research Institute, (Council of Scientific and Industrial Research) Rana Pratap Marg, Post Box No: 436, Lucknow – 226 001, Uttar Pradesh, India
E-mail: chvrao72@yahoo.com

Rawat, A.K.S.
Pharmacognosy and Ethnopharmacology Division, National Botanical Research Institute, Lucknow – 226001, India

Sadowska-Krowicka, Halina

Sairam, T.V.
Customs, Excise and Service Tax Appellate Tribunal (CESTAT) Member, West Block No. 2, R.K. Puram, New Delhi – 110 066
E-mail: tvsairam@rediffmail.com

Shahid, Z.
Department of Pharmacy, Jahangirnagar University, Savar, Bangladesh

Sharma, A.K.
Forest Research Institute, Dehradun, Uttaranchal

Sharma, Anuj
Department of Pathology, Uniformed Services University of the Health Sciences, 4301 Jones Bridge Road, Bethesda, MD 20814, USA

Shilpi, J.A.
Pharmacy Discipline, Life Science School, Khulna University, Khulna – 9208, Bangladesh

Shirwaikar, Annie
E-mail: annieshirwaikar@yahoo.com

Sreelekha, T.T.
Division of Cancer Research, Regional Cancer Centre, Thiruvananthapuram – 695 011, Kerala, India
E-mail: lekhasree64@yahoo.co.in; Phone: 0471-2522378

Srivastava, Sharad
Pharmacognosy and Ethnopharmacology Division, National Botanical Research Institute, Lucknow – 226001, India
E-mail: sharad_ks2003@yahoo.com; Phone: 91-9415082210; Fax: 91-522-2207219

Sunila, E.S.
Amala Cancer Research Centre, Amala Nagar, Thrissur – 680 555, Kerala, India
Tel-91-487-2304190; Fax-91-48-2304030

Thangapazham, Rajesh L.
Department of Pathology, Uniformed Services University of the Health Sciences, 4301 Jones Bridge Road, Bethesda, MD 20814, USA

Van Huyen, Jean-Paul Duong
INSERM U681, Université Pierre et Marie Curie, (UPMC – Paris 6), Institut desCordeliers, Paris, France,Department of Pathology, Hôpital Européen Georges Pompidou, Paris, France

Venugopal, C. Nimita
Amala Cancer Research Centre, Amala Nagar, Thrissur – 680 555, Kerala, India
Tel-91-487-2304190; Fax-91-48-2304030

Vijayan, K.K.
Department of Chemistry, University of Calicut, Thenjipalam, Kerala, India

Warrier, Rajasekharan
Louisiana State University Health Sciences Center and Children's Hospital of New Orleans (LSUHSC; Department of Pediatrics), 200 Henry Clay Avenue, New Orleans, Louisiana 70118, USA

Chapter 1

Mechanisms of Apoptosis Induced by Garlic-Derived Components

D. Karunagaran* and Suby Oommen

Rajiv Gandhi Centre for Biotechnology, Thiruvananthapuram, Kerala–695 014

ABSTRACT

The anticancer properties of garlic have been recognized for centuries and organosulfur compounds of garlic are believed to account for these properties. Major organosulfur compounds derived from garlic include allicin, ajoene, diallyl sulfide (DAS), diallyl disulfide (DADS) and diallyl trisulfide (DATS). We found that allicin inhibited the growth of cancer cells of murine and human origin. Allicin induced the formation of apoptotic bodies and a typical DNA ladder in cancer cells. Furthermore, activation of caspases-3,–8, and–9 and cleavage of poly (ADP-ribose) polymerase were induced by allicin. Our results provide a mechanistic basis for the antiproliferative effects of allicin and partly account for the chemopreventive action of garlic extracts. To understand the antiproliferative and apoptotic effects of allicin metabolites such as DAS, DADS and DATS, cancer cells of diverse origin were treated with these drugs at various concentrations for a fixed time interval. DAS, DADS and DATS were shown to inhibit the proliferation of these cell lines in a cell type specific manner. DAS, DADS and DATS treated cells were analyzed for their effects on the regulation of key proteins that are involved in apoptosis such as p53 and Bax. Further studies are needed to understand the mechanisms of apoptosis induced by garlic components.

Introduction

Garlic (*Allium sativum*), a member of the Liliaceae family, is one of the earliest documented plants for its varied uses and texts of ancient times endorsed its usage in

* *Present address*: Indian Institute of Technology, Chennai – 600036; E-mail: karuna@iitm.ac.in

medicine and also for religious purposes [1]. Egyptians, Greeks, Chinese and Indians used garlic for centuries for treating various ailments such as heart disease, arthritis, pulmonary complaints, abdominal growths (particularly uterine), diarrhoea, and worm infestation [1, 2].

Extensive research on garlic points to the fact that major biological effects of garlic can be attributed to the innumerable chemical compounds present within garlic [3, 4]. Garlic is rich in organosulfur compounds and more than 33 different organosulfur compounds are present within garlic (Figure 1.1). Many of the organosulfur compounds, the major active principles in garlic, inhibit the proliferation of cancer cells and some of them induce apoptosis in tumor cells of different tissue origin [5-9]. Allicin is one of the major organosulfur compounds produced in freshly crushed garlic and is responsible for its characteristic odour. It is biologically very

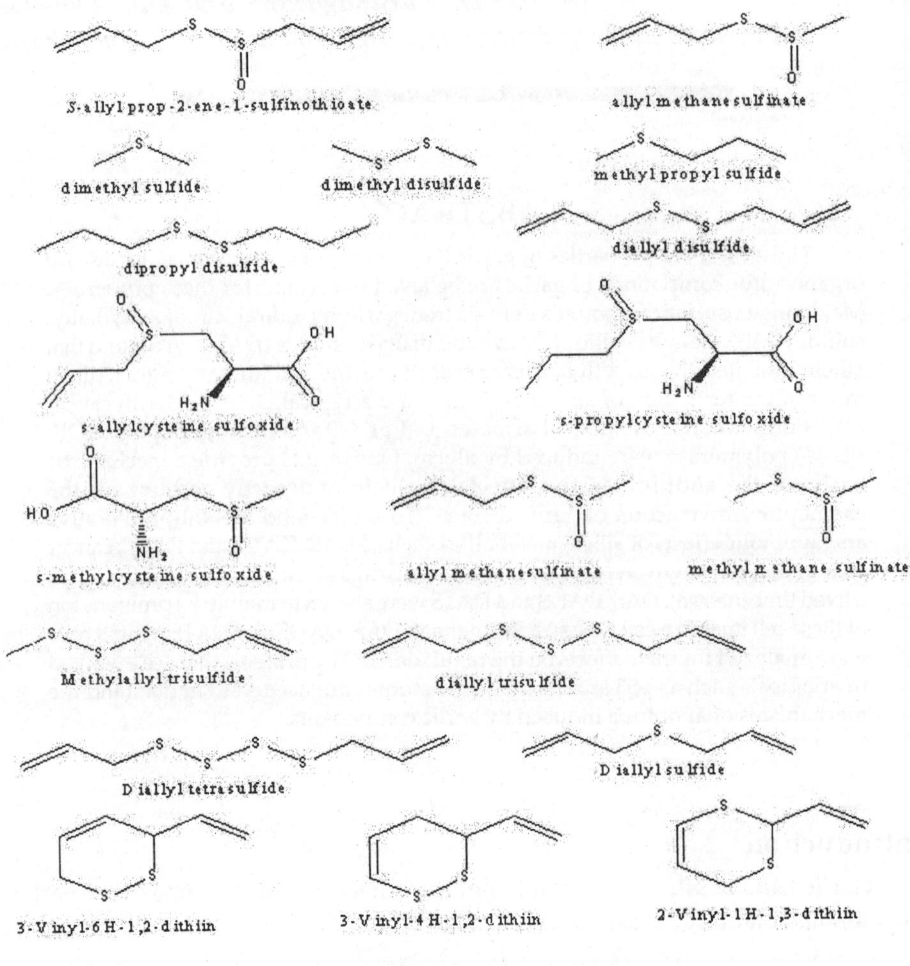

Figure 1.1: Structures of Major Organosulfur Compounds Derived from Garlic

active but is highly unstable and decomposes into mostly diallyl disulfide (DADS), diallyl trisulfide (DATS), ajoene, S-allyl mercapto cysteine, S-allyl cysteine and vinyl dithiines [5, 9-12]. Our group has recently reported that allicin inhibits the growth of cancer cells of murine and human origin [13]. Allicin induced the formation of apoptotic bodies, nuclear condensation and a typical DNA ladder in cancer cells. Furthermore, activation of caspases-3,–8 and–9 and cleavage of poly (ADP-ribose) polymerase were induced by allicin [13]. These results demonstrating allicin-induced apoptosis of cancer cells are novel since allicin has not been shown to induce apoptosis previously. We continued this work essentially focusing on the metabolites of allicin such as DAS, DADS and DATS. Our preliminary data suggest that DATS can efficiently induce apoptosis of cancer cells and is a more effective inducer of apoptosis than DADS and DAS. However, the mechanism of apoptosis is not clear at present.

Materials and Methods

Cell Culture and Maintenance

SiHa cells (human cervical cancer cell line) were obtained from Dr. Sudhir Krishna, National Centre for Biological Sciences, Bangalore, India. L-929 (murine fibrosarcoma), SW480 (human colon cancer) and HeLa (human cervical cancer) cell lines were obtained from the National Centre for Cell Science, Pune, India. The cells were grown in monolayer culture in Dulbecco's Modified Eagle's Medium (Life Technologies Inc, USA) containing 10 per cent fetal bovine serum (Sigma, USA) and antibiotics (100 U/ml penicillin and 100 µg/ml streptomycin) in a humidified atmosphere of 5 per cent CO_2 at 37°C.

Reagents and Antibodies

Allicin (Flavourcin™ 1500) was a gift from Brittania Natural Products Limited, UK, (presently known as Overseal Foods Limited) and involved alliin synthesis and converting this to allicin with allinase (purified from garlic) immobilized on an inert support [14, 15]. Purified allicin (1 mg/mL in 50 mM phosphate buffer, pH 4.5) used by us was stable (due to the low pH and conditions used in the manufacturing process that involved immediate removal of the reactants after product formation preventing its contact with other components) with 20 per cent loss after 3 weeks at ambient temperature and no loss of activity at 4°C up to 10 weeks. Antibodies to caspases-8 and–9, and poly (ADP-ribose) polymerase were purchased from Cell Signaling Inc, USA. Enhanced chemiluminescence (ECL) detection kit was procured from USB, Amersham, UK.

Cell Viability Assay

Cell viability assays were carried out as described with slight modifications [16]. Briefly, cells were seeded at a density of 3×10^4 cells/well into 24-well plates. After 24 h, allicin was added to the medium at various concentrations and incubated for 24 h as indicated. At the end of the incubation, 50 ìL of 3-(4-5 dimethylthiozol-2-yl) 2-5diphenyl-tetrazolium bromide (MTT) (2 mg/ml) per well was added and the formazan crystals formed were solubilized in acidified isopropanol after aspirating the medium. The extent of MTT reduction was measured spectrophotometrically at 570 nm and the cell survival was expressed as percentage over the untreated control.

Terminal Deoxynucleotidyl Transferase Mediated Biotin dUTP Nick End Labeling (TUNEL) Assay

To detect apoptotic cells, *in situ* end labelling of the 3'OH end of the DNA fragments generated by apoptosis associated endonucleases was performed using the Dead End apoptosis detection kit (TUNEL assay) from Promega (Madison, USA). Briefly, the cells were grown in cover slips and treated with allicin for 24 h. The cells were washed in phosphate buffered saline and fixed by immersing the slides in 4 per cent paraformaldehyde for 25 min. All the steps were performed at room temperature, unless otherwise specified. They were then washed twice by immersing in fresh phosphate buffered saline for 5 min. Cells were permeabilised with 0.2 per cent Triton X-100 solution in phosphate buffered saline for 5 min, washed twice in phosphate buffered saline, and then covered with 100 µl of equilibration buffer and kept for 5-10 min. The equilibrated areas were blotted around with tissue paper and 100 µL of terminal deoxynucleotidyl transferase (TdT) reaction mix was added to the sections on the slide and were then incubated at 37°C for 60 min inside a humidified chamber for the end labelling reaction to occur. Immersing the slides in 2X SSC for 15 min terminated the reactions. The slides were washed thrice, by immersing in fresh phosphate buffered saline, for 5 min to remove unincorporated biotinylated nucleotides. The endogenous peroxidase activity was blocked by immersing the slides in 0.3 per cent H_2O_2. After washing, Horseradish-peroxidase-labeled streptavidin solution was applied, and the slides were incubated for 30 min. After incubation, the color was developed with the peroxidase substrate (hydrogen peroxide) and the stable chromogen (Diaminobenzidine). The slides were then mounted and examined with a light microscope.

DNA Fragmentation Assay

SiHa cells were seeded in 60 mm petridishes at a seeding density of 4×10^5 cells/plate and treated with allicin or tetradecanoyl phorbol acetate or without any treatment for 48 h. Tetradecanoyl phorbol acetate treated cells were taken as positive control. The cells were harvested and washed with phosphate buffered saline. The oligonucleosomal DNA fragments were isolated and analysed as described previously [16]. DNA in the gels was visualized under ultraviolet light after staining with ethidium bromide.

Western Blot Analysis

The cells treated with or without allicin were washed with phosphate buffered saline and lysed in ice-cold radioimmunoprecipitation buffer (10 mM Phenyl Methyl Sulfonyl Fluoride, 1 µg/mL of aprotinin, 100 mM EGTA, 100 mM sodium orthovanadate and 100 mM Dithiothreitol). Whole cell extracts (60 µg protein) were resolved on sodium dodecyl sulphate–poly acrylamide gel electrophoresis, transferred to a nitrocellulose membrane, probed with corresponding antibodies to caspase-8 or–9, or poly (ADP-ribose) polymerase and detected by Enhanced Chemiluminescense (ECL) as per the manufacturer's protocol (USB, Amersham, U. K.).

Results

Allicin-mediated Inhibition of Cell Growth

L-929, SW480 and HeLa cells were treated with or without allicin for 24 h as indicated and the cell viability assayed by MTT (expressed as percentage over control) decreased with increase in the concentration of allicin (Figure 1.2). Most of the cancer cells taken up in the present study were killed with 100 µM concentration of allicin (data not shown). We carried out all the experiments using aliquots of a single batch of allicin showing similar pattern and extent of growth inhibition over a range of

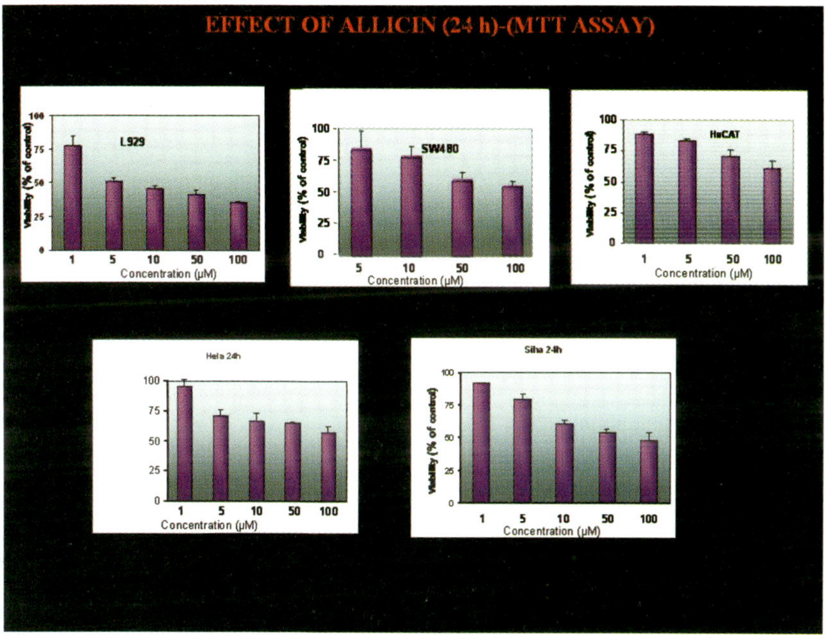

Figure 1.2: Inhibition of Cell Viability of Allicin-treated Cancer Cells

A. HeLa, SW480 and L-929 grown in 96-well plates were treated with or without the indicated concentrations of allicin and incubated for 24 h. At the end of the incubation, MTT was added and the cell viability was assessed by MTT assay with quadruplicate samples as described in Materials and Methods. The results are expressed as the mean percentage over control and experiments were repeated three times with similar results and the error bars indicate standard deviations. The differences among the mean values were analyzed using 1-way ANOVA and the average mean values of cell survival differed significantly as a function of concentration of allicin ($P < 0.001$).

B. Viability of SiHa cells treated with or without allicin and incubated for 24/48 h was assessed by MTT assay with quadruplicate samples as described above. The experiments were repeated three times with similar results and the error bars indicate standard deviations. The one-way ANOVA analysis revealed that the average mean values of cell survival differed significantly as a function of concentration of allicin ($P < 0.001$).

allicin concentrations by MTT assay. DNA synthesis as measured by the incorporation of labeled thymidine was also decreased by allicin in a concentration dependent manner in cancer cells (data not shown). These results indicate that allicin inhibits the proliferation of cancer cells in a concentration and time-dependent manner.

DNA Fragmentation is Induced by Allicin

The degradation of DNA into multiple internucleosomal fragments of 180-200 base pairs is a distinct biochemical hallmark for apoptosis. To confirm whether the effects induced by allicin in cancer cells involve DNA fragmentation, it was assessed by agarose gel electrophoresis and TUNEL assays. For DNA fragmentation assay, the nuclear DNA isolated from cells was separated by agarose gel electrophoresis and stained with ethidium bromide and a typical ladder formation was observed upon 24 h treatment with 1 μM allicin or 50 ng/mL tetradecanoyl phorbol acetate (positive control) in SiHa cells, whereas the untreated cells did not show a typical ladder (Figure 1.3). Allicin also induced DNA fragmentation in a similar way in L-929 cells (data not shown). SiHa cells without allicin did not show a positive TUNEL reaction whereas the cells treated with allicin (50 μM) incorporated the labeled nucleotide into DNA (Figure 1.4).

Activation of Caspases and Poly (ADP-ribose) Polymerase Cleavage are Induced by Allicin

We analyzed the cell extracts for the cleaved forms of caspase-9 (35 and 37 kDa) by Western blotting, which significantly increased with allicin treatment compared to the control in SiHa cells (Figure 1.5A). We also detected the cleaved caspase-8 (18 kDa) upon treatment with allicin in SiHa cells but not in control (Figure 1.5B). Furthermore, we examined the cleavage of a well-characterized caspase-3 substrate, poly (ADP-ribose) polymerase, from its 116 kDa intact form into 89 kDa fragment by Western blotting. Poly (ADP-ribose) polymerase was processed to its predicted cleavage product of 89 kDa after allicin treatment, but the processing was absent in the untreated cells (Figure 1.5C). These results suggest the involvement of poly (ADP-ribose) polymerase cleavage and activation of caspase-3,–8 and –9 during allicin-induced apoptosis in SiHa cells.

Taken together, the above results suggest that allicin inhibits the growth of cancer cells and the antiproliferative effects of allicin are mediated through the induction of apoptosis characterized by DNA fragmentation. Moreover, allicin-induced apoptosis is caspase-dependent, as shown by the activation of caspases-3,–8, and–9. To understand the antiproliferative and apoptotic effects of allicin metabolites such as DAS, DADS and DATS, cancer cells of diverse origin were treated with these drugs at various concentrations for a fixed time interval. DAS, DADS and DATS inhibited the proliferation of these cell lines in a cell type specific manner (Data not shown). DAS, DADS and DATS treated cells were analyzed for their effects on the regulation of key proteins that are involved in apoptosis such as p53 and Bax. p53 was up regulated by all the three compounds (unpublished results). Further studies are needed to understand the mechanisms of apoptosis induced by garlic components.

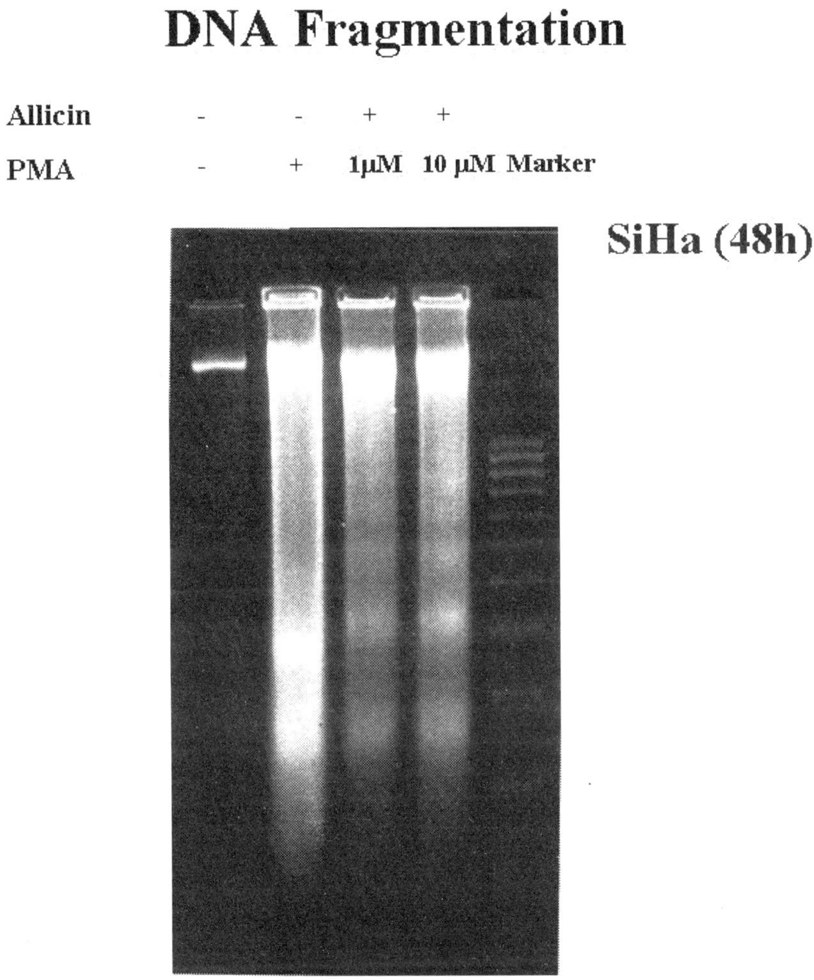

Figure 1.3: Allicin Induced DNA Fragmentation

SiHa cells grown in 60 mm petridishes were treated for 24 h with allicin (1 or 10 μM) or tetradecanoyl phorbol acetate (50 ng/ml) as positive control or left untreated (0). M denotes molecular weight marker. The cells were harvested and the oligonucleosomal DNA fragments were isolated, separated by gel electrophoresis and analysed as described under Materials and Methods. The results were similar when another experiment was carried out under the same conditions.

Discussion

The demonstration that garlic components induce apoptosis is interesting since apoptosis has been shown to be a major mechanism by which anticancer agents act. However, the unstable nature of allicin raises the question whether all the effects of allicin observed by us and others are due to allicin itself or its metabolites [10, 17].

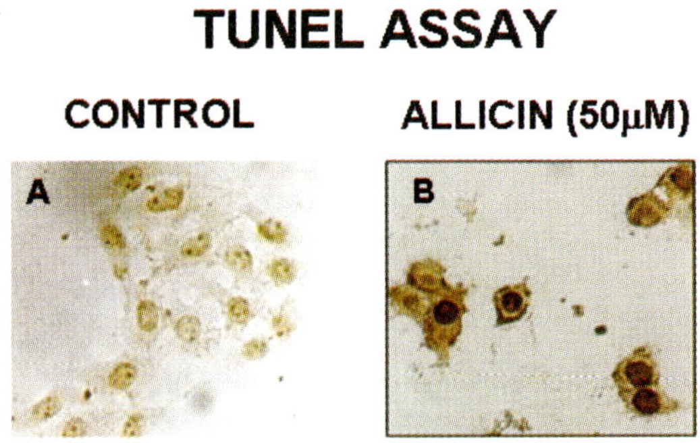

Figure 1.4: Changes in TUNEL Reactivity Induced by Allicin

SiHa cells were grown in cover slips and treated with or without allicin for 24 h. The cells were fixed, permeabilised with 0.2 per cent Triton X-100, end-labelled with terminal deoxynucleotidyl transferase reaction mix and the TUNEL reactivity was visualized as described in Materials and Methods. TUNEL reactivity of SiHa cells without (control) or with 50 μM allicin is shown. Bar = 25 μm.

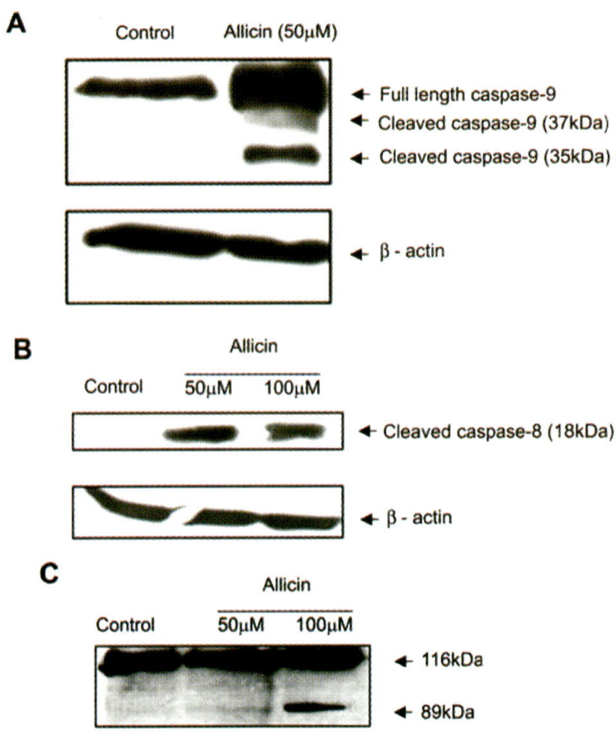

Figure 1.5: Cleavage of Caspases and Poly (ADP-ribose) Polymerase by Allicin

SiHa cells treated with or without allicin for 24 h were lysed, resolved on sodium dodecyl sulphate–poly acrylamide gel electrophoresis and Western blotting was carried out to detect the cleaved products of activation of caspase-9 or–8, or poly (ADP-ribose) polymerase shown respectively, in A, B and C. The experiments were repeated at least two times with similar results and β-actin was used as loading control.

There is evidence that allicin is formed from its metabolite, diallyl disulfide, in human liver microsomes indicating that allicin may also be acting intracellularly [18]. In agreement with the present results, allicin inhibited the proliferation of a tumorigenic lymphoid cell line [19] and purified allicin, but not its precursor, allicin, inhibited the growth of human breast, endometrial and colon cancer cell lines [10]. Antiproliferative effects of allicin were attributed to cell cycle arrest and its ability to decrease intracellular glutathione levels rather than its antioxidant activity [10]. Diallyl disulfide induces apoptosis of human leukemia HL-60 cells and triggers the generation of hydrogen peroxide, activation of caspase-3, degradation of poly (ADP-ribose) polymerase, and fragmentation of DNA [6]. Diallyl trisulfide also induces apoptosis of HL-60 cells although this was initially mistaken to be an effect of allicin [20, 21]. Other products of allicin transformation, ajoene and S-allylmercaptocysteine, also induce apoptosis in human promyeloleukemic and erythroleukemia cell lines, respectively [5, 22].

Our results support the notion that apoptosis is a potential mechanism by which allicin exerts its antiproliferative effects. However, allicin did not induce DNA degradation and poly (ADP-ribose) polymerase cleavage in MCF-7 (breast cancer) and HT-29 (colon cancer) cells [10]. MCF-7 cells are known to be deficient in caspase-3 [23] but whether that accounts for the failure of allicin to induce apoptosis in these cells is not known. Allicin-induced apoptosis is presumably regulated differently in cells with different genetic background and changes in the expression of proteins that regulate apoptosis in tumor cells could also account for the failure of allicin to induce apoptosis in certain cells. In fact, tumor cells often evade apoptosis by expressing several anti apoptotic proteins such as Bcl-2, down regulation and mutation of pro apoptotic genes and alterations of p53, PI3K/Akt or NF-κB pathways that give them survival advantage [24]. It is relevant to point out that ajoene activates NF-κB [5] and decreases Bcl-2 expression [25]. Diallyl sulfide increases the level of p53 and Bax, but decreases Bcl-2 in H460 non small cell lung cancer cells [26]. It will be of interest to study whether such pro and anti apoptotic proteins play any role in allicin-induced apoptosis.

Our results provide a mechanistic basis for the antiproliferative effects of allicin and its metabolites thus partly accounting for the chemo preventive action of garlic extracts reported by earlier workers [10, 19, 27, 28]. Further studies are still needed to understand the various mechanisms regulating the antiproliferative effects and apoptosis induced by allicin and other garlic components.

Acknowledgements

The authors are grateful to Simon Cuthbert, Overseal Foods Limited, UK, for the supply of pure allicin and Drs. Ruby John Anto, Gopal Srinivas and Santhosh Kumar, for technical advice and help. Suby Oommen is a recipient of a Senior Research Fellowship from the Council of Scientific and Industrial Research, Government of India. This study was supported by research grants from Science, Technology and Environment Committee, Government of Kerala (to D. K.) and program support to the Rajiv Gandhi Centre by the Department of Biotechnology, Government of India.

References

1. Rivlin RS: Historical perspective on the use of garlic. *J Nutr* 2001, 131, 951S-954S.
2. Rivlin RS, Budoff M, Amagase H: Significance of garlic and its constituents in cancer and cardiovascular disease. *J Nutr* 2006, 136, v.
3. Sparnins VL, Barany G, Wattenberg LW: Effects of organosulfur compounds from garlic and onions on benzo[a]pyrene-induced neoplasia and glutathione S-transferase activity in the mouse. *Carcinogenesis* 1988, 9, 131-134.
4. Wargovich MJ, Woods C, Eng VW, Stephens LC, Gray K: Chemoprevention of N-nitrosomethylbenzylamine-induced esophageal cancer in rats by the naturally occurring thioether, diallyl sulfide. *Cancer Res* 1988, 48, 6872-6875.
5. Dirsch VM, Gerbes AL, Vollmar AM: Ajoene, a compound of garlic, induces apoptosis in human promyeloleukemic cells, accompanied by generation of reactive oxygen species and activation of nuclear factor kappaB. *Mol Pharmacol* 1998, 53, 402-407.
6. Kwon KB, Yoo SJ, Ryu DG, Yang JY, Rho HW, Kim JS, Park JW, Kim HR, Park BH: Induction of apoptosis by diallyl disulfide through activation of caspase-3 in human leukemia HL-60 cells. *Biochem Pharmacol* 2002, 63, 41-47.
7. Pinto JT, Lapsia S, Shah A, Santiago H, Kim G: Antiproliferative effects of garlic-derived and other allium related compounds. *Adv Exp Med Biol* 2001, 492, 83-106.
8. Shirin H, Pinto JT, Kawabata Y, Soh JW, Delohery T, Moss SF, Murty V, Rivlin RS, Holt PR, Weinstein IB: Antiproliferative effects of S-allylmercaptocysteine on colon cancer cells when tested alone or in combination with sulindac sulfide. *Cancer Res* 2001, 61, 725-731.
9. Sigounas G, Hooker JL, Li W, Anagnostou A, Steiner M: S-allylmercaptocysteine, a stable thioallyl compound, induces apoptosis in erythroleukemia cell lines. *Nutr Cancer* 1997, 28, 153-159.
10. Hirsch K, Danilenko M, Giat J, Miron T, Rabinkov A, Wilchek M, Mirelman D, Levy J, Sharoni Y: Effect of purified allicin, the major ingredient of freshly crushed garlic, on cancer cell proliferation. *Nutr Cancer* 2000, 38, 245-254.
11. Sundaram SG, Milner JA: Impact of organosulfur compounds in garlic on canine mammary tumor cells in culture. *Cancer Lett* 1993, 74, 85-90.
12. Welch C, Wuarin L, Sidell N: Antiproliferative effect of the garlic compound S-allyl cysteine on human neuroblastoma cells in vitro. *Cancer Lett* 1992, 63, 211-219.
13. Oommen S, Anto RJ, Srinivas G, Karunagaran D: Allicin (from garlic) induces caspase-mediated apoptosis in cancer cells. *Eur J Pharmacol* 2004, 485, 97-103.
14. Eilat S, Oestraicher Y, Rabinkov A, Ohad D, Mirelman D, Battler A, Eldar M, Vered Z: Alteration of lipid profile in hyperlipidemic rabbits by allicin, an active constituent of garlic. *Coron Artery Dis* 1995, 6, 985-990.

15. Rabinkov A, Wilchek M, Mirelman D: Alliinase (alliin lyase) from garlic (Alliium sativum) is glycosylated at ASN146 and forms a complex with a garlic mannose-specific lectin. *Glycoconj J* 1995, 12, 690-698.
16. Anto RJ, Maliekal TT, Karunagaran D: L-929 cells harboring ectopically expressed RelA resist curcumin-induced apoptosis. *J Biol Chem* 2000, 275, 15601-15604.
17. Miron T, Rabinkov A, Mirelman D, Wilchek M, Weiner L: The mode of action of allicin: its ready permeability through phospholipid membranes may contribute to its biological activity. *Biochim Biophys Acta* 2000, 1463, 20-30.
18. Teyssier C, Guenot L, Suschetet M, Siess MH: Metabolism of diallyl disulfide by human liver microsomal cytochromes P-450 and flavin-containing monooxygenases. *Drug Metab Dispos* 1999, 27, 835-841.
19. Scharfenberg K, Wagner R, Wagner KG: The cytotoxic effect of ajoene, a natural product from garlic, investigated with different cell lines. *Cancer Lett* 1990, 53, 103-108.
20. Zheng S, Yang H, Zhang S, Wang X, Yu L, Lu J, Li J: Initial study on naturally occurring products from traditional Chinese herbs and vegetables for chemoprevention. *J Cell Biochem Suppl* 1997, 27, 106-112.
21. Zheng S, Yang H, Zhang S, Wang X, Yu L, Lu J, Li J: Erratum. *J Cell Biochem* 2000, 77, 125.
22. Sigounas G, Hooker J, Anagnostou A, Steiner M: S-allylmercaptocysteine inhibits cell proliferation and reduces the viability of erythroleukemia, breast, and prostate cancer cell lines. *Nutr Cancer* 1997, 27, 186-191.
23. Saunders PA, Cooper JA, Roodell MM, Schroeder DA, Borchert CJ, Isaacson AL, Schendel MJ, Godfrey KG, Cahill DR, Walz AM *et al*: Quantification of active caspase 3 in apoptotic cells. *Anal Biochem* 2000, 284, 114-124.
24. Igney FH, Krammer PH: Death and anti-death: tumour resistance to apoptosis. *Nat Rev Cancer* 2002, 2, 277-288.
25. Ahmed N, Laverick L, Sammons J, Zhang H, Maslin DJ, Hassan HT: Ajoene, a garlic-derived natural compound, enhances chemotherapy-induced apoptosis in human myeloid leukaemia CD34-positive resistant cells. *Anticancer Res* 2001, 21, 3519-3523.
26. Hong YS, Ham YA, Choi JH, Kim J: Effects of allyl sulfur compounds and garlic extract on the expression of Bcl-2, Bax, and p53 in non small cell lung cancer cell lines. *Exp Mol Med* 2000, 32,127-134.
27. Milner JA: Garlic: its anticarcinogenic and antitumorigenic properties. *Nutr Rev* 1996, 54, S82-86.
28. Siegers CP, Steffen B, Robke A, Pentz R: The effects of garlic preparations against human tumor cell proliferation. *Phytomedicine* 1999, 6, 7-11.

Chapter 2
Music Therapy: An Introduction

T.V. Sairam*
Customs, Excise and Service Tax Appellate Tribunal (CESTAT) Member
West Block No. 2, R.K. Puram, New Delhi – 110 066

"Music exalts each Joy
Allays each Grief
Expels Diseases
Softens every Pain
Subdues the rage of
Poison and the plague...."

–John Armstrong (1709-1779), The Art of Preserving Health, Book IV

The Rhythms in Life

Music is an intrinsic part of every one of us–irrespective of the fact whether we are singers or listeners. In the words of Kabir, "Nada is music which plays in the body without strings." Rhythm is the first organizing structure in the infant's experience. Modern science acknowledges that pulse and rhythmic patterns found in our heart-beat, in our breathing and in our body movements.These are just a few indicators of rhythms with which all our life-processes are intrinsically linked. There is an inherent rhythm everywhere–in and around us. If we could focus our attention, our body rhythms become transparent to us. We could feel how our breathing cycles, heart beats and our baro-receptor feedback loops are made of resonance and rhythms which simply go on and on, till the Death deprives us of them.

As far as melody goes, it is built in our laughter, cry, screams or songs–all following again a fixed rhythmic pattern. A whole range of emotions could be

E-mail: tvsairam@rediffmail.com.

captured and communicated through a wide range of rhythms, tones and melodies drawn from diverse cultural milieux and musical styles, schools and systems.

As in the case of any biological system, the nature too is made of cycles and rhythms; seasons change in a cyclic manner and life functions in a cycle of births, growth and death; a cycle without a start or an end. Within the human body itself, life-processes are carried out in a pure rhythmic fashion. Various kinds of rhythms *viz.*, endogenous rhythm, muscular rhythm, pain wave rhythm, pulse-breath frequency, rhythms involved in the processes relating to blood circulation, digestion, respiration, sleep, etc., are well known to the World of Science and Medicine.

All biological processes including our breathing, food-intake and excretion, energy exchange, metabolism, circulation, action of nerves, reproduction–follow a basic pattern in an orchestrated manner. It is interesting to note that scientists have discovered a musical symphony in the process by which chromosomes condense and segregate during mitosis (nuclear division). It is likened to a musical symphony produced by an orchestra in which several instruments working individually or in unison make an attempt to produce a collective piece of elegance and beauty–as one may come across in a Bach or a Beethoven, in a Mozart or a Mendelssohn. As a conductor ensures that each musical instrument enters the symphony at the appropriate time, with a wave of the baton so the conductors of the so-called mitotic symphony called 'checkpoints' prevent errors in chromosome segregation that can lead to disease such as Down's syndrome or cancer. (David Cortez and Stephen J Elledge 2000).

The Rhythmic Expansion

Rhythms cannot be confined to intracellular functions alone; complexities of periodic rhythms grow right from cellular levels to the tissue levels and onwards to organs and to the entire organism. The nada yogis visualize their impact even beyond the confines of their bodies on the firm belief of their influence over the Universe. The present-day Physicists are discovering that the foundation of the Universe is not just matter, particles or quartz, but movement of energy–the vibrations.

Some common rhythms in the body such as heart rate and breathing cycle could be directly experienced as we focus our awareness on them. This awareness is more pronounced particularly when one feels excruciating pain–as in toothache, when a wave of pain sweeps over the affected area, occurring in an interval of say, 15 to 30 seconds. The rhythmic pattern here is one and the same as the one, which forms our sleep cycles during the night.

Musical Rhythms and Body Rhythms

It is an age-old practice in all primitive societies wherein by drumming at the rate of 4½ beats per second, shamanic state of consciousness is induced. Recent researchers like Landereth (1974), Harrer (1977) have confirmed that slow beats modify heart rate and breathing cycle in a significant way. Listening to musical rhythms do have an impact on the brain wave rhythms, which are responsible for our level of consciousness: a stage of alertness (with the predominance in beta waves) or a state of relaxation or deep sleep (with the predominance in alpha, theta or delta waves). A musical-harmonic order called 'rhythmic functional order in humans' is responded to be intensified even when a person is sleepy. It has been experimentally found by this author in a workshop conducted at Delhi on the 22nd December 2001 before an enlightened audience, comprising of diplomats, civil servants, yoga teachers and music lovers that by manipulating the rhythmic pace a *tabla* or a *manjira* could lead one to a relaxed state. The literature on music therapy is fast building up confirming that long term musical involvement reaps cognitive rewards–in terms of linguistic skills, reasoning and creativity for enhancing social adjustments, love and peace. Music exercises the brain and playing the instruments for instance, involves vision, hearing, touch, motor planning, emotion, symbol-interpretation–all of which go to activate different areas of brain-functioning. It has been observed that some Alzheimer patients could play music even long after they have forgotten their near and dears. In the deepest and most general level, the forms of music stimulate the forms of adaptation (that is, assimilation and accommodation) which are deeply rooted in our autonomic nervous system. These intimate connections between our life-processes and music can remain despite illness or disability and are never dependent on our musical skill or mastery. Because of this, the emotional, cognitive and developmental needs of people with a wide range of problems arising from such varied causes such as learning difficulties, mental and physical ailments, physical or sexual abuse, stress, terminal illness etc., could be rationally addressed by selecting appropriate music.

Every one of us responds to music–from the new born to the patients at their death-beds and from physically or mentally strong to those who are the weaklings or impaired.

Music Therapy: A Rediscovery

It is strange that the subject of music therapy has not witnessed a revival in India in recent years. This is particularly, surprising for a nation, which had in the past, made great strides in recognizing the therapeutic impact of rhythms, resonance and melodies for the well-being of Body, Mind and Spirit. Those ragas which are therapeutic as in the ancient text of *Raga Chikitsa* were even codified and celebrated.

Music is interred with the very existence of man. It has been an inseparable companion not only to the primitive aboriginal man who feared Nature's fury but also to the contemporary man who is under constant threat by his own species. In the words of Carlyle, "music is a kind of inarticulate, unfathomable speech, which leads us to the edge of the infinite and let us for a moment gaze in that".

Even the Science that usually shows skepticism over the very existence of God is dumb before the power of music. No scientific work could question its impact on mind and consciousness or could deny its role in soothing and pacifying one's mind or in elevating one's moods. On the other hand, a formidable body of research has been built, all confirming its therapeutic, prophylactic and audio-analgesic role. In this process, even those who have sole faith in modern medicine have started coming out openly in acknowledging music as a 'complementary medicine'. Having recognized its significant role in a wide range of disorders including epilepsy, mental ailments, speech-related disorders, and terminal illness such as cancer and AIDS, music is increasingly regarded as medicine. The patients who have undergone the musical treatment would vouchsafe that they had experienced a *neo*-sense of dignity with music, during their struggle for survival. Even while awaiting one's death–as in hospitals or in hospices–the music has lent its dignity in such a way that the passage to the other world could appear more smooth and less painful.

With the publication of *Medicina Musica* by Richard Browne in 1729, music came to occupy the pride of place not only in restaurants and bars but also in shopping malls, street junctions, automobile and railway coaches etc. Its importance was recognized particularly in those places where one's patience undergoes its test *e.g.*, in queues, in waiting halls, in ICU's and CCU's, and in hospices. Several endroits, such as operation theatres, street-corners, examination halls, board rooms etc where tempers and anxiety run amok have also witnessed a sea-change after introduction of musical rhymes and rhythms.

The ancient Indian civilization, which had prescribed meditation for 'taming' the mind so as to reach into higher realms of consciousness, had also devised ways and means to tap the inherent power lying in music for holistic health. The esoteric concepts and practices of Nada Yoga or Laya Yoga not only take into account the gross resonance, captured within the sensory limitations of the human ears, *viz.*, 20 to 20,000 Hz., but also the subtle, *anahata* which is totally beyond one's sensory reach, but can be perceived by mastering the techniques in yoga.

Music or nada reveals a distinct yin-yang pattern, a characteristic common to all living systems in the universe. Here, the sound and silence–the otherwise two opposing phenomena, which stultify each other, is yoked together under a mystic canopy for their mutual interaction in producing synergy. While the acoustically driven recognizes it as a mere sound (or a tone of such-and-such frequency range), a musical *connoisseur* may find it as a marvel. For the *nada yogi*, however, it may even represent the very manifestation of God or Brahman. The synergy arising out of this strange combination of sound and silence is however considered to be the very building block that constitutes the entire Universe.

The Western Note and the Indian Swara: Affinities and Differences

In the Westerner's eyes (or, rather, ears), a note is just a note. Nothing more, nothing less. It has to be mathematically correct and mechanically precise. Take for example the amount of care and concern that go into tuning a piano. The Indian system of *ragas* on the other hand encompasses not only swaras (lit. "self-shining"), but even their partials, those stacks of sub-ordinate vibrations (semi-tones), which appear for an acute observer of resonance. In fact, it is the selective application of such harmonics to appear themselves at appropriate places, that lends a raga, its unique identity in an otherwise virtual ocean of ragas. In other words, it is just not a mere thread of tonal vibration, but a stack of sub-ordinate vibrations that go into the spinning of a raga wick. The subtle way in which the sub-ordinate vibrations in a swara encounter their counterparts in the preceding or succeeding swaras determines the *pakad*, a short cut involved in identifying a raga by presenting a musical phrase and not a sentence. It is not enough if a student is offered a notation or the solfa-syllables to master a raga. As the selected harmonics cannot be properly reflected in these, the Indian system of music is dependent on guru-sishya parampara and which again makes the Indian system of raga unique in the world of music. It is these partials in *swaras* that elevate the Indian *raga* from being a mere mechanistic melody to a lofty divine form.

Apart from lending an Indian touch to the music, it is these partials which have paved way for effective meditation. In the realm of yoga, the concentration on the *swayambhu swaras* especially during *rechaka* (exhalation) and *kumbhaka* (the interval between the incoming and outgoing breath) has heightened one's experience of one's own consciousness.

Therapeutic Traditions in Ancient Civilizations

Long before acoustics came to be studied in Europe, the ancient civilizations of the Arabs, Greeks and Indians were already aware of the prophylactic and therapeutic role of musical sounds and vibrations. While the Greek legends glorify the music that healed Ulysses from his deadly wounds, the Arabian writer Ibn Sina had recorded the therapeutic role of music in his various treatises on medicine. The Indian musician Tan Sen is said to have cured the Emperor Akbar's hypertension with his recipe: the raga yaman. It was widely known that depending on its nature, a raga could induce or intensify joy or sorrow, anger or peace and capture and communicate a whole range of emotions. All these could be done by manipulating the pace or gait or by exploiting certain swaras or ragas through altering or their methods of rendering as in meend or glissando, staccato, iteration, progression etc.

Indian Therapeutic Music: A Musical Alchemy

Indian music is a combination of experiences, both emotional and intellectual. While a listener's emotional hunger is met with by selecting the melodies laced with required *bhavas*, his intellectual thirst is quenched by the mathematical precision involved in the complex and elaborate *tala system*. It is also a well-known fact that the Indian classical music attaches importance to serenity and thoughtful state of mind as its primary aim. In other words it caters both to emotions and intelligence *a la fois*, thus enabling balancing of the analytical mind (*mastish*) and emotional or intuitive mind (*buddhi*). In other words, by listening to certain kind of music one is able to achieve equanimity, a quality propagated in several schools of yoga.

Music emanating from certain instruments is also regarded for their therapeutic value. The credit here goes to the unique texture or timbre (tone colour). For instance, in South India, sweet strains from veena have been believed to ensure a smooth and safe passage for the baby's arrival from the wombs of its mother. Certain ragas are also considered as having an 'equalizing effect' on the mind. For example, there has been a practice of concluding the concerts, *bhajans, kalakshepams* etc with the raga Madhyamavati. It is a raga, which takes the first three notes in the cycles of fifths and fourths (*samvada dvaya*) and naturally has a high degree of *rakti*. When sung at the end, it is no doubt, imparts a state of equilibrium and tranquility in a listener, who would have been exposed to a variety of emotions emanating from a number of ragas.

Therapeutic Indian Ragas

To cure insomnia, one listens to bits and pieces of Nilambari raga; likewise martial fervours are believed to be instilled in people by making them listen to pieces in Bilahari or Kedaram; Sriraga, when sung or listened, after a heavy lunch is said to aid in digestion and assimilation; While Saama raga is to restore mental peace, Bhupalam and Malayamaarudham when sung before the dawn serves as an agreeable invitation to people–including the Lord of the Seven Hills–to wake up from their slumber. Relief from paralysis is reported to be there by listening to pieces of Dvijaavanti Raga. Those who are prone to depression are often recommended with a dose of lilt in Bilahari to overcome their melancholy. Nadanamakriya, yet another raga, is supposed to 'soften' the adamant people and even hardened criminals. Some of the ragas are taken here for a musical analysis to uncover their secrets.

The Probable Therapeutic Components in Some Ragas

Kalyani (Yaman): A Remedy for High Blood Pressure

As we have already noticed, it is the intuitive use of resonance hidden in the tones that lend individuality to ragas. Not only that, according to this writer, it is the way the swaras are selectively used which has a definite impact on mind and moods. For instance the soothing touch inherent in the tivra *madhyam* in the raga kalyani (yaman is the Hindustani equivalent) which is interspersed with the other six swaras which are all *shuddha* render a compassionate personality to this raga, which could be the reason for its acknowledged role in bringing down one's (high) blood pressure. The other ragas identified for similar effects are: ahirbhairav, anandabhairavi, bhairavi, bhupali, darbari, durga, kalavati, puriya, todi, etc.

Malkauns (Hindolam): A Remedy for Low Blood Pressure

For those who suffer from low blood pressure, the morning raga, malkauns (whose Carnatic equivalent is hindolam) is prescribed. The oscillations in Gandhar, Daivat and in Nishad one comes across in this raga, according to this writer, could be the reason behind elevation of one's spirit as well the blood pressure. He finds magic in the pivotal note, the Madhyam, which makes it a feminine raga. The glides one notice in the swara combinations such as 'Ni-Da-Da-Ma' and in 'Ma-Ga', according to this writer, could be a reason for its application in improving one's self-confidence.

Bageshri: A Remedy for Sleep Disorders

A romantic, late night Hindustani raga, introduced to Carnatic system by Sri Muthuswamy Dikshitar is prescribed for sleep disorders and insomnia. This writer is of the view that the occasional inclusion of Pancham, besides the sharpness (*Komal-type*) in Gandhar and Nishad could be the secret for its soporific role!

Bilahari: A Remedy for Depression

Recommended for depression, this raga is ideal for starting the day. This writer feels that this raga should be sung/heard at the very early hours of dawn by those who suffer from dejection and depression. Any prayer song made in this raga could prove quite beneficial in uplifting one's moods. Other ragas such as bhupalam, kedaram and Malaya marutham, could prove equally effective in overcoming the bad effects of depression.

Durbari: An Anti-Stress Raga

A majestic, late night raga, Durbari is considered ideal for soothing nerves and reducing tension. It is often used in devotional music as it brings peace and tranquility. According to the present writer, smooth glides in all its seven notes (it is a septatonic raga) could be the major reason for smoothening the flow of nerve impulses. He pointed out that the Emperor of Music Tan Sen, administered this raga to the Emperor of Hindustan, Akbar the Great to make him recover from his stress and mental tension in governance. Other stress busters such as durga, kalavati, hamsadhwani, shankarabharanam, tilak kamod etc also promise to relieve those who are stressed by the constant expectations of people and society alike.

Shiva Ranjani: For Intellectual Excellence

An ideal raga for the night, which is accredited with the improvement in one's intelligence quotient, this writer feels that that the common man gets the taste of this raga from the least expected source of all: the Bollywood films! It may also be seen that any 'filmi abasement' of this raga leads to a hit song as in the films, Mera Naam Joker ('Jaane Kahaan Gaye Woh Din') and Ek Duje Ke Liye ('Sola Baras Ki') and in many others. At one point of time, every producer in the North and in the South used to insist that at least one song should be composed in this raga so that at least one becomes a hit!

Madhyamavati: The Leveller

Madhyamavati is the raga often chosen by the Carnatic Vidwans for ending their Katcheries (concerts) with *mangalam*. The reason is quite simple. This raga has certain unique qualities to equalize the upheaval of emotions, often brought in by singing or listening to various ragas that heighten them. Akin to Madhyamat Sarang, this writer feels that perhaps the repeated oscillations at Rishabh in this raga could be the cause for equalizing the mind. Another favourite raga for *mangalam* is Saurashtram.

Tambura and the Importance of Drone in Music

Tambura or tanpura, the Indian drone instrument is just not a drone of achala swaras, the tonic and the fifth spilling out monotony all the way! It is conceived to balance the expanding pitches in a *raga* by repeated basic pitches, which acts as a constant reminder to the performer to maintain the purity of the pitch despite the flow of several consonant and dissonant *swaras* that may constitute a *raga*. Further, the harmonics emanating from the heart of this instrument over a period of time–say 15 to 20 minutes a day–also assure harmony and peace all around–an event better experienced than explained in a seminar like this! Bikshandarkovil Subbarayar, a Carnatic Vidwan who lived in the late 19th Century, was known for sending his two tamburas to the stage much ahead of his arrival, so that the concert hall is afloat with harmonics and semitones that prepare the mind of the audience to be well-attuned to the relevant *shruti*. There's no doubt, when the actual concert began, a great degree of compatibility was already established between the artiste and his audience!

Music Therapy: Procedure and Practices

Though no hard and fast rules regarding the music treatment sessions have been laid down, a daily session at a fixed timing is recommended by some Western therapists. Basically, it is the convenience and the need of patients that counts. The session could last for anywhere between 1 to 2 hours and with a few intervals for optimum results. Higher frequency is always better and would in no way, be harmful unlike other medications or drugs, which exhibit significant side-effects. While undergoing music therapy, one should however, avoid an empty stomach.

In a typical therapeutic session, the patient is provided with an instrument or a piece of notation to go on improvising the value of the piece. In the true traditions of *mano dharma sangita,* the patient is encouraged to carry on whatever he feels like doing with them till an emotional bond develops between the patient and the musical piece. It should be made clear to the patient that his musical outputs will never be judged and that he is absolutely free to make the way he wants to sound his music. All that, patient has to attempt to do is to make the sound as pleasant as possible. He is also persuaded to use his vocal chords the way he wants– which could range from mere murmurs to loud shouts. It also creates a 'musical and emotional' environment that accepts everything the patient tries to formulate. There's no rejection whatsoever. As the patient's response to the challenges increases, it also provides experience for socialization, improves his self-confidence and communication. Rhythm instruments have been found to be useful for this type of therapeutic goals, particularly in the case of hyperactive patients. The therapist can also prescribe speech, movement, drama etc to enhance the value of such methods. Familiar songs or tunes of the patients provide better effect than the unfamiliar ones. In the west, the therapist works usually with piano where the potentials of rhythm, melody and harmony are combined with a very wide range of fluctuations of pitch or loudness. A co-therapist may also work with a therapist to help support the client if necessary and both therapists may use their voices or other instruments as appropriate. It has been clinically found that creative endeavor in music has comforted disabled children, trauma victims and individuals under geriatric care in a significant way.

Music, the Custom-made

In the developed world, an individual-based music programme is often customized, after studying the individual constitution of the patient and his problems. Once a programme is formulated, it is also necessary to review it periodically and incorporate changes so as to suit the changed conditions in the patient. Music is thus improvised uniquely for each patient and for each session. Audio recording allows the therapist to monitor the music process from session to session. Particular songs, bits, pieces or styles of music may also become part of the therapy process.

Creative Music Therapy

An approach in which co-creative sessions between the therapist and the patient, aimed at activating the innate musicality, using a variety of standard and specialized instruments has also become popular in recent times, particularly in the West. Combining aesthetic sensibilities with ongoing analytical assessment, such improvisational music has helped patients to overcome their physical, emotional and cognitive barriers. Such improvisational, creative music is administered for helping disabled children, victims of accidents and trauma, individuals under psychiatric or geriatric care and self-referred adults seeking to overcome their emotional problems and stress. Known as Nordoff Robbins System, this approach has its growing popularity in U.S.A, U.K., Germany, Australia, Scotland and Japan.

Music with Guided Imagery

As the musical melody progresses, the therapist explains imaginative events, situations, characters which are further elaborated by the patient. Several symphonies in the Western classical system, particularly those of Beethoven, Bach, Haydn, Vivaldi, Tchaikovsky etc could be utilized by the therapists for activating the imagination of the patient *vis a vis* the melody played, which not only induces satisfaction in the patient but also greatly helps in overcoming his problems such as depression, trauma and other psychological ailments. Such method called 'Bonny Method' is also reported to have considerable impact in lowering one's heart rate.

How does Music Heal?

Though the mechanism of healing is still a mystery to modern science, there is a great deal of belief that music stimulates the pituitary glands, whose secretions affect the nervous system and the blood flow. It is also believed that for healing with music, the cells of the body have to be vibrated. It is through these vibrations, it is said that the diseased person's consciousness could be changed effectively to promote health. Several psychiatrists have confirmed the usefulness of music therapy for neurosis. Lively music is found to be useful for depression, while melodious music played on string instruments has been found useful for anxiety neurosis patients. Faster music is however reported to be preferred by the patients of mania. European experiments have endorsed that a fifteen-minute session of soothing melodies can lull a patient into a sense of well-being before a painful operation. Music is found to nudge some patients into making voluntary movements, which they cannot do otherwise.

Music Therapy Practices: Conducive Environs

Many therapists recommend that the patient should have a comfortable place for treatment without much noise or other disturbances. He should be seated in a most convenient way although yoga postures such as *padmasana* or *vajrasana* are often recommended. Simple steps involved are: (1) Close the eyes (2) Play or mutter soft/slow music, (3) Focus on the breathing process (for instance, by simply placing hands on abdomen one becomes aware of the movement of that part of the body during breathing), (4) One could use meaningful mantras such as "I'm good", "The Environment around is gracious and kind", "God is kind and protective", etc. Phrases such as "I'm loved", "I love me", I'm good" etc. Such assertions are said to result in erasure of depression. As one absorbs music, one absorbs all positive vibrations from Nature, which are conducive to good health and well-being.

The Duration of Therapy

There cannot be any hard and fast rules on the duration of musical inputs. The prescribed music can be played even when the person is in deep sleep or coma. As rhythms are linked to the heartbeat, more music one receives should do wonders. However, instead of playing the music continuously, it can be given with some short intervals of gaps to make it more effective. Duration of therapy could be flexible, depending on the need of each patient and his response to it. Individual duration of therapy can however be determined through trial and error as one develops experience. There is a general consensus that an hour's dose of appropriate music at a fixed time of the day every day with intermittent intervals should be ideal. As the improvement in ailments takes place, there would be a need for changing the musical inputs by the therapist. The first step would however involve the correct diagnosis followed by the selection of appropriate raga or melody to suit the individual requirement.

Vibroacoustic and Vibrotactile Gadgets

Several gadgets such as vibrating platforms, beds, chairs, leg-rests and what not are commercially available in the West which extend a "physical experience" of 25-80 Hz sine wave tones. Thanks to these gadgets, the people with hearing impairment could physically experience (as vibration through their bodies) the middle to low frequency content of music and other sounds. Hearing impaired people can thus enjoy making and experiencing music. The physical experience of vibrations is said to be an effective therapeutic treatment for a variety of ailments such as autistic disability in children, Alzheimer's disease, Asperger's syndrome in adults and children, brain damage, emotional disturbance, Huntington's disease, learning impairments, Parkinson's disease etc. It is considered ideal for sensory impairment and terminal care. It has also been found that various low frequency sine tones will have localized effects within the body. They are said to be helpful in speech correction and in restoration of metabolic and physiological deficiencies. A frequency range from 25 to 45 Hz is said to be useful for ailments connected with feet, ankle, calves, knees, upper thighs and sacrum; a range between 45 to 60 Hz is said to be affecting coccyx, sacrum and lumbar region, where as 60 to 80 Hz is reported to affect thoracic cavity, shoulders, neck and head region.

Vibroacoustic Harp Therapy (VAHT)

A relatively new concept, VAHT refers to amplification of live harp music through vibrotactile pads, tables or cushions. It is found that bass tones, most pronounced in VAHT are the most relaxing for the clients. Glissandos which refer to the smoothness with which the notes are made to glide, is also said to produce a desirable effect on the body.

The Gift of Music

There is a growing awareness in the West that certain music can provide physiological as well as psychological benefits. Several experiments conducted on the music of Wolfgang Amadeus Mozart have revealed that many of Mozart's sonatas result in increased joie de vivre and quality of life, regardless of one's age or health conditions. Dr. Oliver Sacks, a neurologist, acknowledges the role of music in many a neurological disorder such as Parkinson's and Alzheimer's because of its unique capacity to organize and re-organize cerebral functions, when it has been greatly damaged. Design music sessions using music improvisations, receptive music listening, song-writing, guided imagery, learning through music have proved to be useful in ensuring emotional well-being besides improving communication and cognitive skills through musical responses.

Musical Experience

Musical experience is unique in the sense that it can impart an experience of extraordinary freedom to rise beyond limitation of one's physical beings. In other words, one's consciousness level could be increased to the next higher realm, with the appropriate dose of music.

Meditative music where melody and rhythms is combined with inspirational words and expressions (lyrics) as in *bhajans, kirtans, Veda* recitations etc do enhance meditation and concentration and enable the mind to focus inwards. This form of internalisation or inward looking brings about its own advantages such as strength and security and peace and tranquility to those who are mentally challenged. Through music and by letting one's mind go after it, one experiences a deep state of relaxation, which cannot be even guaranteed, with the help of chemical or synthetic drugs without their accompanying side-effects.

Conclusion

There is a growing body of literature, which recognizes the utilization of music therapy as an effective and respected treatment option. It is a well-acknowledged scientific fact that expressive music activities like singing or playing instruments improve coping mechanism and self-confidence. For the terminally ill, music provides greatest solace. Besides a comforting environment, it is found to be of great help in pain management. A combination of touch therapy, imagery and music provides an environment for a peaceful passage. Thus, music therapy has established itself as a dependable health care system using music and music activities. It is increasingly being accepted as a complementary healing system, especially in the advanced countries, where cost of medical cover has gone beyond the reach of the common man. In combination with other healing methods such as acupuncture, anesthesia, medication, surgery, yoga etc. music is found to be greatly efficacious. Regardless of differences due to age, disability or musical upbringing, it has proved useful to one and all.

Soothing and organizational properties of music helps the mentally handicapped. Limitless creative opportunities available in singing or playing instruments provide avenues for their self-expression, which is, otherwise, unavailable to them.

Music exercises aid in organizing one's thought processes and help in overcoming one's inhibitions and restrictions. The creative process of music takes over one's mind and emotion and leads to the feeling of wholeness and completeness with the Universe in all levels of existence: physical, moral or intellectual. It helps in overcoming all forms of inadequacies or frustrations in life.

Music as a therapy, is not exclusive for just a disease; it is meant for all patient groups. From the terminally ill to the temporary sufferer, it suits everybody as it involves no side effects Alzheimer patients, chronic pain sufferers, premature infants, terminal patients etc all respond to the healing power of music. Symptoms of anxiety, depression and pain in terminally ill are overcome by the healing power of music.

Thanks to music, multiple handicap patients gain a variety of skills. It provides a solid foundation for learning various skills including speech, language, self-care and adaptation.

In long term care settings, music is used to exercise a variety of skills. Cognitive games help with long and short term memory recall. Music, combined with movement as in modern gym and aerobic sessions, improve physical capabilities. Music by itself or in combination with other media such as art, aroma or dance offer unlimited scope for experience for the sensory-deprived, which is often caused by coma, injury or degenerative diseases.

Musical Opportunities

It is the birthright of every child to be trained in singing and music. Every citizen should have an easy access to music–and certainly not to noise–during social interactions. In earlier days, the aristocrats in India like Zamindars used to entertain their tenants and labourers with performers and musicians like Yakshaganbayalata, Kathakali, Sadir Katchery, Moothu etc. In the temples, concerts could be arranged on festival days where musicians and instrumentalists using powerful and far-reaching sounds as for example, in nadaswaram, drums, cymbals and the like which touch the nooks and corners of the village even without any amplifier facilities. In some Western countries, low paid workers and those who are to work in noisy factories are given free passes to attend musical concerts. There is a real joy when people attend to live music. Even in factories and offices, melodious music has already started creating conducive atmosphere of harmony and *bon homie* reducing tension among the clients and the employees. Psychiatric and medical hospitals, hospices, outpatient clinics, rehabilitation facilities, day care treatment centres, community health centres, drugs and alcohol programmes, senior centres, nursing homes, correctional facilities, schools and colleges and all such areas where humans interact can improve their functioning with music, providing a better quality of life to one and all.

References

Sairam TV: 2004 *Raga Therapy* Chennai: Nada Centre for Music Therapy.

Sairam, TV: 2004 *Medicinal Music* Chennai: Nada Centre for Music Therapy.

Sairam TV: 2006 *Music Therapy: The Sacred and the Profane.* Chennai: Nada Centre for Music Therapy.

Note: The information provided here is offered as a service and is not meant to replace any medical treatment.

Chapter 3

Application of Traditional Knowledge of Medicinal Plants by Tribes of Some Part of Rajasthan

G.S. *Paliwal*[1] *and Poonam Paliwal*[2]

NRO: NAEB, Ministry of Environment and Forests, B-1/9, Janakpuri, New Delhi – 110 058

[2]Department of Botany, I.P. College, Bulandshahr (U.P.), E-mail: paliwalgk1@rediffmail.com

Beginning with the study of plants used by tribes for food and shelter, the study of ethnobotany now also includes parameters like conservational practices used by the tribal communities, ethnopharmacology, ethnopharmacognosy, ethno gynecology etc. Thus it is no wonder that Technical Knowledge on traditional medicines is considered to be one of the most vital information for the modern drug hunters. Such information is taken as valuable leads in developing desirable therapeutic aids. Quite a good number of examples may be cited where plant products used by the present civilized world have been developed through indigenous knowledge. This list would include reserpine, quinine, digoxin, ephedrine, cocaîne, emetin, khellin, colchicine, artemisinine, gugulipid etc. These have been derived from plants which played important ethnomedical roles in the tribal societies. It is of interest to find that *Lobelia inflata* smoked earlier by the Indian tribes, is now used as a substitute for tobacco. Similarly, *Podophyllum peltatum,* formerly used by the tribes to remove skin warts is now used in treating uterine warts in modern system of medicine [1]. Moreover, out of 120 active compounds currently isolated from higher plants and used in modern medicine, 74 per cent have a positive correlation between the modern therapeutic use and the traditional use of the plants from which they have been derived or extracted. Several other tribal medicines have also been incorporated in the organized system of medicine and some more miraculous medicines known to the tribal communities are still well-guarded secrets of certain families, awaiting exploitation on a large scale.

About the Area

Rajasthan is where all the country's similes and metaphor appear to have come together. Sand dunes, wooden hills and amazing lakes, palaces and rugged forest, harsh sunlight and the cool evening breeze are all present in abundance. It is among the richest states in the country as far as handicrafts are concerned, showing the spirit of the inhabitants to be imaginative and gainfully busy.

It is located in the western part of India and is the largest State of the Republic of India in terms of area. It is encircled by Punjab and Haryana in the north and north-east, Uttar Pradesh in the east, Madhya Pradesh in the south-east and Gujarat in the south. The western boundary of the state is part of the Indo-Pak international territory running to an extent of 1,070 km. The tropic of Cancer passes through south of Banswara town, presenting an irregular rhomboid shape. The State has a maximum length of 869 km from west to east and 826 km from north to south with a total area of 342,239 sq km which is 11 per cent of the country's total geographical land. It is divided into 32 districts and falls between 23°30′ and 30°11′ latitudes and 69° 29′and 78° 17′ longitudes. It has a population of 56,473,122 (Approximately, 56.5 million) as per Census of 2001 with more than 34,526 villages and 222 cities and towns.

Geographically the entire State is bisected into two main regions by the Aravallis, one of the oldest mountain ranges in the world which run from north-east to south-west for about 688 km. The north western region has districts like Barmer, Jodhpur, Jaisalmer and Bikaner and constitute Marwar, which also encloses in it the Great Indian desert, Thar, covering western three fifth portion. The south-eastern region has the former Mewar state (comprising Udaipur and Chittorgarh), Kota, Sawai Madhopur, Alwar, Bharatpur, Dhaulpur etc. Chambal is the main river of Rajasthan which originates from the Vindhyan hills and flows through Kota and Bundi districts and passes on to Uttar Pradesh to join river Yamuna. Kali Sindh, Parbati, Banas, Mej and Parvan are the tributaries of Chambal and river Mahi with its tributaries *viz.* Anas, Som etc. also form a network in the area. Several man-made artificial lakes are spread all over the State. These are used for irrigation, bathing and for supply of drinking water. The Luni river originates from Pushkar lake and travels the marshes of Kutchch through the Marwar region.

Climatically, the south-eastern part of the State is semiarid, pleasant almost throughout the year and being recipient of comparatively higher rainfall, is also rich in forest and agricultural wealth. In contrast to this, the north-western part is dry. The western three-fifth part is sandy, arid plain called Marusthali. The climate of the desert zone is characterized by extremes of temperature, low rainfall, high evapotranspiration, low relative humidity and comparatively high wind velocity.

Rajasthan is very rich in minerals. The forest is spread unequally in different directions and mostly edapho-climatic factors determine the climax forest. 9.39 per cent area of the State is covered with forest which can be classified into three categories:

1. The reserved forest area, 38.67 per cent of the total forest.
2. The protected forest area, 55.77 per cent of the total forest.
3. The un-classified forest area, 5.56 per cent of the total forest.

The vegetative cover can be divided into the following seven types:

1. Dry tropical thorny forest
2. Mixed deciduous type forest
3. Dry evergreen forest
4. Dry deciduous forest
5. Salar forest
6. Dry teak forest
7. Dhak forest.

About the Tribes

The tribes are generally called Adibasi, Girijan, Vanvasi, Janjati, Vanyajati, Adim jati, aboriginals etc. Such distinct ethnic groups are mentioned as Scheduled Tribes, in Article 342 of the Constitution of India.

India has been rightly called as a "Melting Point" of races and tribes. It is one of the richest countries from ethnomedicinal and biodiversity point of view due to the presence of multiethnic groups of ancient lineage. The country presents a colorful mosaic of about 500 tribal communities representing 7.76 per cent of the total population, spread over 19 per cent of the total area of the nation [1]. The tribal population of Rajasthan is 12.44 per cent, which is nearly two times that of the national average. The main tribes of Rajasthan are the Bhils and Meenas that were the original inhabitants of the area. Meenas constitute the largest tribe (49.88 per cent of the total tribal population), followed by Bhils (44.01 per cent), Garasias (2.8 per cent), Saharias (0.98 per cent), Damors (0.75 per cent), Dhanka (0.3 per cent), Naikra (0.22 per cent) etc. The tribes show a wide distribution throughout the State and command considerable knowledge of the flora and fauna of their environment and ecosystem. In fact, these are the pillars on which the social, cultural, economic and political platforms of the State have been raised. They have evolved a way of life which is woven around forest ecology and resources with their primitive technology, limited skills, deep traditional knowledge and ritual practices. Their life style revolves round the forest. Further their knowledge about medicinal usage of plants has survived and continued only by oral communications from generation to generation. The field studies among such societies for advancing our knowledge on medicinal plants are of great significance. This vast knowledge of tribes which has been validated over a long period is now getting appropriate place in new curriculum of scientific research. The present paper is in keeping with this approach and deals with the traditional knowledge on medicinal plants used by the tribes of some parts of the Rajasthan, especially the Banswara, Baran, Udaipur and Dungarpur districts. In Rajasthan a few such studies have been carried out which deserve attention [2-7].

Methodology

The floristic survey of ethnomedicinal plants occurring in tribal areas of Rajasthan was conducted to assess the potential of the plant resources for modern medicine. The information on medicinal plants is based on the observations, participation with tribes and exhaustive interviews with local physicians practicing indigenous system of medicine, village headmen, priests or bhopas.

Generally two types of interviews were conducted, firstly with individuals and secondly with groups of individuals. Interviews were taken at different sites as and when situation demanded. A group of tribal people was taken to the forest and specimens of ethnomedicinally important plants were collected along with notes. The samples of such plants were identified using the earlier floristic works [8-10].

Results

All in all, through our above attempts, we have succeeded to a reasonable extent, in deriving information especially as to how the tribes have been utilizing the plant wealth of the forest in the vicinity of their villages, for their own welfare. This has really widened the horizon of the knowledge since the village people have been using, either whole plants or their specific organs for curing 15 kinds of diseases (Table 3.1) like fever, cough, skin diseases, cardiovascular problems, gastrointestinal troubles, problems of male and female reproductive system, etc. along with the botanical names, Common/ Vernacular names and Family name (Table 3.2). This also reveals that different parts of the plants such as the roots and other underground parts, flowers, flower buds, fruits, seeds, gums, resins are variously utilized by the tribal people for curing the ailments. This has been segregated disease-wise into different sections. As much as 128 ways are listed in the Table in which tribes of this region are using approximately 77 plant species belonging to 45 families of angiosperms. Along with 40 families of dicotyledons, members of 5 families of monocotyledons *viz.* Arecaceae, Cyperaceae, Liliaceae, Musaceae and Poaceae are used by the tribal people for treatment of diseases. It is clear that approximately 20 plant species of both dicots and monocots are consumed by the tribes for the treatment of more than one kind of disease. Species like *Allium cepa, A. sativa, Acacia nilotica, Albizia lebbek, Ficus benghalensis, F. religiosa, Terminalia chebula* are commonly used for treating more than four types of ailments, hence valued very highly by the bhopas or persons practicing indigenous system of medicine in these Districts of Rajasthan.

It has also been observed during the screening of results that the tribal people are more aware of the diseases related to skin, male reproductive system, female reproductive system and poisoning and the nature as well as utility of plants growing in their vicinity, hence using an array of plant species for these diseases.

Conclusion

It can be concluded from the above observations that the tribal population living in and around the forest, which is heavily dependent upon forest for its daily needs related to fuel wood, food, fodder etc., is able to maintain their health and problems related to diseases with their time-tested wealth of information on medicinal plants. This work is a small step to record this vast knowledge which lies scattered with the indigenous people, who with rapid urbanization are being either marginalized or drawn into the cultural renaissance and under either circumstances are in danger of losing their unique lifestyles.

Table 3.1: Use of Plants for Medicinal Purposes

Sl No.	*Ailments*	*Number of Species Being Used*
1	Fever	05
2	Cough	05
3	Eye ailment	05
4	Ear troubles	03
5	Dental troubles	05
6	Tuberculosis	05
7	Skin diseases	14
8	Brain-related problems	08
9	Stomach diseases	09
10	Piles	06
11	Heart diseases	03
12	Male reproductive system	19
13	Female reproductive system	19
14	Remedies against poison consumption	16
15	Diabetes	06

Table 3.2: Statement of Utilization of Various Plant Species for Curing Ailments

Sl.No.	*Botanical Name*	*Family*	*Common/ Vernacular Name*	*Part Used*
		Fever		
1.	*Cordia dichotoma* var. wallichii (C.) Maheshwari	Ehretiaceae	Lasora	Bark
2.	*Cynodon dactylon* (L.) Pers	Poaceae	Dub	Entire plant
3.	*Moringa oleifera* Lamk.	Moringaceae	Sahjan	Roots
4.	*Nyctanthes arbor-tristis* L.	Oleaceae	Harsingar	Leaves
5.	*Terminalia chebula* Retz.	Combretaceae	Harad	Fruit powder
		Cough		
1.	*Adhatoda vasica* Nees	Acanthaceae	Vasak, Arusa	Leaves
2.	*Allium sativum* L.	Liliaceae	Lahsun	Extract of bulb
3.	*Cordia dichotoma* var. wallichii (C.) Maheshwarii	Ehretiaceae	Lasoda	Fruit with seeds
4.	*Ficus religiosa* L.	Moraceae	Peepal	Fruits
5.	*Terminalia belirica* (*Gaertn.*) Roxb.	Combretaceae	Bahera	Fruit, seed-coat

Contd...

Table 3.2–Contd...

Sl.No.	*Botanical Name*	*Family*	*Common/ Vernacular Name*	*Part Used*
		Eye Ailments		
1.	*Acacia nilotica* (L.) Willd.	Mimosaceae	Babool	Leaves
2.	*Albizia odoratissima L.f.*	Mimosaceae	Kala siris	Leaves
3.	*Allium cepa* L.	Liliaceae	Pyaj	Extract of bulb
4.	*Boerhaavia diffusa* L.	Nyctaginaceae	Punarnava	Root
5.	*Ficus benghalensis* L.	Moraceace	Burh, vat	Latex
		Ear Troubles		
1.	*Allium cepa* L.	Liliaceae	Pyaj	Extract of bulb
2.	*A. satvium* L.	Liliaceae	Lahsun	Extract of bulb
3.	*Acacia nilotica* (L.) Willd.	Mimosaceae	Babool	Leaves
		Dental Troubles		
1.	*Albizia lebbek* (L.) Benth.	Mimosaceae	Kala siris	Leaves
2.	*Euphorbia neriifolia auct*, pl. non. L.	Euphorbiaceae	Chhota thuhar	Extract of entire plant
3.	*Ficus benghalensis* L.	Moraceae	Bargad, Bad	Latex, Fruit
4.	*Helianthus annuus* L.	Asteraceae	Surajmukhi	Seed oil
5.	*Syzygium aromaticum* (L.) Merr. and Perry	Myrtaceae	Laung	Bud, Clove oil
		Tuberculosis		
1.	*Adhatoda vasica* Nees	Acanthaceae	Vasak, Arusa	Leaves
2.	*Allium sativum* L.	Liliaceae	Lahsun	Bulb
3.	*Dendrocalamus strictus* (Roxb.) Nees	Poaceae	Laathibans	Alcoholic extract
4.	*Elettaria cardamomum* Maton	Zingiberaceae	Chhoti elaichi	Alcoholic extract
5	*Tinospora cordifolia* (Willd.) Miers. ex Hook. F. and Thoms.	Menispermaceae	Giloe	Alcoholic extract
		Skin Diseases		
1.	*Albizia lebbek* (L.) Benth.	Mimosaceae	Siris	Bark
2.	*Allium cepa* L.	Liliaceae	Pyaj	Extract of bulb
3.	*A. satvium* L.	Liliaceae	Lahsun	Extract of bulb
4.	*Annona squamosa* L.	Annonaceae	Sharipha	Leaves
5.	*Azadirachta indica* A. Juss.	Meliaceae	Neem	Leaves, Bark
6.	*Buchnania lanzan* Spreng.	Anacardiaceae	Chironji	Seeds
7.	*Crotalaria juncea* L.	Fabaceace	Sanai	Leaves
8.	*Cynodon dactylon* (L.) Pers	Poaceae	Doob	Entire plant

Contd...

Table 3.2–Contd...

Sl.No.	Botanical Name	Family	Common/ Vernacular Name	Part Used
9.	*Dalbergia sissoo* Roxb.	Fabaceace	Sheesham	Oil, Leaves
10.	*Datura stramonium* L.	Solanaceae	Dhatura	Fruits
11.	*Ficus religiosa* L.	Moraceae	Peepal	Bark
12.	*Mangifera indica* L.	Anacardiaceae	Aam	Leaves
13.	*Nicotiana tabacum* L.	Solanaceae	Tambaku	Leaves
14.	*Terminalia chebula* Retz.	Combretaceae	Harad	Fruits, Leaves
		Brain Related Diseases		
1.	*Acorus calamus* Linn.	Araceae	Bach	Powder
2.	*Albizia lebbek* (L.) Benth.	Mimosaceae	Siris	Seeds
3.	*Bacopa monnieri* (L.) Pennell	Scrophulariaceae	Nira-Brahmi	Plant extract
4.	*Cynodon dactylon* (L.) Pers.	Poaceae	Doob	Entire plant
5.	*Evolvulus alsinoides*	Convolvulaceae	Shankh-pushpi	Extract
6.	*Moringa oleifera* Lamk.	Moringaceace	Sahjan	Flower buds
7.	*Pongamia pinnata* (L.) Pierre	Fabaceace	Karanj	Seeds
8.	*Terminalia chebula* Retz.	Combretaceae	Harad	Fruits, Seeds
		Stomach Diseases		
1.	*Acacia nilotica* (L.) Willd.	Mimosaceae	Babool	Bark, Seeds
2.	*Albizia lebbek* (L.) Benth.	Mimosaceae	Siris	Extract of Leaves and twigs
3.	*Boerhaavia diffusa* L.	Nyctaginaceae	Punarnava	Root
4.	*Cinnamomum tamala* (Buch. Ham.)	Lauraceae	Tejpat	Bark
5.	*Euphorbia tirucalli* L.	Euphorbiaceae	Sehund	Latex
6.	*Ficus religiosa* L.	Moraceae	Peepal	Aqueous extract of the bark
7.	*Operculina turpethum* (L.) Silva Manso	Convolvulaceae	Nisoth	Root, bark
8.	*Terminalia bellirica* (Gaertn.) Roxb.	Combretaceae	Baheda	Fruit, Seed
9.	*T. chebula* Retz.	Combretaceae	Harad	Fruit, Seed
		Piles		
1.	*Allium cepa* L.	Liliaceae	Pyaj	Bulb
2.	*Cynodon dactylon* (L.) Pers.	Poaceae	Doob	Stem
3.	*Ficus benghalensis* L.	Moraceae	Vat, Bargad	Latex, aerial roots
4.	*Plumbago zeylanica* L.	Plumbaginaceae	Chitrak	Root, milky juice
5.	*Pyrus pyrifolia* (Burm.F.) Nakai	Rosaceae	Nashpati	Fruit pulp
6.	*Thespesia populnea* (L.) Soland. ex. Corr.	Malvaceae	Paras Peepal	Seed, Young buds, flowers

Contd...

Table 3.2–Contd...

Sl.No.	*Botanical Name*	*Family*	*Common/ Vernacular Name*	*Part Used*
		Heart Diseases		
1.	*Bacopa monnieri* (L.) Pennel	Scrophulariaceae	Nira-Brahmi	Whole plant extract, leaves
2.	*Terminalia arjuna* (Roxb.) W. and A.	Combretaceae	Arjun	Bark
3.	*Tinospora cordifolia* (Willd.) Miers. ex Hook. F. and Thoms	Menispermaceae	Giloe	Stem extract
		Ailments of the Male Reproductive System		
1.	*Acacia nilotica* (L.) Willd.	Mimosaceae	Babool	Bark, Thorn
2.	*Acorus calamus* Linn.	Araceae	Bach	Rhizome
3.	*Albizia lebbek* (L.) Benth.	Mimosaceae	Siris	Bark
4.	*Allium cepa* L.	Liliaceae	Pyaj	Bulb
5.	*Asparagus racemosus* Willd.	Liliaceae	Shatavar	Root Juice
6.	*Butea monosperma* (Linn.) Taub.	Fabaceace	Palash, chhola	Gum
7.	*Catharanthus roseus* (L.) G. Don	Apocynaceae	Sada Vahar	Roots
8.	*Ceiba pentandra* L.	Bombacaceae	Semal	Roots
9.	*Chlorophytum borivilianum* Sant.	Liliaceae	Safed musli	Rhizome
10.	*Curculigo orchioides* Geartn.	Hypoxidaceae	Kali musli	Stem
11.	*Ficus benghalensis* L.	Moraceae	Vat, Bargad	Bark,Latex
12.	*F. religiosa* L.	Moraceae	Peepal	Bark,Latex
13.	*Hygrophila auriculata* (Schum.)	Acanthaceae		Leaf, Seed, Root
14.	*Mucuna prurita* Hook.	Fabaceace	Kaunch, Kavanch	Seed
15.	*Peganum harmala* L.	Zygophyllaceae	Gokhru	Seeds
16.	*Phoenix sylvestris* (L.) Roxb.	Arecaceae	Khajuri	Fruits
17.	*Rhinacanthus nasuta* Kurz	Acanthaceae	Palak juhi	Leaves, roots, seeds
18.	*Tamarindus indica* L.	Caesalpiniaceae	Imli	Fruit pulp
19.	*Terminalia chebula* Retz.	Combretaceae	Harad	Fruit
		Ailments of the Female Reproductive System		
1.	*Acacia nilotica* (L.) Willd.	Mimosaceae	Babool	Bark powder, Seed powder
2.	*Acorus calamus* Linn.	Araceae	Bach	Stem extract
3.	*Anogeissus pendula* Edgew	Combretaceae	Dhaura, Dhav	Bark

Contd...

Table 3.2–Contd...

Sl.No.	Botanical Name	Family	Common/ Vernacular Name	Part Used
4.	*Azadirachta indica* A. Juss.	Meliaceae	Neem	Gum of the stem
5.	*Butea monosperma* Taub.	Fabaceace	Palash, Chhola	Gum of the stem, Bark
6.	*Crocus sativus* L.	Iridaceae	Kesar	Petal, steman
7.	*Crotalaria juncea* L.	Fabaceace	Sanai	Seeds
8.	*Cyperus scariosus* R. Br.	Cyperaceae	Nagarmotha	Rhizome
9.	*Phyllanthus embilica* Linn.	Euphorbiaceae	Anola, Amla	Fruit
10.	*Ficus benghalensis* L.	Moraceae	Vat, Bargad	Arial root, young leaves
11.	*Ficus glomerata* Roxb.	Moraceae	Gular	Fruit
12.	*F. religiosa* L.	Moraceae	Peepal	Fruit
13.	*F. rumphii* Blume	Moraceae	Pakhar	Fruit
14.	*Musa paradisiaca* L.	Musaceae	Kela	Fruit
15.	*Drypetes roxburghii* Wall.	Euphorbiaceae	Putranjiv	Bark
16.	*Tectona grandis* L.f.	Verbenaceae	Sagwan	Secondary wood
17.	*Terminialia bellerica* (Gaertn.) Roxb.	Combretaceae	Behda	Fruit, Seed
18.	*T. chebula* Retz.	Combretaceae	Harad	Fruit, Seed
19.	*Tribulus terrestris* L.	Zygophyllaceae	Gokhru	Fruit, Leaves, root
	Remedies against Poison Consumption			
1.	*Albizia odoratissima* Benth.	Mimosaceae	Kali siris	Gum of the stem
2.	*Allium cepa* L.	Liliaceae	Pyaj	Bulb extract
3.	*Brassica juncea* (L.) Gaertn. and Coss.	Brassicacaeae	Rai	Seeds
4.	*Butea monosperma* Taubert.	Fabaceace	Palash	Stem gum
5.	*Cordia dichotoma* var. wallichii (C) Maheshwari	Ehretiaceae	Lasoda, Labheda	Fruit
6.	*Gossypium hirsutum* L.	Malvaceae	Kapas	Seeds
7.	*Heliotropium indicum* L.	Boraginaceae	Hatta Juri	
8.	*Leptadenia pyrotechnia* (Forsk.) Dence	Asclepiadaceae	Khip	Stem
9.	*Malus pumila* Mill.	Rosaceae	Seb	Fruit pulp
10.	*Mangifera indica* L.	Anacardiaceae	Aam	Fruit pulp, Leaves
11.	*Michelia champaca* L.	Magnoliaceae	Champaca	
12.	*Piper nigrum* L.	Piperaceae	Kali mirch	Fruit
13.	*Salvadora persica* L.	Salvadoraceae	Pilu	Leaf, Root, Fruit
14.	*Sesamum indicum* L.	Pedaliaceae	Til	Seed, leaves
15.	*Tephorsia purpurea* (L.) Pers.	Fabaceace	Sarphonka	Leaf, Leaf powder
16.	*Tinospora cordifolia* (Willd.) Miers. ex Hook. F. and Thoms	Menispermaceae	Giloe	Aerial stem extract

Contd...

Table 3.2–Contd...

Sl.No.	Botanical Name	Family	Common/ Vernacular Name	Part Used
		Diabetes		
1.	*Aegle marmelos* (L.) Corr.	Rutaceae	Bael	Fruit pulp
2.	*Azadirachta indica* A. Juss.	Meliaceae	Neem	Fruit, seed
3.	*Ficus glomerata* Roxb.	Moraceae	Gular	Fruit
4.	*Gossypium hirsutum* L.	Malvaceae	Kapas	Seed
5.	*Pterocarpus marsupium* Roxb.	Fabaceace	Bijasal	Gum, Flower, Seeds
6.	*Syzygium cumini* (L.) Skeels	Myrtaceae	Jamun	Fruit, seed

References

1. Singh V and Pandey RP: Ethnobotany of Rajasthan, India 1998, Scientific Publishers, Jodhpur.
2. Mishra R and Dixit RD: Vajradanti–An ethnobotanical study. *J Res Ind Med* 1973, 8, 3.
3. Mishra R and Dixit RD: Studies on ethnobotany of some less known medicinal plants of Ajmer Forest Division. *Nagarjun* 1976, 14, 12.
4. Billore KV and Bhatt GK: Ethno-botanical lore from Ajmer Forest Division, Rajasthan. *Sachitra Ayurved* 1978.
5. Billore KV and Audichya KC: Some oral contraceptive family planning tribal way. *J Res Ind Med Yoga and Homeo* 1978, 13, 2.
6. Mishra R and Billore KV: Some ethnobotanical lores from Banswara district. *Nagarjun* 1983, 26, 10.
7. Mishra R, Billore KV, Yadav BBL and Chaturvedi DD: Some ethnomedicinal plants-lore from Ajmer Forest Division (Rajasthan). *J Econ Tax Bot* 1992, 16, 2.
8. Mathur CM: Forest types of Rajasthan. *Indian For* 1990, 86, 1-10.
9. Singh U, Wadhwani AM and Johri BM: Dictionary of Economic Plants in India. 1983, ICAR. New Delhi.
10. Sharma NC: Studies on the flora of Banswara District of Rajasthan. 1984, Kalyani Publishers. New Delhi.

Chapter 4

An Experimental Evaluation to the Anticancer Activity of Homeopathic Medicines

Ramadasan Kuttan*, Girija Kuttan, E.S. Sunila, K.C. Preethi, C. Nimita Venugopal and K.B. Hari Kumar

Amala Cancer Research Centre, Amala Nagar, Thrissur – 680 555, Kerala, India

There are only a few experimental evidences on the activity of homeopathic drugs in clinical, laboratory animal and cell culture to support the effectiveness of these drugs in patients. For example, in clinical studies *Arsenicum album* was reported to reduce the arsenic induced toxicity [1]. Pathak *et al.*, reported the effectiveness of Ruta 6 against human gliomas in brain in human patients [2] and there are reports on the Ruta as an alternative drug for intracranial cysticercosis [3]. Carbon tetrachloride induced hepatic damage was found to be prevented by *Lycopodium clavatum* [4]. Homeopathy was reported as a supportive therapy in cancer [5]. Moreover *Chelidonium* and *Lycopodium* have been reported to ameliorate para dimethylamino azobenzene induced hepatocarcinogenesis [6,7]. *Hydrastis* at different potencies increases the average life span of ascites tumour bearing animals [8]. There are only few reports on the action of homeopathic drugs in the *in vitro* cell culture system. *Podophyllum* has been shown to inhibit adhesion of neutrophil to serum-coated micro plates [9]. *Traumeen S*, a homeopathic formulation used in human to relieve trauma and inflammation has been shown to inhibit the production of Interleukin-beta, TNF-alpha and Interleukin-8 by human T-cells and monocytes in culture [10].

The aim of the present study is to evaluate the action of homeopathic drugs in cancer using transplanted tumours and chemically induced cancers and to find out the possible mechanism of action of homeopathic drugs useful in cancer.

Anti-cancer activity of the homeo drugs was studied using two different transplantable tumour models; ascites and solid tumour and drugs were administered

---

* Tel: 91-487-2304190; Fax–91-487-2304030;
E mail–amalaresearch@rediffmail.com, amalaresearch@hotmail.com.

simultaneously and after tumour development. The oral administration of *Hydrastis* 1M (100µL/dose/day) for 10 consecutive days significantly increased lifespan of ascites tumour bearing animals. The increase in the lifespan was found to be 69.4 per cent when compared to control, which did not get any treatment. Solid tumour was induced by subcutaneous injection of 1 million Daltons Lymphoma Ascites tumour cells through the hind limb of mice.

One group of animals received *Hydrastis* 200c (10µL/dose/day) for 12 consecutive days. *Hydrastis* 200c treated animals had significant reduction in tumour volume when compared to that of control animals. Reduction in tumour volume of *Hydrastis* 200c treated group was 53.1 per cent on day 19th and 95.8 per cent on 31st day.

There was also a significant reduction in tumour volume when the animals were treated with *Hydrastis*1M after the tumour development. It was found that 9 out of 15 animals did not increase their tumour volume when the drug treatment was initiated. All the animals in the control group increased their tumour volume and died by the 55th day. However, in the treated group only 4 animals died by the 70th day and 6 animals by the 95th day while all other animals remained tumour free by 120th day and thereafter.

The anticarcinogenic activity of the *Ruta* 200c was checked against the chemical carcinogen N-nitroso diethyl amine (NDEA), which induces liver cancers. Liver morphology of control animals, which were treated with NDEA, showed a number of tumour nodules on the surface with variable shapes, normal morphology was completely lost, necrotic mass was seen at places, and some tumour nodules showed irregular protuberances from their surfaces. The livers of vehicle treated animals also exhibited same morphological characters as the control. The livers of *Ruta* 200c treated animals showed fewer incidences of tumour nodules. It retained the normal morphology of the liver with smaller necrotic masses seen in the large lobe of some animals. The tumour incidence was very low in the liver of *Ruta* treated animals.

Administration of *Ruta* 200c was ineffective in controlling the increased liver weight induced by NDEA. The activity of the enzyme γ-glutamyl transpeptidase (γ-GT), a marker of cellular proliferation was found to be significantly elevated in the serum and the liver of all the NDEA treated animals. Serum γ-GT activity was 79.09 ± 6.70 U/L for control group as compared to the normal, which was 22.25 ± 1.99 U/L. Almost similar increases in γ-GT was observed in the liver tissue also. Administration of *Ruta* 200c significantly lowered the elevated levels of γ-GT (55.44 per cent). The level of one of the major cellular antioxidant glutathione (GSH) was elevated in the blood after NDEA administration (35 ± 3.94 nmol/mL). The administration of *Ruta* 200c reduced the GSH levels to almost normal level (21.58 ± 2.36). The treatment of NDEA also elevated the activities of three major markers of hepatic function *viz.* alkaline phosphatase (ALP), Glutamate pyruvate transaminase (GPT) and Glutamate oxaloacetate transaminase (GOT) both in the serum and the liver. The elevated levels of these marker enzymes were decreased considerably by the administration of homeopathic drug *Ruta* 200c. For example, the serum the ALP activity was 64.71 ± 6.03 KA units for control group, which was reduced to 29.92 ± 3.84 KA units, which was almost same as normal after treatment with *Ruta* 200c. ALP activity of the liver also showed a similar pattern. Similarly the level of total bilirubin, which is increased in both the serum and the tissue by NDEA, was decreased by the treatment with *Ruta* 200c.

Histopathological evaluation of the livers of NDEA alone treated animals showed extensive areas of necrosis, haemorrhage and multiple foci of carcinomatous changes. Hepatocytes were in degenerating condition. Vehicle treated group also showed similar changes. In animals treated with *Ruta* there was no carcinomatous change of the liver. It showed foci of hemorrhage and mild necrosis. The results collectively indicate that administration of *Ruta* 200c effectively prevented the NDEA induced hepatocarcinogenesis in rats.

In another model the effect of *Phosphorus*1M was studied against 3 methyl cholanthrene induced sarcoma in mice. The administration of *Phosphorus* 1M (100µL/dose/day) was found to significantly delay the sarcoma induction produced by 3-MC (200µg/ animal/dose subcutaneously). By the end of 16th week all the animals in the control group treated with 3MC developed sarcoma. Only 4 out of 20 animals treated with *Phosphorus* 1M developed sarcoma by 16th week. At the end of 30th week only 5 out of 20 animals treated with *Phosphorus* 1M developed sarcoma. The *Phosphorus* 1M also elevated the survival rate of the animals harboring sarcoma. All the animals in the control group died by the end of the 20th week. At the end of the 30th week, 14 out of 20 of the *Phosphorus* 1M treated animals were found to be alive. The results indicated the significant inhibition of 3-MC induced sarcoma by *Phosphorus* 1M.

To examine the possible mechanism through which these homeo drugs may act, the effect of these drugs on the induction of apoptosis in DLA cells were studied. The results indicated that most of the mother tinctures as well as some potentiated preparations induced apoptosis as seen by their morphological features. DNA isolated from cells treated with potentiated preparations produced typical DNA laddering after electrophoresis indicating apoptosis. *Thuja, Hydrastis, Lycopodium* and *Carcinosinum* produced apoptosis at 30c potency while 200c potencies of *Ruta, Thuja* and *Carcinosinum* produced apoptosis as seen by DNA laddering pattern.

The expression of proapoptotic genes p53, Caspase 3 and antiapoptotic gene Bcl-2 was checked after treatment with *Ruta* 200c, *Thuja* 200c and *Carcinosinum* 200c. There was no expression of p53 and Caspase 3 when DLA cells were incubated with *Ruta* and *Thuja*. However *Carcinosinum* was found to induce significant expression of p53, a proapoptotic gene. It is also possible that the potentiated preparation of homeopathic drugs may be acting directly on the expression of the apoptotic genes through interaction with high affinity receptors.

It could be postulated that homeopathic drugs may be acting directly at cellular genes. Other possible mechanism includes immunomodulatory action of homeo drugs. More studies are needed in order to elucidate the actual mechanism of action of homeo drugs.

eferences

. Philippe Belon, Pathikrit Banerjee, Sandipan Chaki Choudhury, Antara Banerjee, Surjyo Jyoti Biswas, Susanta Roy Karmakar, Surajit Pathak, Bibhas Guha, Sagar Chatterjee, Nandini Bhattacharjee, Jayanta Kumar Das and Anisur Rahman Khuda-Bukhsh: Can administration of potentized homeopathic remedy, Arsenicum album, alter antinuclear antibody (ANA) titer in people living in high-risk arsenic contaminated areas? I. A correlation with certain hematological parameters. *Evid Based Comp and Altern Med* 2006, 3, 99-107.

. Pathak S, Multani AS, Banerji P and Banerji P: Ruta 6 selectively induces cell death in brain cancer cells but proliferation in normal peripheral blood lymphocytes: A novel treatment for human brain cancer. *Int J Cancer* 2003, 23, 975-982.

. Banerji P and Banerji P: Intracranial cysticercosis: an effective treatment with alternative medicines. *In Vivo* 2001, 15, 181-184.

. Sur RK, Samajdar K, Mitra S, Gole MK and Chakrabarthy BN: Hepatoprotective action of potentized *Lycopodium clavatum* L. *Br Homeopath J* 1990, 79, 152-156.

. Rajendran ES: Homeopathy as a supportive therapy in cancer. *Homeopathy* 2004, 93, 99-102.

. Pathak S, Das JK, Biswas SJ and Khuda-Bukhsh AR: Protective potentials of a potentized homeopathic drug Lycopdium-30, in ameliorating azo dye induced hepatocarcinogenesis in mice. *Mol Cell Biochem* 2006, 285, 121-131.

. Biswas SJ, Pathak S and Khuda-Bukhsh AR: Efficacy of a potentized homeopathic drug, Carcinosin-200, fed alone and in combination with another drug, Chelidonium 200, in amelioration of p-DAB induced hepatocarcinogenesis in mice. *J Altern Comp Med* 2005, 11, 839-854.

. Maliekal TP: Antineoplastic effects of 4 homeopathic medicines. *Br Homeopath J* 1997, 86, 90-91.

. Chirumbolo S, Signorini A, Bianchi I, Lippi G and Bellavite P: Effects of *Podophyllum peltatum* compounds in various preparations, dilutions on human neutrophil functions *in vitro*. *Br Homeopath J* 1997, 86, 16-26.

0. Porozov S, Cahalon L, Weisesr M, Branski D, Lider O and Oberbaum M: Inhibition of IL-1 beta and TNF-alpha secretion from resting and activated human immunocytes by homeopathic medication Traumeel S. *Clin Dev Immunol* 2004, 11, 143-149.

Chapter 5

Molecular Mechanisms Underlying Immunomodulatory Effects of *Viscum album* Preparations

***Fabienne Prost*[1]*, Jean-Paul Duong Van Huyen*[1,2]**
***Sriramulu Elluru*[1,3]*, Sandrine Delignat*[1]*, Jagadeesh Bayry*[1]**
***Michel D. Kazatchkine*[1] *and Srini V. Kaveri*[1]**

[1]*INSERM U681, Université Pierre et Marie Curie, (UPMC–Paris 6), Institut des Cordeliers, Paris, France*

[2]*Department of Pathology, Hôpital Européen Georges Pompidou, Paris, France*

[3]*Universite de Technologie, Compeiegne, France*

ABSTRACT

Viscum album extracts (VA extracts) consist of aqueous extracts from *Viscum album* or European mistletoe growing on different host trees. Biologically active components of VA extracts include Mistletoe lectins and viscotoxins. The treatment with VA extracts or with purified ML has been shown to be associated with tumor regression in several *in vivo* experimental tumor models. The mechanisms underlying the anti-tumoral activity of VA or ML are complex and involve apoptosis, angiogenesis and immunomodulation. However, the detailed mechanisms of action of VA extracts still remain unclear. This review provides an account of the current status of the understanding of the VA-associated immunomodulation in various cell types including lymphoblastoid, monocytic or endothelial cell lines.

Keywords: Viscum album, Cytotoxicity, Apoptosis, Endothelium, Immunomodulation, Immune system, Angiogenesis.

* Tel: + 33 1 55 42 82 64, Fax: + 33 1 55 42 82 62; E-mail: srini.kaveri@umrs681.jussieu.fr.

Introduction

Viscum album (VA) preparations consist of aqueous extracts from *Viscum album* or European mistletoe plants growing on different host trees [1-3]. Mistletoe lectin (ML) I, II, and III belong to the ribosome-inactivating protein (RIP) family of type II. RIP of type II are composed of an N-glycosidase (A chain) and a galactoside-recognizing lectin (B-chain) connected by a disulfide bridge [4].

The entire preparations used therapeutically consist in addition to mistletoe lectins and viscotoxins, several enzymes, peptides (for eg., viscumamide), amino acids, thiols, amines, polysaccharides, cyclitoles, lipids, phytosterols, triterpenes, flavonoids, phenylpropanes and minerals. Several studies have reported the clinical usefulness of preparations consisting of VA extracts in cancer patients [5-7]. Treatment with VA extracts or by purified ML has also been shown to be associated with tumor regression in several *in vivo* experimental models of tumoral implantation [8-10].

It is well established that the cytotoxicity of VA extracts is dependent on the induction of apoptosis. Experimental anti-tumoral effect of VA extracts may be supported by the direct cytotoxic properties of ML towards tumor cell lines [1, 11, 12]. However, the mechanisms underlying the VA extract-induced apoptosis have not been fully elucidated [10, 13-20]. More recently, several studies have demonstrated that VA extracts and purified ML have immunomodulatory properties [14, 17, 18, 21-27]. VA preparations or purified ML have been shown to induce activation of transcription and secretion of pro-inflammatory cytokines such as IL-1, IL-6 and TNFα in human PBMC, and endothelial cells [17, 22, 24, 26]. Moreover, several studies have shown that VA extracts exert immunomodulatory properties *i.e.* enhancement of NK cell activity or modulation of TH polarization [28, 29]. However, the *in vitro* cytotoxic properties of VA extracts towards cancer cell lines, raise the question concerning the interaction of VA preparations with the survival of cell implicated in the immune and inflammatory systems *i.e.* lymphocytes, monocytes and endothelial cells (EC). To address this question, we have conducted several *in vitro* studies on the interaction of VA extracts with various established cell lines (monocytic and lymphoblastoid cell lines, EC lines...) or primary cultures (normal murine splenocytes, HUVEC).

VA Extracts are Cytotoxic Towards Human Cell Lines Derived from T and B Lymphocytes, and from Monocytes *in vitro*

Several authors have established that the cytotoxicity of VA extracts could greatly differ depending on the type of preparation and the investigated cell. The induction of cell necrosis by VA extracts has been reported in human peripheral blood lymphocytes (PBL), human peripheral blood monocytes (PBM), murine thymocytes, human monocytic THP1 cells and mononuclear leukemia cells MOLT4 [14, 16-18].

In one study, we compared the cytotoxic properties of VA Qu FrF, Qu Spez, M Spez and VA P in a large representative panel of lymphoblastoid cell of T and B origins and in monocytic cell lines [19, 30]. The induction of cell toxicity by various VA extracts was assessed *in vitro* in the human T cell lines CEM and Jurkat, B lymphoblastoid lines Raji, BC36, BC28, BC41, WW2-LCL, and in HL-60 and MM-6 monocytic cell lines [19, 30]. Cell death was measured by the uptake of propidium iodide followed by FAC Scan analysis. VA Qu FrF, Qu Spez and M Spez induced a dose-dependent cell death in both T cell lines, and in monocytic cell lines. Cell toxicity was associated with a dose-dependent inhibition of cell proliferation. As expected VA P was devoid of cytotoxicity in all tested cell lines. This may be in part explained by the low concentrations of cytotoxic ML in VA P preparations.

Cell toxicity induced by VA extracts in various tumoral cell lines demonstrated the involvement of apoptosis [13-17, 31]. The molecular mechanisms are not fully understood and conflicting results have been published. Concerning lymphoblastoid cells, using Fas-resistant HuT78.B1 T cell line, we have demonstrated that Fas pathway is not involved in VA Qu FrF apoptosis as previously reported by others [32]. We have also shown that VA QuFrF induces a dramatic decrease in the amount of anti apoptotic proteins Bcl-2 and Bcl-X proteins in T lymphocytes [19], a finding consistent with the release of cytochrome c from mitochondria induced by ML I [13].

At the concentrations studied, nearly all B lymphoblastoid cell lines were resistant to all VA preparations (only BC41 cell line was fully sensitive to the three preparations). Our findings clearly confirm that cell lines of B lymphocyte origin are refractory to the cell death induced by VA extracts. Our findings were similar to those results obtained by Bantel *et al.*, [13]. To attain an optimal level of apoptosis, the B lymphocyte cell line, BJAB, required approximately 1000-fold higher amounts of ML I than that required by Jurkat cells [13]. Currently, the molecular mechanisms of such resistance of cell lines of B-cell origin is unknown.

Results from preliminary experiments conducted in our laboratory may provide new insight into the interaction of VA extracts with the immune system. These preliminary *ex vivo* experiments suggest that VA preparations may induce cell proliferation in normal C57BL6 murine splenocytes as measured by cellular incorporation of tritiated Thymidine. However, these data clearly show a balance between inhibition or induction of proliferation and induction of apoptosis that varied depending on the preparation used, the concentration and the incubation time (Figure 5.1). The results emphasize the need to design the adequate schedule to achieve immunostimulation in both *in vivo* and *in vitro* experiments.

Viscum album Extracts from Different Host Trees Induce Apoptosis on Both Immortalized Human Venous Endothelial Cell Lines and Huvec

In addition to its gate-keeping role between blood and tissue, the endothelium plays a pivotal role in several biological processes. EC actively participate in the regulation of blood flow and coagulation, in initiation and enhancement of inflammation, and in angiogenesis that is fundamental to reproduction, development and repair [33, 34]. The contribution of an EC-mediated effect in the anti-tumoral properties of VA extracts thus needs to be investigated. In this respect, we assessed the interactions between VA extracts and EC.

Our *in vitro* study focused on the ability of VA extracts to induce EC death. Using primary human venous endothelial cell HUVEC and the immortalized human venous

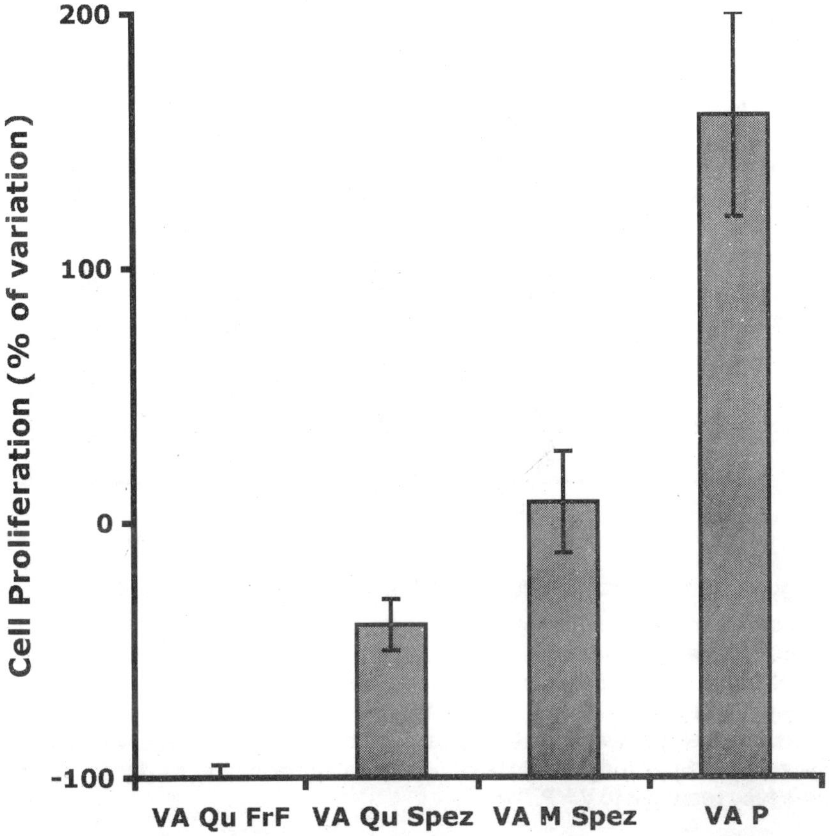

Figure 5.1: Modulation of Proliferation of Murine Splenocytes by VA Extracts

Murine splenocytes were obtained from normal C57BL6 mice (6 mice). Cells were cultured for 72h in the presence of 50 µg/ml of VA Qu FrF, Qu Spez, M Spez and P. After 48h, [^{3}H]thymidine (0.5 µCi) was added to the medium. The cells were then cultivated for further 24h. The splenocytes were then collected and the incorporated [^{3}H]thymidine was measured. The results are represented as a percentage of variation as compared to untreated controls. After 72h of culture, VA Qu FrF and Q Spez strongly inhibited murine splenocyte proliferation, whereas VA P dramatically induced cell proliferation.

endothelial cell lines IVEC and EA-hy926, we have shown that VA extracts induce EC death in a dose–and time-dependent manner [20]. Figure 5.2 depicts the cytotoxic properties of VA extracts towards EA-hy926 as assessed by the uptake of PI. Three VA extracts induced a potent and dose mortality of EA-hy926 as assessed by the uptake of PI. While, VA M Spez had less cytotoxic properties, VA Qu FrF and VA Qu Spez were the most effective preparations. However, EA-hy926 cells were insensitive to VA P at any tested concentration. Similar results were obtained with the IVEC cell lines. Other authors have also reported the sensitivity of various EC lines to VA extracts [35].

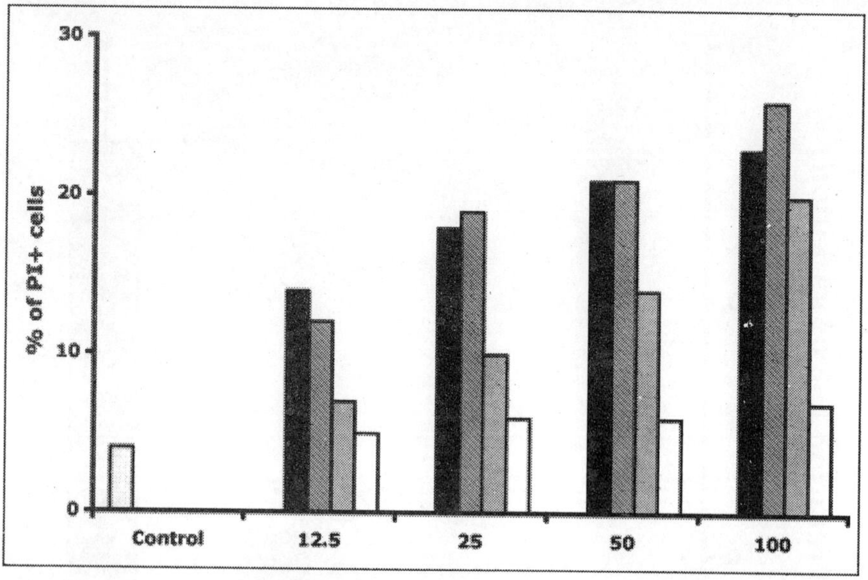

Figure 5.2: VA Extracts Induce Cell Death in Endothelial Cell Line EA-hy926

Sub-confluent endothelial cells from the human cell line EA-hy926 were cultured for 48h in the presence of increasing concentration of VA extracts: VA Qu FrF (black bars), Qu Spez (hatched bars), M Spez (grey bars) and P (open bars), or were left untreated (Control). Cell death was then quantitated by measuring the uptake of PI and expressed as a percentage of dye-positive cells. VA Qu FrF, Qu Spez and M Spez induced dose-dependent cell toxicity in EA-hy926 cells. EC were fully resistant to VA P.

We then demonstrated that VA-mediated EC death involves apoptosis, using various methods *i.e.* DNA ladder formation, AnnexinV labeling, and western blot analysis for poly (ADP)-ribose polymerase (PARP) cleavage. Figure 5.3A illustrates the cytological aspect of HUVEC incubated with high concentrations of VA Qu FrF [20]. Numerous typical apoptotic bodies were observed. We then performed DNA ladder experiments. As illustrated in Figure 5.3B, DNA obtained from HUVEC cultured in the presence of VA extracts exhibited the typical fragmentation pattern of apoptosis. The involvement of apoptosis in the EC cell death induced by VA extracts was also confirmed by V labeling with FACS analysis. The percentage of EC undergoing apoptosis (An V+/PI-) increased in a time–and dose-dependent manner for VA extracts. Western blot analysis also demonstrated that the cleavage of PARP is involved in VA-induced HUVEC apoptosis.

Are VA Extracts Anti-angiogenic?

Angiogenesis is the process by which new blood vessels are formed by sprouting pre-existing vessels [33, 34, 36, 37]. Tumor angiogenesis plays an important role in tumor progression and metastasis. Clinical applications of research on angiogenesis

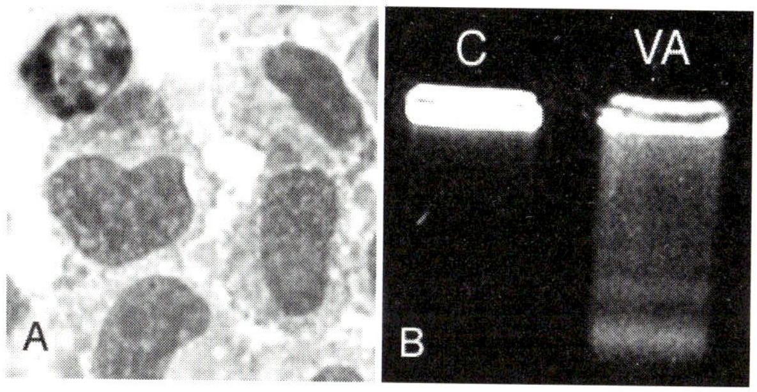

Figure 5.3: VA Qu FrF Induces HUVEC Apoptosis

Sub-confluent HUVEC were cultivated with VA Qu FrF at 50 µg/ml for 48h. Panel A illustrates the features of EC under cytologic examination, with the presence of typical apoptotic body. Panel B confirmed the involvement of apoptosis with a typical pattern of DNA laddering (VA), as compared to untreated cells (C).

have emerged towards the diagnosis, prognosis or therapy of neoplasia [38, 39]. The mechanisms involved in tumor angiogenesis consist of a wide range of phenomena including enhanced division of endothelial cells (EC) within the tumor, up-regulation of cell adhesion molecules and production of angiogenic factors [33, 34].

The role of VA extracts in the process of angiogenesis is thus of interest to understand some of the molecular mechanisms involved in the anti-tumoral properties of VA extracts. Figure 5.3 illustrates our preliminary results obtained in capillary tube formation experiments using EA-hy926 cell line. EC were seeded on matrigel and incubated with various concentrations of VA extracts. A well-organized capillary tube network was observed in control treatment (Figure 5.4A). In contrast, the capillary tube formation was abrogated in the presence of VA Qu Spez as above 12.5 µg/mL (Figure 5.4B). Thus, these preliminary results suggest that VA extracts inhibit *in vitro* angiogenesis. *In vivo* anti-angiogenesis effect of VA extracts have also been examined

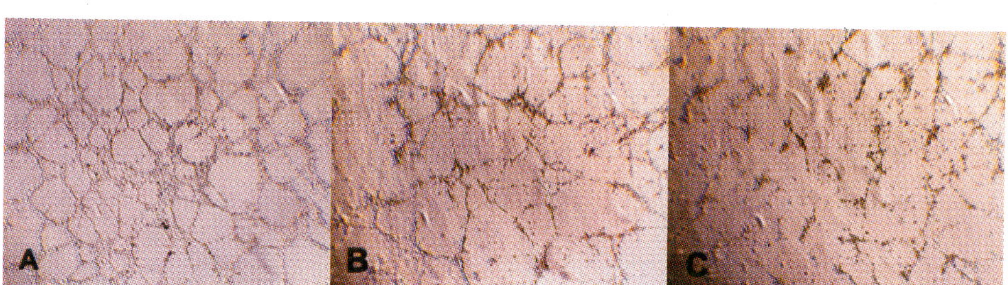

Figure 5.4: VA Qu Spez Inhibits Capillary Tube Formation

EA-hy926 cells were seeded on Matrigel© which promotes *in vitro* angiogenesis. After 24h, untreated cells formed a well-defined capillary tube network (A). Incubation with VA Qu Spez (25 µg/ml) partially abrogated capillary tube formation (B).

by choriallantoic membrane assays in C57BL6 mice inoculated with B16-BL6 melanoma cells and treated with *Viscum album* L. coloratum agglutinin [10]. In addition, VA *coloratum* extracts suppressed tumor growth *in vivo* and inhibited the number of blood vessels oriented towards the tumor mass [40].

The molecular mechanisms underlying the VA-induced inhibition of angiogenesis have not been fully elucidated. At the level of EC, our results may suggest the implication of VA-associated EC apoptosis, at least in part in its anti-angiogenic properties. Several studies have well demonstrated that EC apoptosis is implicated in the physiological inhibition of angiogenesis. Consistently, Yoon *et al.*, have observed in *in vitro* experiments that VA coloratum extracts inhibit the proliferation of rat EC.

Conclusion

The molecular mechanisms underlying the anti-tumoral activity of VA or ML are complex and involve several inter-related biological phenomena including apoptosis, angiogenesis and immunomodulation. As in the case of other members of RIP II family, VA extracts exert cytotoxic activity towards cell lines derived from both human and rodent origins although to a lesser extent as compared to ricin. VA extracts and purified ML also induce activation of transcription and secretion of pro-inflammatory cytokines in human PBMC and endothelial cells. To address the interactions between immunomodulatory and anti-tumor properties of VA preparations, we have recently investigated the mechanisms underlying the effects of VA extracts on tumoral growth of melanoma implanted in mice. These studies are suggestive of the implication of certain anti-tumoral cytokines. Together, several lines of evidence that have been accumulated in the recent years, in favor of anti-tumoral and immunomodulatory properties of VA extracts, strongly encourage further intensive investigation.

Acknowledgments

The authors thank Rainier Dierdorf, Jean Chazarenc, and Marc Follmer for helpful suggestions. This work was supported by Weleda AG, Switzerland, and by Institut National de la santé et de la Recherche Médicale (INSERM) and Centre National de la recherché Scientifique (CNRS).

References

1. Stirpe F, Sandvig K, Olsnes S *et al.*: Action of viscumin, a toxic lectin from mistletoe, on cells in culture. *J Biol Chem.* 1982, 257, 13271-13277.
2. Olsnes S, Stirpe F, Sandvig K *et al.*: Isolation and characterization of viscumin, a toxic lectin from *Viscum album* L. (mistletoe). *J Biol Chem.* 1982, 257, 13263-13270.
3. Franz H, Ziska P and Kindt A: Isolation and properties of three lectins from mistletoe (*Viscum album* L.). *Biochem J.* 1981, 195, 481-484.
4. Eschenburg S, Krauspenhaar R, Mikhailov A *et al.*: Primary structure and molecular modeling of mistletoe lectin I from *Viscum album*. *Biochem Biophys Res Commun.* 1998, 247, 367-372.

5. Ernst E, Schmidt K and Steuer-Vogt MK: Mistletoe for cancer? A systematic review of randomised clinical trials. *Int J Cancer.* 2003, 107, 262-267.
6. Kienle GS, Berrino F, Bussing A *et al.*: Mistletoe in cancer–a systematic review on controlled clinical trials. *Eur J Med Res.* 2003, 8, 109-119.
7. Mansky PJ: Mistletoe and cancer: controversies and perspectives. *Semin Oncol.* 2002, 29, 589-594.
8. Braun JM, Ko HL, Schierholz JM. *et al.*: Standardized mistletoe extract augments immune response and down-regulates local and metastatic tumor growth in murine models. *Anticancer Res.* 2002, 22, 4187-4190.
9. Burger AM, Mengs U, Schuler JB *et al.*: Anticancer activity of an aqueous mistletoe extract (AME) in syngeneic murine tumor models. *Anticancer Res.* 2001, 21, 1965-1968.
10. Park WB, Lyu SY, Kim JH *et al.*: Inhibition of tumor growth and metastasis by Korean mistletoe lectin is associated with apoptosis and antiangiogenesis. *Cancer Biother Radiopharm.* 2001, 16, 439-44.
11. Ribereau-Gayon G, Jung ML, Baudino S *et al.*: Effects of mistletoe (*Viscum album* L.) extracts on cultured tumor cells. *Experientia.* 1986, 42, 594-599.
12. Maier G and Fiebig HH: Absence of tumor growth stimulation in a panel of 16 human tumor cell lines by mistletoe extracts in vitro. *Anticancer Drugs.* 2002, 13, 373-379.
13. Bantel H, Engels IH, Voelter W *et al.*: Mistletoe lectin activates caspase-8/FLICE independently of death receptor signaling and enhances anticancer drug-induced apoptosis. *Cancer Res.* 1999, 59, 2083-2090.
14. Hostanska K, Hajto T, Weber K *et al.*: A natural immunity-activating plant lectin, *Viscum album* agglutinin-I, induces apoptosis in human lymphocytes, monocytes, monocytic THP-1 cells and murine thymocytes. *Nat Immun.* 1996, 15, 295-311.
15. Hostanska K, Vuong V, Rocha S *et al.*: Recombinant mistletoe lectin induces p53-independent apoptosis in tumor cells and cooperates with ionising radiation. *Br J Cancer.* 2003, 88, 1785-1792.
16 Lavastre V, Pelletier M, Saller R *et al.*: Mechanisms involved in spontaneous and *Viscum album* agglutinin-I-induced human neutrophil apoptosis: *Viscum album* agglutinin-I accelerates the loss of antiapoptotic Mcl-1 expression and the degradation of cytoskeletal paxillin and vimentin proteins via caspases. *J Immunol.* 2002, 168, 1419-1427.
17 Mockel B, Schwarz T, Zinke H *et al.*: Effects of mistletoe lectin I on human blood cell lines and peripheral blood cells. Cytotoxicity, apoptosis and induction of cytokines. *Arzneimittelforschung.* 1997, 47, 1145-1151.
18 Ribereau-Gayon G, Jung M L, Frantz M *et al.*: Modulation of cytotoxicity and enhancement of cytokine release induced by *Viscum album* L. extracts or mistletoe lectins. *Anticancer Drugs.* 1997, 8 Suppl 1, S3-8.

19. Duong Van Huyen J P, Sooryanarayana Delignat S. *et al.*: Variable sensitivity of lymphoblastoid cells to apoptosis induced by *Viscum album* Qu FrF, a therapeutic preparation of mistletoe lectin. *Chemotherapy*. 2001, 47, 366-376.

20. Van Huyen J P, Bayry J, Delignat S *et al.*: Induction of Apoptosis of Endothelial Cells by *Viscum album*: A Role for Anti-Tumoral Properties of Mistletoe Lectins. *Mol Med*. 2002, 8, 600-606.

21. Gorter R W, Joller P, and Stoss M: Cytokine release of a keratinocyte model after incubation with two different *Viscum album* L extracts. *Am J Ther*. 2003, 10, 40-47.

22. Hajto T, Hostanska K, Frei K *et al.*: Increased secretion of tumor necrosis factors alpha, interleukin 1, and interleukin 6 by human mononuclear cells exposed to beta-galactoside-specific lectin from clinically applied mistletoe extract. *Cancer Res*. 1990, 50, 3322-3326.

23. Hajto T, Hostanska K, Weber K *et al.*: Effect of a recombinant lectin, *Viscum album* agglutinin on the secretion of interleukin-12 in cultured human peripheral blood mononuclear cells and on NK-cell-mediated cytotoxicity of rat splenocytes in vitro and in vivo. *Nat Immun*. 1998, 16, 34-46.

24. Hostanska K, Hajto T, Spagnoli GC *et al.*: A plant lectin derived from *Viscum album* induces cytokine gene expression and protein production in cultures of human peripheral blood mononuclear cells. *Nat Immun*. 1995, 14, 295-304.

25. Kovacs E: Serum levels of IL-12 and the production of IFN-gamma, IL-2 and IL-4 by peripheral blood mononuclear cells (PBMC) in cancer patients treated with *Viscum album* extract. *Biomed Pharmacother*. 2000, 54, 305-310.

26. Ribereau-Gayon G, Dumont S, Muller C *et al.*: Mistletoe lectins I, II and III induce the production of cytokines by cultured human monocytes. *Cancer Lett*. 1996, 109, 33-38.

27. Hajto T, Hostanska K and Gabius HJ: Modulatory potency of the beta-galactoside-specific lectin from mistletoe extract (Iscador) on the host defense system in vivo in rabbits and patients. *Cancer Res*. 1989, 49, 4803-4808.

28. Tabiasco J, Pont F, Fournie JJ *et al.*: Mistletoe viscotoxins increase natural killer cell-mediated cytotoxicity. *Eur J Biochem*. 2002, 269, 2591-2600.

29. Yoon TJ, Yoo YC, Kang TB *et al.*: Antitumor activity of the Korean mistletoe lectin is attributed to activation of macrophages and NK cells. *Arch Pharm Res*. 2003, 26, 861-867.

30. Duong Van Huyen JP, Delignat S, Kazatchkine MD *et al.*: Comparative study of the sensitivity of lymphoblastoid and transformed monocytic cell lines to cytotoxic effects of *Viscum album* extracts of different origin. *Chemotherapy*. 2003, 49, 298-302.

31. Büssing A: Induction of apoptosis by the mistletoes lectins: A review on the mechanisms of cytotoxicity mediated by *Viscum album* L. Apoptosis. 1996, 1, 25-32.

32. Elsasser-Beile U, Ruhnau T, Freudenberg N *et al.*: Antitumoral effect of recombinant mistletoe lectin on chemically induced urinary bladder carcinogenesis in a rat model. *Cancer.* 2001, 91, 998-1004.

33. Carmeliet P: Mechanisms of angiogenesis and arteriogenesis. *Nat Med.* 2000, 6, 389-395.

34. Folkman, J: Angiogenesis in cancer, vascular, rheumatoid and other disease. *Nat Med.* 1995, 1, 27-31.

35. Harmsma M, Gromme M, Ummelen M *et al.*: Differential effects of *Viscum album* extract IscadorQu on cell cycle progression and apoptosis in cancer cells. *Int J Oncol.* 2004, 25, 1521-1529.

36. Lucas R, Holmgren L, Garcia I *et al.*: Multiple forms of angiostatin induce apoptosis in endothelial cells. *Blood.* 1998, 92, 4730-4741.

37. Thompson WD, Li WW and Maragoudakis M: The clinical manipulation of angiogenesis: pathology, side-effects, surprises, and opportunities with novel human therapies. *J Pathol.* 2000, 190, 330-337.

38. Folkman J, Browder T and Palmblad J: Angiogenesis research: guidelines for translation to clinical application. 2001, *Thromb Haemost.* 86, 23-33.

39. Keshet E and Ben-Sasson SA: Anticancer drug targets: approaching angiogenesis. 1999, *J Clin Invest.* 104, 1497-1501.

40. Yoon TJ, Yoo YC, Choi, OB *et al.*: Inhibitory effect of Korean mistletoe (*Viscum album* coloratum) extract on tumor angiogenesis and metastasis of haematogenous and non-haematogenous tumor cells in mice. *Cancer Lett.* 1995,97, 83-91.

Chapter 6

A Rasayana, ICHOR-CR, as a Possible Chemoprotectant Against Doxorubicin-Related Toxicity

Renee Vanessa Gardner[1*], Hernan Correa[2], Randall Craver[3], Evangeline McKinnon[4], Halina Sadowska-Krowicka[5] and Rajasekharan Warrier[1]

[1]*Louisiana State University Health Sciences Center and Children's Hospital of New Orleans (LSUHSC; Department of Pediatrics), 200 Henry Clay Avenue, New Orleans, Louisiana 70118, USA*

[2]*Vanderbilt University Medical School (Department of Pathology), Nashville, TN*

[3]*LSUHSC and Children's Hospital of New Orleans (Department of Pathology)*

[4]*LSUHSC and The Children's Research Institute (Department of Pediatric Research), 200 Henry Clay Avenue, New Orleans 70118*

ABSTRACT

Doxorubicin (Doxo)'s use is limited by toxicities such as cardiomyopathy, a progressively debilitating condition without effective treatment. One proposed mechanism of damage is oxidative injury to cardiac myocytes. We tested a Rasayana with antioxidant properties, ICHOR-CR, to see if it could ameliorate acute Doxo-induced cardiomyopathy, using mice.

C57B6/J (B6) mice, given 50 mg/day p.o. of ICHOR on days 1-5, received, on day 5, Doxo at 20mg/kg i.p (x1) (ICHOR/Doxo). Alternatively, mice received only ICHOR or Doxo, or no drug. Mice were sacrificed on day 7 and 11; hearts were weighed and used for histological analysis and antioxidant enzyme assays.

Glutathione peroxidase levels within heart rose 50 per cent above control levels on days 7 and 11, after ICHOR-CR and remained at up to twice levels of controls or Doxo-treated animals, when adjusted for tissue weight. Lipid

* Tel: 504-896-9740; E-mail: rgardn@lsuhsc.edu.

peroxidation was significantly reduced even at day 11, after ICHOR alone (p=0.04). Declines in lipid peroxidation after Doxo/ICHOR approached but did not attain significance. Cardiac damage as assessed by the Billingham scale of cardiotoxicity lessened significantly (p<0.05) after ICHOR/Doxo.

The Rasayana, ICHOR-CR, partially protects against Doxo-mediated acute cardiomyopathy. It remains to be seen whether there is protection against chronic cardiomyopathy.

Keywords: *Doxorubicin, Cardioprotection, Rasayana.*

Introduction

Cardiotoxicity is the dose-limiting side-effect of Doxorubicin (Doxo) and related anthracyclines [1-3]. This toxicity limits the usefulness of this class of drugs, and is a problem of growing concern for oncologists [4]. Cardiomyopathy may take years to fully evolve in patients who have otherwise appeared well and without ill-effects of previously administered anthracyclines [1]. The acute form of cardiomyopathy occurs within 1 year of completion of Doxorubicin therapy; in one study, it was observed in about 10 per cent of patients, recurring in just under 50 per cent of individuals up to 10 years after treatment was discontinued. The chronic form of cardiomyopathy may be seen within 4 weeks to 1-2 years after therapy, while the more recently recognized late or delayed-onset form may occur up to 20 years after completion of therapy [1].

Risk factors for cardiomyopathy have been identified through statistical analyses [5-7], but these predictive factors have failed to prevent ensuing cardiac damage or indicate all individuals at greatest risk. Clinical monitoring strategies, such as frequent measurement of the ejection fraction through use of MUGA scans or conventional ECHOcardiography, have also been ineffective in predicting which patients are likely to experience cardiac damage [5]. Serum levels of cardiac troponin T, a component of the troponin complex in the thin sarcomeric filament of heart, may correlate with severity of Doxo-induced cardiomyopathy [8]. However, in children who may be more sensitive to anthracyclines [9, 10], measurements of cardiac troponin T may be more variable, and their usefulness in this population is unknown [11, 12].

As a result, cardiotoxicity remains a difficult clinical problem, in terms of prevention and treatment. Once present, it is irreversible [13], with a high mortality rate (~20 per cent -61 per cent) [14, 15]. In those initially responding to treatment, progression or recurrence of heart failure is observed in almost 50 per cent. Cardiac transplant may offer the only satisfactory solution to treatment [16].

Prevention of Doxo-associated cardiotoxicity has become the focus of many investigations that are based on a thus far incomplete knowledge of causes of toxicity. One of the most popular theories of pathogenesis of cardiomyopathy is that it is mediated by free radicals, produced upon exposure to Doxo [17]. Antioxidants have then been proposed as a means of protecting against Doxo-mediated cardiac damage [18-20]. The most widely used of these drugs is dexrazoxane (Zinecard) [21, 22]. Its protection against the acute or subacute form of cardiomyopathy has been incomplete [23], and it is not known whether it provides similar protection against chronic or delayed toxicity. Severe, even fatal myelosuppression was reported with its use, although at higher than currently used ratios of dexrazoxane:doxorubicin [24]. Also, possible compromise of antitumor efficacy has been reported in at least one study [23]. Prolonged use of related drugs, razoxane or bimolane, led to an increase in incidence of secondary acute myelogenous leukemia, leading some to fear that dexrazoxane may have a similar association [21]. The high cost of dexrazoxane limits its usefulness for many individuals, especially in developing countries.

ICHOR-CR (ICHOR), a Rasayana in the herbal class of medicines used by the Ayurvedic system of medicine, demonstrated antioxidant activity after irradiation [25]. We have tested the hypothesis that ICHOR, when given in conjunction with Doxorubicin, may offer cardioprotection.

Materials and Methods

Drug and Herb Administration

ICHOR is a mixture of 36 medicinal herbs, formulated by the Cybele Herbal Laboratories in Trichur, India, using precise proportions of herbs as stipulated by the Ayurvedic Pharmacopeia of India [26]. Quality control is achieved by a government-approved laboratory in India, under the supervision of the Department of Indian Systems of Medicine and Homeopathy, established as a separate department in the Ministry of Health and Family Welfare in 1995 (personal communication). Manufacture of the herbal preparation is in compliance with Drugs and Cosmetic Act of 1940 and the Good Manufacturing Practices Law. The drug is supplied as a tablet. It was pulverized and weighed prior to being mixed in water at a concentration of 50 mg/0.2 ml.

Animal Model

For these experiments, we used an *in vivo* murine model of acute Doxo-induced cardiomyopathy [27]. A schema of the experiment is shown in Figure 6.1. Female C57B6/J mice, 12 weeks old, received 50 mg/dose/animal of ICHOR via gavage feeding tube on 5 consecutive days (days 1-5). Equal aliquots (or 0.2 ml) of this emulsion, which was gently agitated to insure even distribution of the herb, were administered to each mouse. On day 5, mice were injected i.p. with 20 mg/kg Doxo mixed in water. Alternately, animals were given Doxo or ICHOR only at the above doses, or no drug or herb. The animals were then sacrificed 6 days after the last drug or drug combination was administered, and their hearts were removed and weighed. The tissue was subsequently used for studies detailed in this section. Experiments were duplicated and the number of mice analyzed for each set of experiments was 9-12/treatment group.

Enzyme Determinations

Heart tissue was homogenized in cold buffer. Buffer was either 50 mM Tris-HCl, pH 7.5, 5 mM EDTA and 1 mM DTT for glutathione peroxidase (Gpx) and superoxide dismutase (SOD) determinations, or Tris-HCl, pH 7.4 with butylated hydroxybutane for the lipid peroxidation assay. Samples were prepared using a ratio of 4-8 ml buffer to 1 g tissue. Homogenates were centrifuged respectively at 11,000 rpm (~10,000 x g)

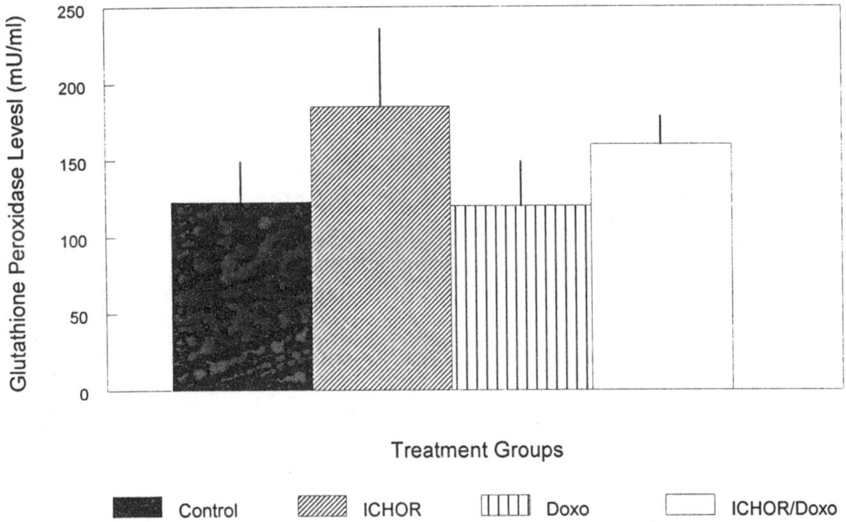

Figure 6.1: Glutathione Levels 6 Days after Last Dose of Doxo +/or ICHOR

Results are given as mU/ml; means ± standard error of the means (S.E.M.). The represented groups are control (no drug or herb), ICHOR (herb only), Doxo (doxorubicin only), and Ichor/Doxo (a combination of drug and herb). Tests were performed three times with an n of 9-10. Differences between ICHOR and Doxo, either given solo or in combination, and control and Doxo groups were significant ($p<0.01$).

or 6500 rpm (3000 x g) at 4°C for 10 to 20 min. Supernatant was removed and used, according to specifications of the kit manufacturers: (1) Cellular Gpx and SOD (Calbiochem, San Diego, CA); and (2) LPO-586 (Oxis International, Inc., Portland, OR) assays. Spectrophotometric absorption readings were taken, as instructed, at λ 340, 586 and 595 respectively for Gpx, lipid peroxidation (LPO; actual measurement made of malonaldehyde (MDA) as a parameter for LPO), and SOD measurements.

Histologic Review

Tissue sections were stained with hematoxylin-eosin and reviewed independently by 3 individuals, including a pathologist. Myocytic damage was evaluated, using the Billingham grading scale [28]. This scale allows scoring of tissue for damage by analyzing percentages of cells having evidence of myofibrillar loss or cytoplasmic vacuolization. Tissue was graded from 0 to 3 (depending upon the percentage of damaged cells): 0, <5 per cent; 1.5, 6-15 per cent; 2.0, 16-25 per cent; 2.5, 26-35 per cent; 3.0, >35 per cent.

Statistics

All experiments were performed in duplicate or triplicate. Measurements of enzymes were corrected for tissue weight. Results are shown as means ± standard error of the means (S.E.M.). Significance was determined by the Student-Newman-Keuls test, using a p value of ≤ 0.05 as an indicator of significance.

Results

Measurement of Mouse and Heart Weights

Mice were weighed at the onset of experiments (day 1) and again on day 7 or 11. The hearts were removed and also weighed prior to homogenization. There were no significant differences in mouse weights among the treatment groups prior to administration of ICHOR or Doxo. However, at the end of the experimental period, mice receiving ICHOR alone or no drug (controls) had negligible changes in weight (ICHOR, +0.21 ± 0.25 g; control,–0.85 ± 0.42 g). However, mice receiving Doxo, whether alone or with ICHOR, suffered weight loss, at times ≥ 10 per cent of initial body weight. The ICHOR/Doxo group registered a loss of 2.4 ± 0.4 g while mice injected with Doxo alone lost 2.2 ± 0.3 g weight. The actual averaged weights of mice were as follows: ICHOR, 19.9 ± 0.5 g; ICHOR/Doxo, 16.4 ± 0.5 g; Doxo, 16.8 ± 0.6 g; and control, 19.5 ± 0.4 g. The differences in weight between control mice or those receiving ICHOR, and those receiving Doxo (with and without ICHOR) were significant ($p<0.001$).

The weights of the animals' hearts followed a similar trend, with control or ICHOR alone groups having hearts that weighed significantly more than the hearts from mice receiving either Doxo alone or in combination with ICHOR: ICHOR, 122.9 ± 6.6 mg; ICHOR/Doxo, 100 mg ± 4.8 mg; Doxo, 98 ± 4.3 mg; and control 122 ± 6 mg ($p<0.05$ for control/ICHOR vs Doxo or Doxo/ICHOR). This data did not change whether the animal was sacrificed on day 7 or 11. Adjustment of heart measurement for mouse weight, *i.e.* ratio of mouse heart to mouse body weights also did not alter this assessment.

Results of Enzymatic Assays

Half the heart was used for the enzymatic assays. SOD levels were measured only on day 7, while Gpx levels were obtained on both days 7 and 11. Results of the assays are displayed as means ± S.E.M. When indicated, the results were corrected for heart weight.

No significant difference in SOD levels was observed 48 h post-ICHOR or –Doxo administration, although mice receiving Doxo alone or with ICHOR had slightly higher levels of SOD than those seen in controls (data not shown). On the other hand, ICHOR administration resulted in an increment of Gpx of 50 per cent above control levels, an increase still evident 11 days after initiation of the experiment. Results are seen in Figure 6.1. Gpx levels measured 123 ± 26 mU/mL for control hearts and 185 ± 51 mU/mL for mice receiving ICHOR alone. When Doxo was given, Gpx levels were comparable to those in control animals (Doxo, 120 ± 29 mU/mL vs. ICHOR/Doxo, 160 ± 19 mU/mL). These values were adjusted for the weight of tissue used. Corrected values are shown in Figure 6.2. While the differences among groups again were not statistically significant, use of ICHOR was responsible for an impressive gain in tissue Gpx content. The respective numbers (in mU/mL/g weight) were: ICHOR only, 1638; ICHOR/Doxo, 2212; Doxo, 1054; control 1103.

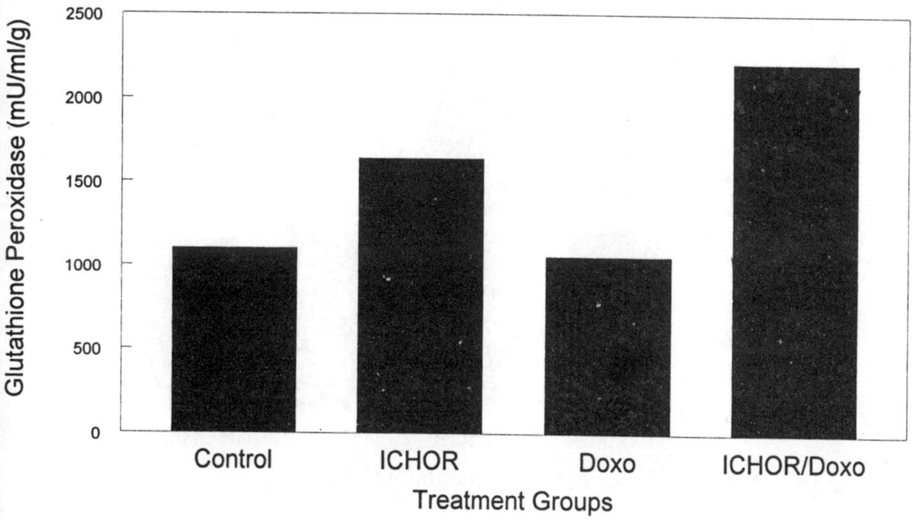

Figure 6.2: Corrected Glutathione Peroxidase Levels 6 Days After Treatments Glutathione peroxidase (Gpx) levels corrected for the weight of heart tissue used for the enzymatic assay are shown as Means ± S.E.M. The unit of measurement was mU/ml/g tissue weight. As noted above, results were obtained 11 days from inception of the experiment (or 6 days from last administration of ICHOR or dose of Doxo). Mean Gpx levels were divided by mean tissue weight to derive the results demonstrated.

Gpx was, as noted, also measured within 48 h of the last dose of ICHOR or Doxo (day 7) (Figure 6.3). At that time point, ICHOR usage itself resulted in almost 2 times the amount of Gpx seen in heart tissue in control animals or after Doxo injection (ICHOR, 10207 mU/mL/g weight vs. 5368 mU/mL/g for controls or 5525 mU/mL/g for Doxo-treated mice). Administration of ICHOR with Doxo did not bring about an increase in Gpx levels (5096 mU/ml/g).

Malonaldehyde (MDA) was used as a marker of lipid peroxidation, with measurements taken in micromoles (μM). Correction was again made for weight of tissue used and the assays were performed on day 11. Results after correction are shown in Figures 6.4a and 6.4b. After ICHOR was used alone, a decline in lipid peroxidation to 30 per cent below control levels was observed: control, 80 ± 12 μM vs. ICHOR 56 ± 12 μM (n=9-10). Doxo use by itself was associated with an increase in MDA levels to 106 ± 11 μM; this is an appreciable although insignificant increase, even at this relatively prolonged time after Doxo administration (6 days). The concomitant use of ICHOR with Doxo resulted in a lowering of MDA levels to 88 ± 11 μM (p=0.08). Differences between the ICHOR only and Doxo only groups were significant (p=0.04). With correction for tissue weight, MDA levels (μM/g) were: control, 656; ICHOR, 459; Doxo, 1082; and ICHOR/Doxo, 880.

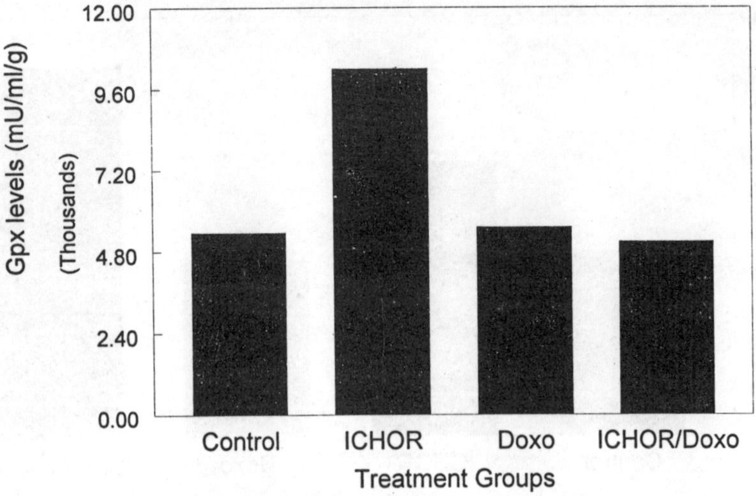

Figure 6.3: Corrected Glutathione Peroxidase Levels at 48 Hours

Corrected Gpx levels are shown in this figure (mU/ml/g tissue weight) after mice were sacrificed 48 hours after last dose of chemotherapeutic agent and ICHOR dose.

Histologic Assessment of Doxo-induced Damage

Myocytic damage after Doxo was indicated by extent of myofibrillar loss and presence of vacuolization within the cytoplasm (Figure 6.5). To achieve consistency and objectivity of pathologic assessment, three independent reviewers evaluated slides in blinded fashion. The Billingham grading scale [28] was used, as previously stated, in the Materials and Methods section. Using this scale, tissue is scored by counting percentages of cells having evidence of damage, including intracytoplasmic vacuolization and myofibrillar loss (Table 6.1). As expected, Doxo significantly damaged heart muscle. ICHOR with Doxo, however, significantly reduced such damage ($p<0.001$), although not to completely normal levels.

Table 6.1: Assessment of Degree of Cardiomyopathy in Various Treated Groups

Treatment Groups	*Percent Cells with Damage*	*Billingham Score*
Control	9 ± 2	1.5
Doxo Only	44 ± 3*@	3
Ichor/Doxo	25 ± 0#@	2

The Billingham grading scale allows assessment of damage based on percentage of cells with myofibrillar loss and cytoplasmic vacuolization. The grading is as follows: Grade 0, <5 per cent; Grade 1.5, 6-15 per cent; Grade 2, 16-25 per cent; Grade 2.5, 26-35 per cent; Grade 3, >35 per cent. Three reviewers independently examined slides of tissue in blinded fashion. These reviewers included a certified Pathologist. Results are given as mean ± S.E.M. There was a minimum of 5 mice in each group. (There was no group receiving Ichor alone). The groups are identified as detailed in Figure 6.1 The asterisk (*) denotes results that are statistically significant for differences between Ichor/Doxo and Doxo groups ($p<0.01$). The sign # indicates statistically significant differences between control and Ichor/Doxo ($p<0.05$). Lastly, @ indicates a result that is significantly different from that of controls ($p<0.001$).

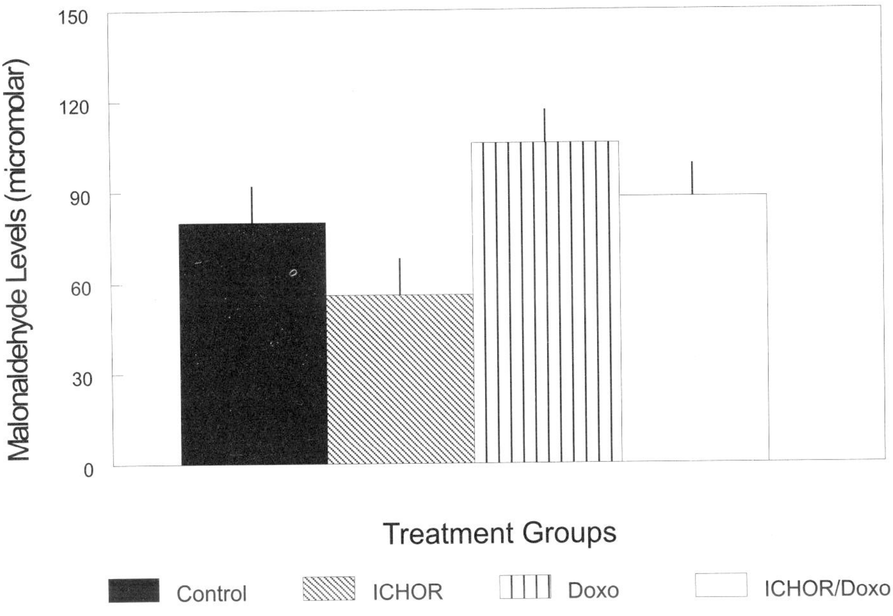

Figure 6.4a: Lipid Peroxidation after ICHOR+/or Doxo

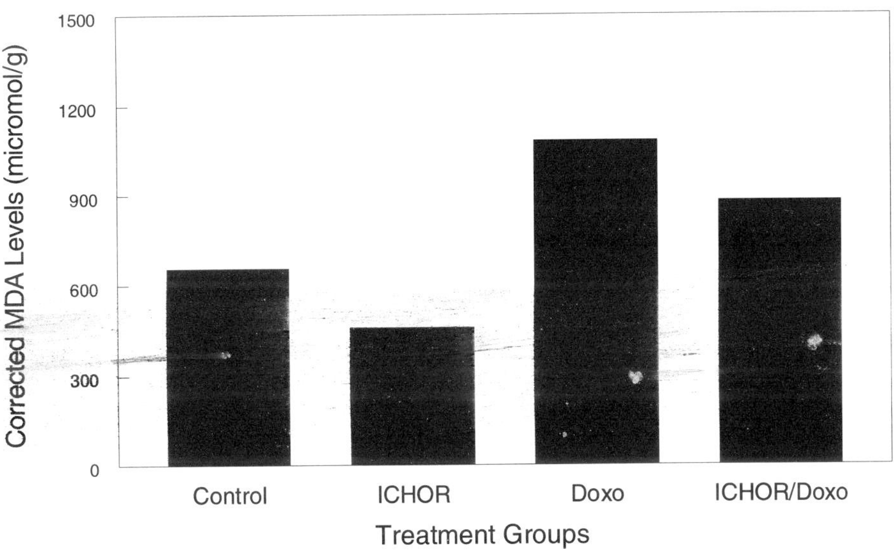

Figure 6.4b: Malonaldehyde (MDA) Levels After Correction for Heart Weight

Level of lipid peroxidation was measured indirectly by assaying malonaldehyde levels in heart tissue obtained 6 days after completion of drug and/or herb administration (n=8).

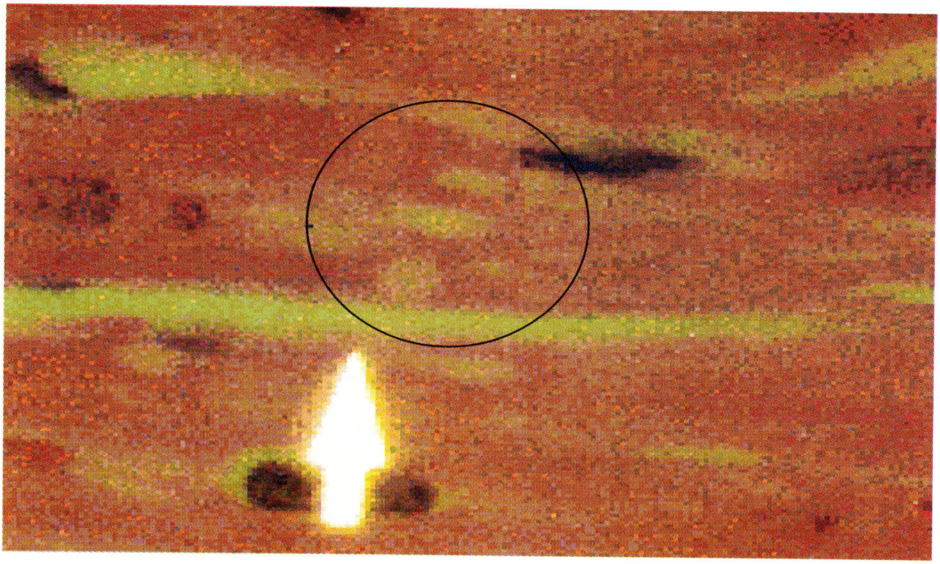

Figure 6.5: (Left) Shows an H&E Stained Section of Murine Cardiac Muscle in which Vacuolization is Seen After Doxorubicin Therapy. The arrow indicates an area of myofibrillar "drop out" while the circle encloses one area of vacuolization.

Discussion

Doxo-associated cardiotoxicity is an important clinical issue that is likely to increase in importance over time. Potential causes of Doxo toxicity have been previously summarized and include (1) inhibition of protein and nucleic acid synthesis [20, 30]; (2) irreversible topoisomerase II inactivation [31]; and (3) mitochondrial dysfunction [32]. Causes of damage are most likely multifactorial. However, the role of free radical formation with lipid peroxidation is a popular and widely, although not universally, accepted theory of damage [17, 33]. It is theorized that oxidative stress causes loss of myofibrils, myocardial vacuolization, and other parameters of damage. This damage can be compounded by a relative deficiency within the myocardium of antioxidative enzymes [34] and by further decrease in endogenous antioxidant levels after Doxo usage [35].

We have presented data that suggest that a Rasayana [25, 35], ICHOR-CR, with previously reported antioxidant properties may offer protection to the heart, when used in conjunction with Doxo, a potent cardiotoxin. We have not attempted to assess the effect of treatments on mortality of the animals. We also have not performed functional assays of damage, since it has been shown by other investigators that cardiac function as measured by ECHOcardiography did not always change sufficiently for early injury to be detected, or for the effects of protective strategies to become evident [37]. We have instead focused on evaluating histopathologic criteria in a model of acute usage, to assess extent of damage.

The degree of elevation of antioxidant enzymes after ICHOR alone was impressive, although not statistically significant. It was also durable, being present 11 days after ICHOR use was initiated (and 6 days after it was discontinued). Admittedly, other antioxidants such as catalase that have an important detoxifying function in heart, or of free radical scavengers, such as metallothionein, were not measured. However, because lipid peroxidation was significantly diminished after ICHOR, we may be seeing the additive effects of individual antioxidant enzymes, acting in concert with one another to prevent or ameliorate Doxo toxicity. Alternately, the herb itself may act directly as an antioxidant, rather than by inducing the production of antioxidant enzymes. Lastly, it is conceivable that ICHOR's augmentation of enzymatic production and, therefore, its protective effects, may have been greatest on day 5, *i.e.* prior to administration of Doxo. Measurements were not obtained at that time. Future experiments will focus on changes in antioxidant levels on days 5-7.

Our results are in agreement with those of other investigators. Joseph and others have previously reported that ICHOR has antioxidant properties [37, 38]. Antioxidants have been proposed as protectants against Doxo-induced damage. Protection has been variably observed after the use of carnitine [37], vitamins E and C [38, 39], probocol [40], metallothionein [18] and melatonin [41]. The partial protection seen in our experiments is consistent with that observed in other antioxidant trials.

ICHOR has a very real salutary effect on heart, as shown by the results of our histopathologic analysis. While there was some variability in the level of protection offered by ICHOR, significant reduction of cardiomyopathic changes in heart muscle such as vacuolization or myofibrillar loss occurred with the combined treatment. Variability of effect most probably stemmed from incomplete solubility of the herb in its current form with resultant variable dosing to mice.

Experiments need to be performed that examine the impact of ICHOR on chronic cardiotoxicity. As has been shown with vitamin E, we cannot assume that protection against acute cardiotoxicity necessarily infers protection against the more chronic forms of damage [42], especially since there are probable disparities in mechanisms of damage between acute and chronic forms of damage. Long-term negative (or positive) effects of ICHOR's use must also be probed, along with its effect on other organ systems.

Rasayanas have been used in the Ayurvedic system of medicine for hundreds of years, and have been touted as having antiaging and immune restorative properties [35]. They have been reported to be myeloprotective agents, stimulating increases in peripheral blood leukocyte counts, bone marrow cellularity and preserving colony-forming activity after chemotherapy [25, 36]. If also proven to be cardioprotective, it would be a highly desirable product, with no, as yet, reported toxicity, the ability to counter chemotherapy-induced myelosuppression, and offer no interference with chemotherapeutic efficacy. Importantly, its low cost would be especially attractive, potentially benefiting populations, where the utilization of cytokines or dexrazoxane may be contravened by their expense.

Acknowledgement

Work funded by a grant provided by the Ladies' Leukemia League of New Orleans, LA.

References

1. Steinherz LJ, Steinherz PG, Tan TC, Heller G and Murphy L: Cardiac toxicity 4 to 20 years after completing anthracycline therapy. *JAMA* 1999, 266, 1672-1677.
2. Singal PK and Iliskovic N: Doxorubicin-induced cardiomyopathy. *N Engl J Med* 1998, 339, 900-905.
3. Otero FJ, Boor PJ and Sheahan RG: Doxorubicin-induced cardiomyopathy. *Am J Med Sci* 2000, 320: 59-63.
4. Orhan B: Doxorubicin-cardiotoxicity: growing importance. *J Clin Oncol* 1999, 17, 2294-2295.
5. Serrano J, Palmeira CM, Kuehl DW, and Wallace KB: Cardioselective and cumulative oxidation of mitochondrial DNA following subchronic doxorubicin administration. *Biochim Biophys Acta* 1999, 1411, 201-205.
6. Krischer JP, Epstein S, Cuthbertson DD, Goorin AM, Epstein ML, and Lipshultz SE: Clinical cardiotoxicity following anthracycline treatment for childhood cancer: The Pediatric Oncology Group experience. *J Clin Oncol* 1997, 15, 1544-1552.
7. Nysom K, Holm K, Lipsitz SR, Mone SM, Colan SD, Orav EJ, Sallan SE, Olsen JH, Hertz H, Jacobsen R and Lipshultz SE: Relationship between cumulative anthracycline dose and late cardiotoxicity in childhood acute lymphoblastic leukemia. *J Clin Oncol* 1998, 16, 545-550.
8. Abramowicz M: Dexrazoxane for cardiac protection against doxorubicin. *The Medical Letter* 1995, 37, 110-111.
9. Ali MK and Ewer MS: The natural history of anthracycline cardiotoxicity in children. *In:* [Muggia, FM, Green, MD, Speyer, JL (ed.)], *Cancer Treatment and the Heart*, The Johns Hopkins University Press, Baltimore, 1992.
10. Billingham ME: Role of endomyocardial biopsy in diagnosis and treatment of heart disease. [ed. Silver, M.D.], *Cardiovascular Pathology*, Churchill Livingstone, New York, 1992.
11. Boucek RJ Jr, Miracle A, Anderson M, Engelman R, Atkinson J, and Dodd DA: Persistent effects of doxorubicin on cardiac gene expression. *J Mol Cell Cardiol* 1999, 31, 1435-1446.
12. Bristow MR, Billingham ME, Mason JW, and Daniels JR (1978) Clinical spectrum of anthracycline antibiotic cardiotoxicity. *Cancer Treat Rep* 1978, 62, 873-879.
13. Dreyer ZE, Blatt J, and Bleyer A: Late Effects of Childhood Cancer and its Treatment. [ed. Pizza PA and Poplack DG], *Principles and Practice of Pediatric Oncology*, Lippincott, Williams and Wilkins, Philadelphia, 2001.

14. Duroshow JH, Locker GY and Myers CE: Enzymatic defenses of the mouse heart against reactive oxygen metabolites. Alterations produced by doxorubicn. *J Clin Invest* 1980, 65, 128-135.

15. Fink FM, Genser N, Fink C, Falk M, Mair J, Mauer-Dengg K, Hammerer I, and Puschendorf B: Cardiac troponin T and creatine kinase MB mass concentrations in children receiving anthracycline chemotherapy. *Med Pediat Oncol* 1995, 25, 185-189.

16. Ghosh B, Hanevold CD, Dobashi K, Orak JK, and Singh I: Tissue differences in antioxidant enzyme gene expression in response to endotoxin. *Free Radic Biol Med* 1996, 21, 533-540.

17. Grenier MA and Lipshultz SE: Epidemiology of anthracycline cardiotoxicity in children and adults. *Semin Oncol* 1998, 25, 72-85.

18. Hellman K: Anthracycline cardiotoxicity prevention by dexrazoxane: breakthrough of a barrier—sharpens antitumor profile and therapeutic index. *J Clin Oncol* 1996, 14, 332-333.

19. Herman EH, Zhang J, Lipshultz SE, Rifai N, Chadwick D, Takeda K, Yu ZX, and Ferrans VJ: Correlation between serum levels of cardiac troponin-T and the severity of the chronic cardiomyopathyy induced by doxorubicin. *J Clin Oncol* 1999, 17, 2237-2243.

20. Joseph CD, Praveenkumar V, Kuttan G, and Kuttan R: Myeloprotective effect of a non-toxic indigenous preparation Rasayana in cancer patients receiving chemotherapy and radiation therapy. A pilot study. *J Exp Clin Cancer Res* 1999, 18, 325-329.

21. Krischer JP, Epstein S, Cuthbertson DD, Goorin AM, Epstein ML, and Lipshultz SE: Clinical cardiotoxicity following anthracycline treatment for childhood cancer: The Pediatric Oncology Group experience. *J Clin Oncol* 1997, 15, 1544-1552.

22. Kumar VP, Kuttan R, and Kuttan G: Effect of "rasayanas," a herbal drug preparation on immune responses and its significance in cancer treatment. *Ind J Exp Biol* 1999, 37, 27-31.

23. Lipshultz SE: Dexrazoxane for protection against cardiotoxic effects of anthracycline in children. *J Clin Oncol* 1996, 14, 328-331.

24. Lipshultz SE, Colan SD, Gelber RD, Perez-Atayde AR, Sallan SE, and Sanders SP: Late cardiac effects of doxorubicin therapy for acute lymphoblastic leukemia in childhood. *N Engl J Med* 1991, 324, 808-815.

25. Marti JE: Botanical medicines. [ed. Kalasky, K.L.] *The Alternative Health and Medicine Encylopedia*, Gale Research, Detroit, 1998.

26. Morishima I, Okumura K, Matsui H, Kaneko S, Numaguchi Y, Kawakami K, Mokuno S, Hayakawa M, Toki Y, Ito T, and Hayakawa T: Zinc accumulation in adriamycin-induced cardiomyopathy in rats: effects of melatonin, a cardioprotective antioxidant. *J Pineal Res* 1999, 26, 204-210.

27. Nysom K, Holm K, Lipsitz SR, Mone SM, Colan SD, Orav EJ, Sallan SE, Olsen JH, Hertz H, Jacobsen JR, and Lipshultz SE: Relationship between cumulative anthracycline dose and late cardiotoxicity in childhood acute lymphoblastic leukemia. *J Clin Oncol* 1998, 16, 545-550.

28. Olson RD, Mushlin PS: Doxorubicin cardiotoxicity: analysis of prevailing hypotheses. *FASE B J* 1990, 4, 3076-3086.

29. Orhan B: Doxorubicin-cardiotoxicity: growing importance. *J Clin Oncol* 1999, 17, 2294-2295.

30. Otero FJ, Boor PJ, and Sheahan RG: Doxorubicin-induced cardiomyopathy. *Am J Med Sci* 2000, 320, 59-63.

31. Ottlinger ME, Sallan S, and Rifai N: Myocardial damage in doxorubicin-treated children: A study of serum cardiac troponinT. *Proc Am Soc Clin Oncol* 1995, 14, 345a.

32. Rosenoff SH, Olson HM, Young DM: Brief communication: Adriamycin-induced cardiac damage in the mouse: a small-animal model of cardiotoxicity. *J Natl Cancer Inst* 1975a, 55, 191-194.

33. Rosenoff SH, Brooks E, Bostick F, and Young RC: Alterations in DNA synthesis in cardiac tissue induced by adriamycin in vivo—relationship to fatal toxicity. *Biochem Pharmacol* 1975, 24, 1898-1901.

34. Serrano J, Palmeira CM, Kuehl DW, and Wallace KB: Cardioselective and cumulative oxidation of mitochondrial DNA following subchronic doxorubicin administration. *Biochim Biophys Acta* 1999, 1411, 201-205.

35. Singal PK, and Iliskovic N: Doxorubicin induced cardiomyopathy. *N Engl J Med* 1998, 339, 900-905.

36. Singal PK, Olweny CL, Li T: Doxorubicin-induced cardiomyopathy. *N Engl J Med* 1999, 340, 655.

37. Singal PK, Siveski-Iliskovic N, Hill M, Thomas TP, Li T: Combination therapy with probucol prevents adriamycin-induced cardiomyopathy. *J Mol Cell Cardiol* 1995, 27, 1055-1063.

38. Sorensen K, Levitt G, Sebag-Montefiore D, Bull C, Sullivan I: Cardiac function in Wilms' Tumor survivors. *J Clin Oncol* 1995, 13, 1546-1556.

39. Steinherz LJ, Steinherz PG, Tan TC, Heller G, and Murphy L: Cardiac toxicity 4 to 20 years after completing anthracycline therapy. *JAMA* 1999, 266, 1672-1677.

40. Strohm GH, Payne CM, Alberts DS, Peng YM, Moon TE, Bahl JJ, and Bressler R: Cardiotoxic effects of doxorubicin with and without carnitine—usefulness of the mouse model in assessment. *Arch Pathol Lab Med* 1982, 106, 181-185.

41. Tewey KM, Rowe TC, Yang L, Halligan BD, and Liu LF: Adriamycin-induced DNA damage mediated by mammalian DNA topoisomerase II. *Science* 1984, 226: 466-468.

42. Wexler LH, Andrich MP, Venzon D, Berg SL, Weaver-McClure L, Chen CC, Dilsizian V, Avila N, Jarosinski P, Balis FM, Poplack DG, and Horowitz ME: Randomized trial of the cardioprotective agent ICRF-187 in pediatric sarcoma patients treated with doxorubicin. *J Clin Oncol* 1996, 14, 362-372.

43. Yen HC, Oberley TD, Vichitbandha S, Ho YS, St. Clair DK: The protective role of manganese superoxide dismutase against adriamycin-induced acute cardiac toxicity in transgenic mice. *J Clin Invest* 1996, 98, 1253-1260.

44. Zhou Z and Kang YJ: Immunocytochemical localization of metallothionein and its regulation to doxorubicin toxicity in transgenic mouse heart. *Am J Pathol* 2000, 156, 1653-1662.

Chapter 7

Ethnomedicinal Potential of Herbal Drugs on Gastric Dysfunction in Experimental Animals

Ch. V. Rao* and P. Pushpangadan

*Gastropharmacology Laboratory, Ethnopharmacology Division,
National Botanical Research Institute (Council of Scientific and Industrial Research),
Rana Pratap Marg, Post Box No. 436, Lucknow – 226 001, Uttar Pradesh, India
E -mail: chvrao72@yahoo.com

ABSTRACT

As a part of our ongoing study, we have pharmacologically validated some plants traditionally used for treating gastrointestinal disorders. Selected plants *Utleria salicifolia, Cissampelos pareira, Emblica officinalis* Gaerten. (Amalki), *Aegle marmelos, Zingiber officinale* and *Euphorbia hirta* were screened against various validated physical and chemical factors–induced gastric ulceration and diarrhoeal models in experimental animals. Our study demonstrated the scientific potential of *Utleria salicifolia* and *Euphorbia hirta* in treating gastric ulcer. However, *Cissampelos pareira* showed potent antidiarrhoeal activity.

Keywords: Herbal drugs, Ulcer, Diarrhoea

Introduction

The present article deals with the detailed exploration of ulcer protective and antidiarrhoeal activities of traditionally used standardized plant extracts. Gastric hyperacidity and ulcer are very common, causing human suffering. Prolonged anxiety, emotional stress, surgical shock, burns and trauma are known to cause severe mucosal irritation.

Herbal medicines have been used since the dawn of civilization to maintain health and to treat diseases. Herbs, which have been the principal form of medicine in developing countries, are once again becoming popular throughout the developing and developed world. Our ethnic societies had already elaborated their own traditional herbal cures even before the advent of modern medicine. In Ayurveda, peptic ulcer mostly refers to *Amlapitta* or *Parinamasula*. *Amlapitta* is a disease of the gastrointestinal tract, especially of the stomach. *Amlapitta* literally means, pitta leading to sour taste [1]. Apart from the stress laid on food habits and personal hygiene, some herbal drugs have also been mentioned. Numerous epidemiological surveys have shown an inverse relationship between the intake of fruits, vegetables and cereals and the incidence of coronary heart disease, gastrointestinal disorders and cancers. Some medicinal plants or parts thereof–that are relatively high in flavonoids are known to exert the curative action in ulcer and diarrhoea [2]. The rhizomes of *Utleria salicifolia* [3] and *Zingiber officinale* [4], *Euphorbia hirta* whole plant [5], *Cissampelos pareira* roots [6] *Emblica officinalis* Gaerten. [1] and *Aegle marmelos* fruits [7] etc were investigated for the treatment of gastrointestinal disorders *viz.* ulcer and diarrhoea. Plants showing promising activities in the preliminary studies were processed further in large quantities for detailed investigations.

Materials and Methods

Animals

Male Sprague-Dawley rats (150-175 g) were used throughout our study and they were housed three to a cage for the duration of the study. Rats had free access to standard rodent pellet diet (Amrut, India) and were maintained in a temperature and humidity controlled environment on a 12 h dark/light cycle. Animals were fasted for 24 h before the study and water was allowed *ad libitum*.

Plant Materials and Preparation of Extract(s)

Utleria salicifolia and *Zingiber officinale* rhizomes, whole plant of *Euphorbia hirta, Cissampelos pareira* roots, *Emblica officinalis* Gaerten. (Amalki) and *Aegle marmelos* fruits were collected and authenticated by the taxonomist and authentic specimens were prepared for future reference. *Utleria salicifolia* rhizomes were collected from the Parambikulam forests of the South Western Ghats region of Palakkad district of Kerala and the remaining plants were collected from the Botanical Garden of NBRI in May to July 2002. The plant parts were shade dried, coarsely powdered and extracted with 50 per cent ethanol by percolation at room temperature. The extract was separated by filtration and concentrated using rotary evaporator (Buchi, USA) and lyophilized (Labconco, USA). The yield of the extracts are presented in Table 7.1.

Table 7.1: The Per cent Yield (w/w) of Ethanol Extractives

Sl.No.	*Botanical Name*	*Part Used*	*Solvent*	*Per cent (w/w) Yield*
1.	*Utleria salicifolia*	Rhizome	EtOH: H_20 (1:1)	4.2 per cent
2.	*Cissampelos pareira*	Roots	EtOH: H_20 (1:1)	3.4 per cent
3.	*Euphorbia hirta*	Whole plant	EtOH: H_20 (1:1)	4.2 per cent
4.	*Emblica officinalis*	Fruit	EtOH: H_20 (1:1)	9.2 per cent
5.	*Aegle marmelos*	Fruit	EtOH: H_20 (1:1)	11.5 per cent
6.	*Zingiber officinale*	Rhizomes	EtOH: H_20 (1:1)	10.5 per cent

Phytochemical Screening

The selected plants were subjected to preliminary qualitative phytochemical screening. The rhizomes of *Utleria salicifolia* extract (USE) gave positive tests for steroids, alkaloids, terpenoids, saponins, and tannins. High performance thin layer chromatography (HPTLC) studies of the 50 per cent ethanolic extract of *Utleria salicifolia* were carried out using pre-coated silica gel plate (Merck 60 F 254) as the stationary phase and toluene: ethyl acetate: formic acid (5:5:1) as the mobile phase. The extract was spotted using a Camag Linomat IV spotter. These plates were observed at UV 254 nm and were scanned on TLC scanner III using CAT software (Figure 7.1). The extract of *Euphorbia hirta* showed positive test for flavonoids and it was further fractionated with water followed by dichloromethane and diethyl ether to give a flavonoid fraction, which on repeated column and preparative chromatographic separation gave a dark yellow substance (325 mg, 0.325 per cent W/W), R_f: 0.52 (toluene: ethylacetae: formic acid 5:4:1), m.p. 176°C (8). It was identified as quercetin-3-*O*-β-D-rhamnoside and further confirmed by co-TLC (Figures 7.2 and 7.2a).

Experimental Procedure

Test doses in the range of 50, 100 and 200 mg/kg and synthetic antiulcer compound ranitidine in the dose of 50 mg/kg as a positive control were used throughout the experiment. The animals were treated orally twice daily at 10.00 and 16.00 hrs respectively for five days in aspirin, cold restraint stress, pylorus ligation and ethanol-induced acute ulcers. The isolated compound quercetin-3-*O*-β-D-rhamnoside (quercitrin) 100 mg/kg was given orally twice: 20 h and 1 h prior to subjecting the animals to gastric ulcer. Control group of animals received suspension of 1 per cent carboxymethyl cellulose (CMC) in distilled water (10 mL/kg).

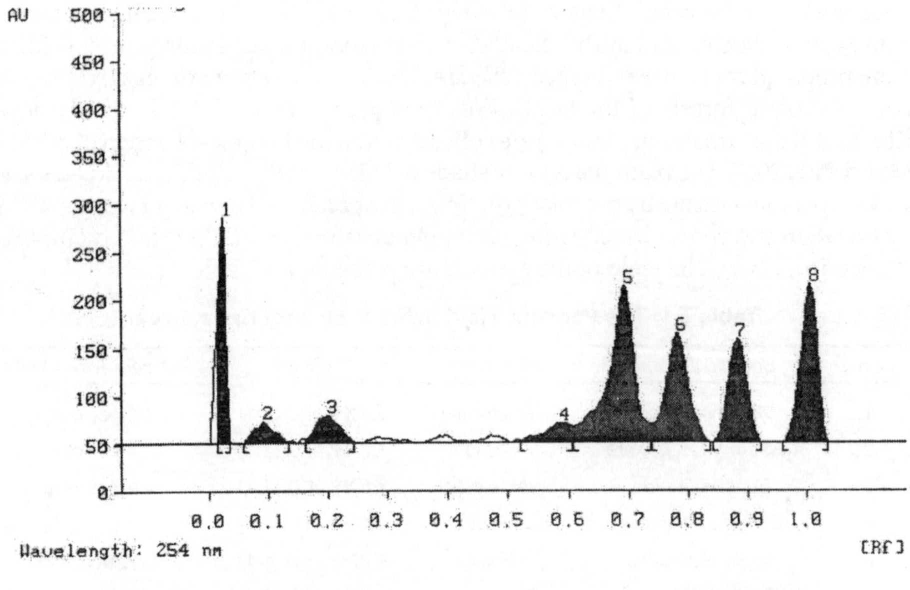

Figure 7.1: HPTLC Fingerprint Profile of *Utleria salicifolia* Extract

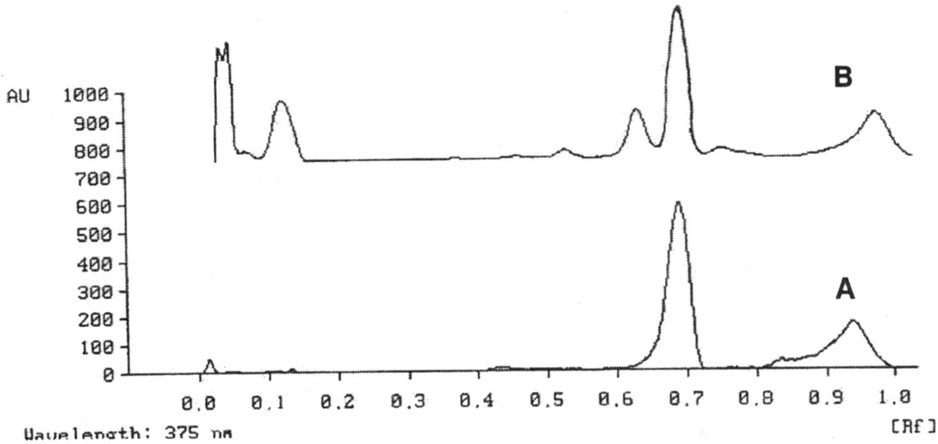

Figure 7.2: HPTLC Densitometric Scan at UV 278 nm of *Euphorbia hirta* A: Quercetin standard; B: 50 per cent Ethanolic extract of *Euphorbia hirta*.

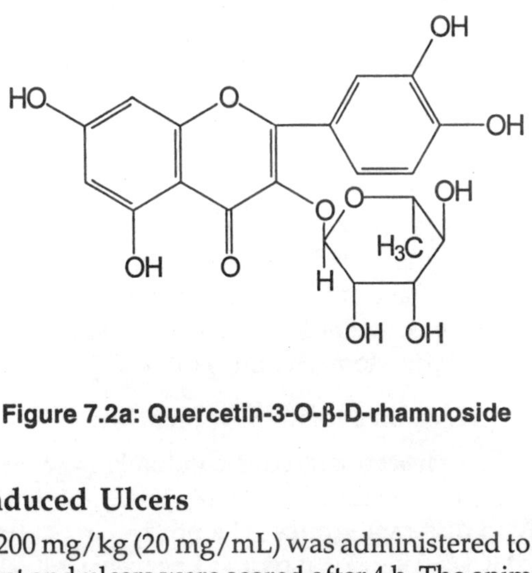

Figure 7.2a: Quercetin-3-O-β-D-rhamnoside

Aspirin (ASP)-induced Ulcers

ASP in dose of 200 mg/kg (20 mg/mL) was administered to the animals on the day of the experiment and ulcers were scored after 4 h. The animals were sacrificed and the stomach was then excised and cut along the greater curvature, washed carefully with 5.0 mL of 0.9 per cent NaCl and ulcers were scored by a person unaware of the experimental protocol in the glandular portion of the stomach. Ulcer index has been calculated by adding the total number of ulcers per stomach and the total severity of ulcers per stomach. The total severity of the ulcers was determined by recording the severity of each ulcer after histological confirmation as follows: 0, no ulcer; +, pin point ulcer and histological changes limited to superficial layers of mucosa and no congestion; ++, ulcer size less than 1 mm and half of the mucosal thickness showed necrotic changes; +++, ulcer size 1-2 mm with more than two-thirds of the mucosal thickness destroyed wih marked necrosis and congestion, muscularis remaining unaffected; ++++, ulcer either more than 2 mm in size or perforated with complete destruction of the mucosa with necrosis and haemorrhage, muscularis still remaining unaffected. The pooled group ulcer score was then calculated according to the method of Sanyal *et al.* [9].

Cold-restraint Stress (CRS)-induced Ulcers

Rats were deprived of food, but not water, for about 18 h before the experiment. On day six, the experimental rats were immobilized by strapping the fore and hind limbs on a wooden plank and kept for 2 h, at 4-6 °C [10]. Two hours later, the animals were sacrificed by cervical dislocation and ulcers were examined on the dissected stomachs as described above.

Pylorus Ligated (PL)-induced Ulcers

Drugs were administered for a period of 5 days as described above and the rats were kept for 18 h fasting and care was taken to avoid coprophagy. Animals were anaesthetized using pentobarbitone (35 mg/kg, ip), the abdomen was opened and pylorus ligation was done without causing any damage to its blood supply. The stomach was replaced carefully and the abdomen wall was closed in two layers with interrupted sutures. The animals were deprived of water during the post-operative period [11]. After 4 h, stomachs were dissected out and cut open along the greater curvature and ulcers were scored by a person unaware of the experimental protocol in the glandular portion of the stomach as mentioned in aspirin induced ulcers.

Ethanol (EtOH)-induced Ulcers

The gastric ulcers were induced in rats by administrating 100 per cent EtOH (1mL/200 g, 1h) [12] and the animals were sacrificed by cervical dislocation and stomach was incised along the greater curvature and examined for ulcers. The ulcer index was scored, based upon the product of length and width of the ulcers present in the glandular portion of the stomach (mm^2/rat).

Evaluation of the Effect on Normal Defecation

Group of six mice each were placed individually in separate cages with filter papers at the bottom. The doses of the extracts (25, 50 and 100 mg/kg) were administered orally to different groups. The nonspecific antidiarrhoeal reference drug diphenoxylate HCl (5.0 mg/kg, p.o.) and 1 per cent CMC (10 mg/kg, p.o.) were administered to two groups and later served as controls [13]. The total number of the faecal matter in each group was assessed every hour for the next 4 h. Percent reduction in the total number of faeces in the treated groups were obtained by comparison with control animals.

Castor Oil-induced Diarrhoea

The method of Awouters *et al.* [14] as modified by Nwodo and Alumanah [15] was used. Briefly, rats fasted for 24 h were randomly allocated to five groups of six animals each. Group I received 1 per cent CMC (10 mL/kg, p.o.), groups II, III and IV received orally the drug extract (25, 50 and 100 mg/kg), respectively. The group V was given diphenoxylate HCl (5.0 mg/kg, p.o.) as suspension. After 60 min each animal was administered with 2 mL of castor oil by orogastric cannula, and placed in a separate cage and observed for 4 h defecation. Transparent plastic dishes were placed beneath each cage and the characteristic diarrhoeal droppings were noted.

Small Intestinal Transit

Animals were divided into four groups of six rats each and each animal was given orally 1 mL of charcoal meal (5 per cent activated charcoal suspended in 1 per cent CMC) 60 min after an oral dose of drugs or vehicle. Group I was administered with 1 per cent CMC (10 mL/kg) and animals in the groups II and III received drug extract (50 and 100 mg/kg). The group IV received atropine sulfate (0.1 mg/kg, i.p.) as standard drug. After 30 min animals were killed by cervical dislocation and the intestine was removed without stretching and placed lengthwise on moist filter paper. The length of the intestine (pyloric sphincter to caecum) and the distance travelled by the charcoal as a percentage of that length were evaluated for each animal, and group means were compared and expressed as percentage inhibition [16].

Statistical Analysis

All the data were presented as mean ± SEM and analyzed by Wilcoxon Sum Rank Test and unpaired Student's t-test for the possible significant interrelation between the various groups. A value of $P < 0.05$ was considered statistically significant.

Results and Discussion

The preliminary HPTLC studies revealed that the solvent system toluene: ethyl acetate: formic acid (5: 5: 1) was ideal and gave well-resolved peaks for *Utleria salicifolia* extract (Figure 7.1). The chromatogram showed spots at Rf 0.10, 0.20, 0.59, 0.69, 0.78 and 0.88 on examination under UV 254 nm. The densitometric scanning at 254 nm gave the percent area of the three major spots at Rfs 0.69, 0.78 and 0.88 as 28.16, 17.17 and 13.79 respectively. However, the preliminary HPTLC analysis of *Euphorbia hirta* revealed that the solvent system toluene: ethyl acetate: formic acid (5: 4: 1) was ideal and gave well-resolved peaks (Figure 7.2). The spots of the chromatogram were visualized at 254 nm and 278 nm and one of the spots with Rf value 0.52 matched with quercetin which was used as the marker compound (Figure 7.2 and 7.2a). Extracts of *Utleria salicifolia* and *Euphorbia hirta* at doses of 50-200 mg/kg, twice a day for 5 days prevented the acute gastric ulcers in a dose related manner. The range of percent protection were PL 14.48-51.03 per cent ($P< 0.01$), ASP 28.80–56.52 per cent ($P< 0.05$), EtOH 13.22–60.74 per cent ($P<0.05$–0.001) and CRS 21.22–77.14 per cent ($P<0.05$–<0.001), respectively. The percent protection of ranitidine ranged from 57.44–80.0 per cent ($P< 0.05$–< 0.001), respectively in various gastric ulcer models in *Utleria salicifolia* (Table 7.2). Pylorus ligation-induced ulcers are due to autodigestion of the gastric mucosa and break down of the gastric mucosal barrier. Synthetic NSAIDs like aspirin cause mucosal damage by interfering with prostaglandin synthesis, increasing acid secretion and back diffusion of H^+ ions [1,2]. The incidence of ethanol-induced ulcers is predominant in the glandular part of stomach which was reported to stimulate the formation of leukotriene C4 (LTC4), mast cell secretory products and reactive oxygen species resulting in the damage of rat gastric mucosa [17]. Ethanol –induced depletion of gastric wall mucus has been prevented by *Utleria salicifolia*. It implies that a concomitant increase in prostaglandins or sulfhydryl compounds contribute to protect the stomach from ethanol injury [2,4]. Stress plays an important role in aetiopathology of gastro-duodenal ulceration. Increase in gastric motility, vagal over activity, mast cell degranulation, decreased gastric mucosal blood flow, and decreased prostaglandin synthesis [3,17] are involved in genesis of stress induced ulcers. Similarly the extract of *Euphorbia hirta* and isolated marker quercetin (100 mg/kg) showed significant protection in various physical and chemical factors induced gastric ulceration in rats as indicated in Table 7.3.

Table 7.2: Effect of *Utleria salicifolia* extract (USE, twice daily for 5 days) on Pylorus Ligation (PL)–Aspirin (ASP)-, Ethanol (EtOH) and Cold Restraint Stress (CRS)-Induced Gastric Ulcers in rats

Treatment (mg/kg)	*Ulcer Index*			
	PL	*ASP*	*EtOH (mm²/rat)*	*CRS*
Control	14.5 ± 2.5	18.4 ± 4.3	24.2 ± 5.5	24.5 ± 3.8
USE 50	12.4 ± 2.6	13.1 ± 2.1	21.0 ± 5.1	19.3 ± 1.4
USE 100	9.1 ± 2.1	10.2 ± 1.6	11.5 ± 4.2	14.6 ± 2.2[a]
USE 200	7.1 ± 1.2[a]	8.0 ± 1.3[a]	9.5 ± 2.5[a]	5.6 ± 1.1[c]
Ranitidine 50	5.1 ± 1.3[b]	7.6 ± 1.5[a]	10.3 ± 2.8[a]	4.9 ± 1.0[c]

Values are mean ± SEM for six rats.

P: [a]<0.05, [b]<0.01 and [c]<0.001 compared to respective control group.

Table 7.3: Effect of *Euphorbia hirta* on Ethanol (EtOH)-, Aspirin (ASP)-, Cold Restraint Stress (CRS)–and Pylorus Ligation (PL)–Induced Gastric Ulcers in Rats

Groups	*Treatment (mg/kg x 5 days)*	*Ulcer Index*			
		ASP	*PL*	*CRS*	*EtOH (mm²/rat)*
I	Control	15.8 ± 1.9	18.9 ± 1.9	24.5 ± 4.1	22.5 ± 5.8
II	*E. hirta* 50	11.4 ± 1.5	15.7 ± 1.7	19.6 ± 3.0	15.6 ± 3.6
III	*E. hirta* 100	7.8 ± 1.3[b]	12.6 ± 1.5[a]	15.1 ± 2.2	10.2 ± 2.7
IV	*E. hirta* 200	4.6 ± 1.1[c]	9.5 ± 1.3[c]	10.4 ± 1.5[b]	6.6 ± 1.5[a]
V	Quercetin 100	5.7 ± 1.2[c]	9.8 ± 1.1[c]	11.0 ± 1.6[b]	8.1 ± 2.3[a]
VI	Ranitidine 50	6.1 ± 1.4[b]	6.9 ± 1.3[c]	4.8 ± 1.0[c]	7.2 ± 2.0[a]

Values are mean ± SEM for eight rats in each group.

P: [a]<0.05, [b]<0.01 and [c]<0.001 compared to respective control group.

The extract of *Cissampelos pareira* roots at 50 and 100 mg/kg doses inhibited defecation by 100 per cent in the initial 2 h on normal defecation in mice. The activity was reduced to 40.0 per cent and 73.0 per cent respectively at the higher doses in the third hour. In the present investigation, ethanolic extract of *Cissampelos pareira* roots showed dose dependent antidiarrhoeal activity in various validated models in rats. Castor oil produced characteristic semisolid diarrhoea dropping in all the animals of the control group. The effect of *C. pareira* roots extract at the dose levels of 25–100 mg/kg caused a dose dependent decrease in the total number of faecal matter (29.2 and 60.0 per cent). Diphenoxylate HCl, a standard antidiarrhoeal drug inhibited the diarrhoea by 70.8 per cent (Table 7.4). The action of castor oil as diarrhoea inductor has been largely studied and it is known, that its most active component is the ricinoleic acid, which produces an irritating activity in small intestine. Prostaglandins contribute to the patho-physiological functions of the gastrointestinal tract and act on the local electrical and mechanical activities of the ileal circular muscles [6]. The effect of *Cissampelos pareira* on castor oil stimulated gastrointestinal transit was also significant and dose dependent. The reduction in the gastrointestinal transit of 53.6 to 61.3 per cent was comparable to the standard antimuscarinic drug atropine sulphate (68.3 per cent) (Figure 7.3). The highest inhibition of gut motility was however obtained with antimuscarinic drug atropine sulphate. These observations demonstrate the antiulcer activity of *Utleria salicifolia*, *Euphorbia hirta* and antidiarrhoeal activity of *Cissampelos pareira*.

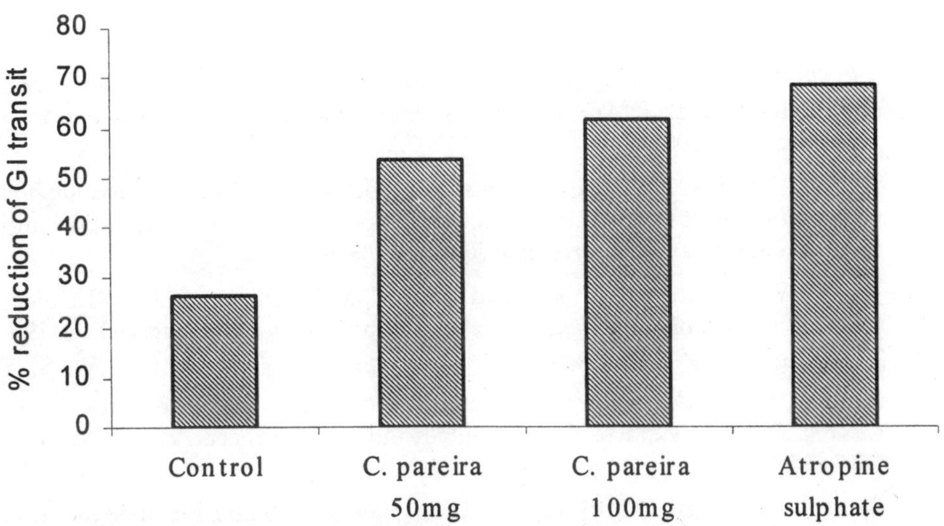

Figure 7.3: Effect of *Cissampelos pareira* (*C. pareira*) Extract on Charcoal Meal-stimulated Gastrointestinal Transit in Rats (n=6)

Table 7.4: Effect of *Cissampelos pareira* (*C. pareira*) Extract on 2 mL Castor Oil-Induced Diarrhoea in Rats

Treatment	*Dose (mg/kg)*	*Total no. of Faecal Matter*	*Reduction Per cent*
Control	–	65	–
C. pareira	25	46	29.2
C. pareira	50	38	41.5
C. pareira	100	26	60.0
Diphenoxylate HCl	5.0	19	70.8

Values are presented as mean values of six rats in each group.

Acknowledgement

This study was supported partially by grants from the Department of Science and Technology, Ministry of Science and Technology, New Delhi.

References

1. Rao Ch V, Sairam K and Goel RK: Experimental evaluation of *Emblica officinalis* fruit on gastrict ulcer and mucosal offensive and defensive factors in rats. *Acta Pharm Turcica* 2001, 93, 155-160.

2. Rao Ch V, Ojha SK, Govindarajan R, Rawat AKS, Mehrotra S and Pushpangadan P: Quercetin, a bioflavonoid, protects against oxidative stress-related gastric mucosal damage in rats. *Nat Prod Sci* 2003, 9, 68-72.

3. Rao Ch V, Ojha SK, Radhakrishnan K, Govindarajan R, Rastogi S, Mehrotra S and Pushpangadan P: Antiulcer activity of *Utleria salicifolia* rhizome extract. *J Ethnopharmacol* 2004, 91, 243-249.

4. Agarwal VK, Rao Ch V, Sairam K, Joshi VK and Goel RK: Effect of *Piper longum* Linn., *Zingiber officinalis* Linn. and *Ferula* species on gastric ulceration and secretion in rats. *Ind J Experimental Biol* 2000, 38, 994-998.

5. Rao Ch V, Rao GMM, Kartik R, Sudhakar M, Mehrotra S and Goel RK: Ulcer protective effect of *Euphorbia hirta* extract in rats. *J Trop Med Plants* 2003, 4, 199-205.

6. Amresh, Reddy GD, Rao Ch V and Annie Shirwaikar: Ethnomedical value of *Cissampelos pareira* extract in experimentally induced diarrhoea. *Acta Pharmacutica* 2004, 54, 27-35.

7. Rao Ch V, Amresh, Kartik R, Aziz Irfan, Rawat AKS and Pushpangadan P: Protective effect of *Aegle marmelos* Correa fruit in gastrointestinal dysfunction in rats. *Pharmaceutical Biol* 2003, 41, 558-563.

8. Mallavadhani UV, Sahu G, Narasimhan K and Muralidhar J: Quantitative Estimation of an antidiarrhoeic marker in *Euphorbia hirta* samples. *Pharmaceutical Biol* 2002, 40, 103-106.

9. Sanyal AK, Pandey BL and Goel RK: The effect of a traditional preparation of copper, tamrabhasma, on experimental ulcers and gastric secretion. *J Ethnopharmacol* 1982, 5, 79-89.

10. Gupta MB, Nath R, Gupta GP and Bhargava KP: A study of the antiulcer activity of diazepam and other tranquillosedatives in albino rats. *Clinical Experimental Pharmacol* 1985, 12, 61-63.

11. Shay H, Komarov SA, Fels SS, Meranze D, Gruenstein M and Siplet H. A simple method for the uniform production of gastric ulceration. *Gastroenterol* 1945, 5, 43-61.

12. Hollander D, Taranawski A, Krause WJ and Gergely H. Protective effect of sucralfate against alcohol-induced gastric mucosal injury in the rat. *Gastroenterol* 1985, 88, 366-374.

13. Melo L, Thomas G and Mukherjee R. Antidiarrhoeal activity of bisnordihydrotoxiferine isolated from root bark of *Strychonus trinervis* (Vell.) Mart. (Longaniaceae). *J Pharm Pharmacol* 1988, 40, 79–82.

14. Awouters F, Niemegeers CJE, Lenaerts FM and Janssen PAJ: Delay of castor oil-induced diarrhoea in rats; a new way to evaluate the prostaglandin synthesis. *J Pharm Pharmacol* 1978, 30, 41-45.

15. Nwodo OFC and Alumanah EO: Studies on *Abrus precatorious* seed II: Antidiarrhoeal activity. *J Ethnopharmacol* 1991, 31, 395-398.

16. Lutterodt GD: Inhibition of gastrointestinal release of acetylocholine by quercetine as a possible mode of action of *Psidium guajava* leaf extracts in the treatment of acute diarrhoeal disease. *J Ethnopharmacol* 1989, 25, 235-247.

17. Rao Ch V, Maiti RN and Goel RK: Effect of mild irritant on gastric mucosal offensive and defensive factors. *Ind J Physiol and Pharmacol* 1999, 44, 185-191.

Chapter 8

Anti-inflammatory, Antinociceptive and Diuretic Activities of *Amoora cucullata* Roxb.

A.K. Das[1], I.Z. Shahid[1], M.S.K. Choudhuri[2], J.A. Shilpi[1] and Firoj Ahmed[1*]

[1]*Pharmacy Discipline, Life Science School, Khulna University, Khulna-9208, Bangladesh*

[2]*Department of Pharmacy, Jahangirnagar University, Savar, Bangladesh*

ABSTRACT

The crude methanolic extract of the leaves of *Amoora cucullata* Roxb. was investigated for its possible anti-inflammatory activity using carrageenan induced rat paw oedema model and cotton pellet implantation method in rat. The extract was also studied for its antinociceptive activity using acetic acid induced writhing model in mice. At the doses of 200 and 400 mg/kg body weight, the extract showed significant anti-inflammatory activity in both models. At the same doses, the extract also significantly reduced the number of acetic acid-induced abdominal constriction (writhing) in mice. The crude extract also showed significant diuretic activity in albino mice.

Keywords: *Amoora cucullata, Anti-inflammatory, Antinociceptive and Diuretic activities.*

Introduction

Amoora cucullata Roxb., syn.: *Aglaia cucullata,* (Roxb.) Pellegr. (Meliaceae) is a tall tree mostly grown in coastal forests of Bengal, Burma, Malay peninsula, Andamans and Borneo. In Bangladesh, it grows in the Sundarbans mangrove forest located in the southern region of the district of Khulna. Locally it is known as 'Amur', 'Latmi

* Tel.: 880-41-720171-3, Ext. 252; Fax: 880-41-731244; E-mail: firoj72@yahoo.com

and 'Natmi'. In the local traditional medicinal practice, the leaves are used in the treatment of inflammation [1]. The juice of the leaves is antibacterial and extensively used for the treatment of dysentery, skin diseases and in cardiac diseases [2]. In view of the above, the present study was undertaken to evaluate the anti-inflammatory, antinociceptive and diuretic activities of the methanolic extract of the leaves of *Amoora cucullata*.

Materials and Methods

Plant Material and Extraction

The leaves of *A. cucullata* were collected in January 2003 from the Sundarbans Mangrove Forest, Khulna, Bangladesh and were identified at Forestry Discipline, Khulna University. The dried leaves of *A. cucullata* were pulverized into a fine powder. The powdered material (400 g) was extracted with 90 per cent aqueous methanol. The extract was filtered and evaporated using rotary vacuum evaporator to obtain the methanol extract in 14 per cent yield.

Animals

Swiss-albino mice of either sex, weighing 22-25 g, bred in the animal house of the Department of Pharmacy, Jahangirnagar University, Savar, Bangladesh were used for antinociceptive and diuretic activity test. Wistar rats of either sex, weighing 180-200 g, were purchased from the Animal Resources Branch of the International Center for Diarrhoeal Diseases and Research, Bangladesh (ICDDR, B) and were used for anti-inflammatory activity tests. All the animals were acclimatized one week prior to the experiments. The animals were housed under standard laboratory conditions (relative humidity 55–65 per cent, room temperature 25.0±2.0°C and 12 hours light: dark cycle). The animals were fed with standard diet (ICDDR, B formulated) and had free access to tap water.

Drugs

Carrageenan (Sigma Chemicals, USA), aspirin (Square Pharmaceuticals Ltd, Bangladesh), furosemide (Square Pharmaceuticals Ltd, Bangladesh).

Anti-inflammatory Activity

Carrageenan-induced Hind Paw Oedema in Rats

Anti-inflammatory activity of *A. cucullata* was tested using the carrageenan-induced rat paw oedema model as described by Winter *et al.* [3]. Experimental animals (Wistar rats) were randomly divided into four groups with six animals in each group. Control group received vehicle (1 per cent Tween 80 in water) at the dose of 10 mL/kg body weight. Positive control group received aspirin (standard drug) at the dose of 150 mg/kg and the test groups were treated with *A. cucullata* extract at the doses of 200 and 400 mg/kg. The drugs were administered orally 1 h prior to the injection of 0.1 mL of 1 per cent freshly prepared suspension of carrageenan into the left hind paw of each rat. The paw volume was measured by using a plethysmometer (Ugo Basile 7140, Italy) every hour for 5 h after the carrageenan injection.

Cotton Pellet Implantation

Wistar rats were anaesthetized and 10 mg of the sterile cotton pellets were inserted in each axilla of rats. *A. cucullata* extracts (200 and 400 mg/kg), aspirin (150 mg/kg), and control vehicle (1 per cent Tween 80 in water, 10 mL/kg) were administered orally for seven consecutive days starting from the day of cotton pellet implantation. The animals were anaesthetized again on the 8th day and cotton pellets were removed surgically, freed from extraneous tissue. These pellets were incubated at 37°C for 24 h and dried at 60°C to constant weight [4].

Antinociceptive Activity

The antinociceptive activity was studied using acetic acid induced writhing model in mice [5]. The animals were divided into control, positive control and test groups with ten mice in each group. The animals of test groups received test substance at the doses of 200 and 400 mg/kg body weight. Positive control group was administered aspirin (standard drug) at the dose of 100 mg/kg body weight and vehicle control group was treated with 1 per cent Tween 80 in water at the dose of 10 mL/kg body weight orally 45 min before intraperitoneal administration of 0.7 per cent acetic acid. After an interval of five minutes, the mice were observed for specific contraction of body referred as 'writhing' for 15min.

Diuretic Activity

Diuretic activity of the extract was investigated using the method as described [6]. The test animals were randomly chosen and divided into five groups having ten mice in each. Twenty-four hours prior to the experiment, the test animals were placed in metabolic cages with the withdrawal of food and water. Group-1 or the control group received vehicle (1 per cent Tween 80 in water) at a dose of 10 mL/kg body weight orally. Group-2 was provided with urea solution at a dose of 500 mg/kg. Group-3 was provided with standard diuretic drug furosemide at a dose of 0.5 mg/kg. Group-4 and group-5, the test groups were treated with the methanol extract of *A. cucullata* leaves at the doses of 200 and 400 mg/kg respectively. From the graduated urine chamber of metabolic cage, the urinary output of each group was recorded 5 h after the above treatments. Collected urine was centrifuged and then estimated for sodium and potassium using digital flame photometer (Elico Pvt. Ltd., model CL 22D). Chloride was estimated by the Schales and Schales method reproduced by Godkar [7].

Statistical Analysis

Student's *t*-test was used to determine a significant difference between the control group and experimental groups.

Results

Anti-inflammatory Activity

Carrageenan-induced Rat Paw Oedema

In the carrageenan induced rat paw oedema model of anti-inflammatory activity, the methanolic extract of leaves of *A. cucullata* showed a significant inhibitory effect on the oedema formation from the first hour to fifth hour. The highest inhibitory effect was found during the third hour where the inhibition was 24.59 per cent ($P<0.001$)

and 40.98 per cent ($P<0.001$) at the doses of 200 and 400 mg/kg respectively. These findings were comparable to standard drug aspirin where the inhibition was 51.23 per cent (Table 8.1).

Table 8.1: Effect of Methanolic Extract of *A. cucullata* on Carrageenan-induced Rat Paw Oedema

Animal Group/Treatment	*Time After Carrageenan Injection*				
	1 hr	*2 hr*	*3 hr*	*4 hr*	*5 hr*
	Oedema Volume x 1000 (ml) (Percent inhibition)				
Control 1 per cent Tween 80 10 ml/kg; p.o.	15.0±0.47	164.5±1.61	244.5±1.82	272.0±1.92	231.0±1.23
Positive control Aspirin 150 mg/kg; p.o.	10.54±1.23** (29.71)	100.5±2.34* (38.91)	119.25±1.92* (51.23)	172.8±1.72* (36.47)	155.4±2.11* (32.72)
Test group-1 AC extract, 200 mg/kg; p.o.	12.86±0.52* (14.26)	133.8±0.98* (18.68)	184.38±1.43* (24.59)	224.4±1.66* (17.51)	194.7±1.76* (15.71)
Test group-2 AC extract 400 mg/kg; p.o.	11.43±1.04* (23.80)	113.3±1.10* (31.13)	144.30±2.21* (40.98)	192.6±1.72* (29.18)	170.5±1.27* (26.18)

Values are expressed as mean ± SEM (Number of animals, n=6); * indicates $P<0.001$, ** indicates $P<0.05$ vs. control; AC: *A. cucullata;* p.o.: per oral

Cotton Pellet Implantation

In the cotton pellet implantation model for anti-inflammatory activity, the extract showed a marked reduction in the weight of the cotton pellet in test animal compared to control (Table 8.2). At the doses of 200 and 400 mg/kg, the extract exhibited 23.31 per cent and 34.41 per cent reduction of the weight of the cotton pellets respectively which was comparable to that of the standard drug aspirin where the reduction was 41.79 per cent. These results were statistically significant ($P<0.001$).

Table 8.2: Effect of Methanolic Extract of *A. cucullata* on Cotton Pellet-Induced Granuloma Pouch in Albino Rat

Animal Group/ Treatment	*Mean Weight of Granuloma Pouch (mg)*	*Inhibition (per cent)*
Control 1 per cent tween-80 solution in water; p.o.	19.84 ± 0.75	–
Positive control Aspirin 150 mg/kg; p.o.	11.55 ± 0.24*	41.79
Test group-1 AC extract 200 mg/kg; p.o.	15.22 ± 0.31*	23.31
Test group-2 AC extract 400 mg/kg; p.o.	13.01 ± 0.26*	34.41

Values are expressed as mean ± SEM (Number of animals, n=6); * indicates $P<0.001$ vs. control; p.o.: per oral; AC: *A. cucullata*

Antinociceptive Activity

Table 8.3 shows the effect of the methanolic extract of *A. cucullata* on acetic acid induced writhing in mice. At the doses of 200 and 400 mg/kg, the extract produced 32.00 and 51.34 per cent writhing inhibition in test animals, respectively. The results were statistically significant (*P*<0.001) and were comparable to the standard drug aspirin, which showed 63.64 per cent writhing inhibition at the dose of 100 mg/kg.

Table 8.3: Effect of Methanolic Extract of *A. cucullata* on Acetic Acid Induced Writhing in Mice

Animal Group/Treatment	*Number of Writhes*	*Inhibition (per cent)*
Control 1 per cent tween-80 solution in water; p.o.	18.7 ± 0.52	–
Positive control Aspirin 100 mg/kg; p.o.	6.80 ± 0.69*	63.64
Test group-1 AC extract 200 mg/kg; p.o.	12.70 ± 0.70*	32.00
Test group-2 AC extract 200 mg/kg; p.o.	9.10 ± 1.00*	51.34

Values are expressed as mean ± SEM (Number of animals, n=10); * indicates *P* <0.001 vs. control; p.o.: per oral; AC: *A. cucullata*

Diuretic Activity

The effect of the methanolic extract of *A. cucullata* leaves on the urination of mice was observed for 5 h which revealed that the extract has a marked diuretic effect in the test animals. This was comparable to that of standard drug furosemide and diuretic agent urea (Table 8.4). Electrolyte loss showed similar ratio (Na^+/K^+ excretion ratio was 1.48 and 1.45 at the doses of 200 and 400 mg/kg respectively) as that of the loop diuretic furosemide (1.47).

Table 8.4: Effect of Methanolic Extract of *A. cucullata* on Urine Excretion Parameters in Mice

Treatment	*Dose (mg/kg; p.o.)*	*Volume of Urine (ml)*[b]	*Concentrations of Ions (m.eq.l^{-1})*			
			Na^+	*K^+*	*Cl^-*	*Na^+/K^+*
Group-1 (Control)	–	2.75±0.08	75.67±1.25	49.75±1.18	77.56±1.24	1.52
Group-2 (Urea)	500	3.81±0.09	113.67±1.36**	76.56±1.27**	86.75±1.38*	1.48
Group-3 (Furosemide)	0.5	4.75±0.13	125.86±1.75**	85.46±1.67**	94.39±1.49*	1.47
Group-4 (ME)	200	4.36±0.07	117.50±1.18**	79.34±1.87**	91.76±1.68*	1.48
Group-5 (ME)	400	4.88±0.05	132.75±1.56**	91.23±1.79**	97.59±1.87*	1.45

ME: Methanolic extract of *A. cucullata*; Values are expressed as mean ± SEM (Number of animals, n =10); * indicates *P* <0.01, ** indicates *P* < 0.001 vs. control; [b] Collected for 5 hours after treatment.

Discussion

Since *A. cucullata* belongs to the coastal forests, part of the plant constituents may be polar in nature. Methanol was used which has a wide range of solubility in both polar and non-polar region. To avoid any solvent effect on the experimental animals, the solvent was removed by evaporation to dryness using a rotary vacuum evaporator.

Carrageenan induced rat paw oedema model is one of the most widely used primary test for the screening of new anti-inflammatory agents [3]. The oedema formation is a biphasic event. The initial phase, observed during the first hour, is attributed to the release of histamine and serotonin [8] and the delayed oedema is due to the release of bradykinin and prostaglandins [9,10]. These results tend to suggest that the inhibitory activity of the extracts observed in the first phase of carrageenan induced inflammation may be due to inhibition of early mediators, such as histamine and serotonin. The action on the second phase may be due to the inhibition of bradykinin and prostaglandins.

The results of the cotton pellet implantation model for anti-inflammatory activity further support the anti-inflammatory activity of the crude extract.

Inhibition of prostaglandin synthesis could give rise to analgesic activity. So the extract was further investigated for its possible anti-nociceptive activity. Antinociceptive activity of the methanolic extract of *A. cucullata* leaves was tested by acetic acid induced writhing model in mice. Acetic acid induced writhing model represents pain sensation by triggering localized inflammatory response. Acetic acid, which is used to induce writhing, causes algesia by liberation of endogenous substances, which in turn excite the pain nerve endings [11]. Increased levels of PGE_2 and PGF_{2a} in the peritoneal fluid have been reported to be responsible for pain sensation caused by intraperitoneal administration of acetic acid [12]. On the basis of the result of acetic acid induced writhing test, it can be concluded that the methanolic extract of *A. cucullata* possesses antinociceptive activity.

Diuretic activity may be very useful in a number of conditions like hypertension, hypercalciuria, cirrhosis of liver etc. Furosemide, used as the standard drug in this experiment belongs to the loop or high-ceiling diuretics, which act by inhibiting $Na^+/K^+/Cl^-$co-transport of the luminal membrane in the ascending limb of the loop of Henle and have the highest efficacy in mobilizing Na^+ and $Cl^-$from the body. The extract was able to increase the volume of urine with statistical significance along with a considerable Na^+ and Cl^-load which was comparable to that of furosemide. The diuretic action of the extract may be due to its action on the kidney. The extract may also contain a high proportion of osmotically active compounds or their metabolites that lead to an increased urine volume. Further studies may be carried out to identify whether these actions are associated with the same agent or a number of agents that are responsible for such activities.

In conclusion, it can be suggested that the crude extract of *Amoora cucullata* may possess anti-inflammatory, anti-nociceptive and diuretic effects, which correlate well with the traditional use of the plant. Therefore, further studies are essential to find out the active principles responsible for these activities.

References

1. Shahid IJ: Phytochemical and Pharmacological screening of *Amoora cucullata* Roxb. *In*: B. Pharm. Project report, Pharmacy Discipline, Khulna University, Bangladesh 2003, 13-15.
2. Kirtikar KR and Basu BD: Indian Medicinal Plants, 2nd edition, International Book Distributors, India 1999, 553-554.
3. Winter CA, Risley EA, Nuss CW: Carrageenan-induced oedema in hind paw of rats-an assay for anti-inflammatory drugs. *Proc Soc Exp Biol Med* 1962, 111, 544.
4. D'Arcy PF, Howard EM, Muggletone PW and Townsend SB: The anti-inflammatory action of griseofulvin in experimental animals. *J Pharm Pharmacol* 1960, 12, 659.
5. Koster R, Anderson M, De Beer EJ: Acetic acid for analgesic screening. *Fed Proc* 1959, 18, 412.
6. Lipschitz WL, Hadidian Z, Kerpesar A: Bioassay of diuretics. *J Pharmacol Exp Therap* 1943, 79, 97-110.
7. Godkar PB: Text Book of medical laboratory technology. Bhalani Publishing House, Mumbai 1994.
8. Vinegar R, Schreiber W, Hugo R: Biphasic development of carrageenan oedema in rats. *J Pharmacl. Exp Therap* 1969, 166, 95-103.
9. Di Rosa N, Giroud JP, Willoughby DA: Studies of the mediators of acute inflammatory response reduced in rats in different sites by carrageenan and turpentine. *J Pathol Bacteriol* 1971, 104, 15-29.
10. Flower BA, Moncada S, Vane JR: Analgesic, antipyretic and anti-inflammatory agents: drugs employed in the treatment of gout. *In*: Gilman AG, Goodman LS, Rall TW, Murad F, (Eds), Goodman and Gilman's the Pharmacological Basis of Therapeutics, 7th edition, Mcmillan Publishing, New York 1985, 674-715.
11. Taesotikul T, Panthong A, Kanjanapothi D, Verpoorte R, Scheffer JJC: Anti-inflammatory, antipyretic and antinociceptive activities of *Tabernaemontana pandacaqui* Poir. *J Ethnopharmacol* 2003, 84, 31-35.
12. Derardt R, Jougney S, Delevalcee F, Falhout M: Release of prostaglandins E and F in an algogenic reaction and its inhibition. *Eur J Pharmacol* 1980, 51, 17–24.

Chapter 9

The Role of Ethnomedical Leads in Drug Discovery

V. George* and J. Anil John

Phytochemistry and Phytopharmacology Division,
Tropical Botanic Garden and Research Institute,
Pacha-Palode, Thiruvananthapuram, Kerala, India
**E-mail: georgedrv@yahoo.co.in*

Introduction

With the advent of the new millennium, there has been an unprecedented boom in the herbal drug industry. Unlike in the past, during the last few years, large pharmaceutical companies, including multinationals, have entered in to the commercial production of herbal drugs. The rapid increase in popularity of herbal drugs has been caused by a general change in the life style and social attitude of the people, especially the younger generation, towards things 'natural'. In almost all societies and cultures, developed and underdeveloped, such changes are visible especially in their preference for organically produced food items such as fruits, vegetables, cereals, pulses and other articles of daily use such as soft drinks, toiletries, cosmetic products developed from naturally occurring substances. This desire for adopting a 'green' life style for a healthy living and the general disillusionment towards allopathic medicines in particular due to their toxicity and side effects have helped to boost the herbal drug industry from its former status of a small scale family business to that of a medium to large scale pharma business in India and elsewhere. The global herbal drug industry runs into several billion dollars. Countries with long traditions of use of herbs for healing such as India, China and the Middle East should have been the major beneficiaries and players in the global drug scenario. However, but for China, the other traditional herbal users could not take advantage of this newly found marketing opportunity mainly because of the lack of scientific validation of their products. On the other hand, technologically advanced countries such as Germany, Japan, France etc. have taken advantage of the new situation and they are exporting sizable quantity of scientifically validated herbal products to other nations. India, with her vast floristic wealth, ancient health care practices, immense traditional knowledge on the use of plants in food and medicine, scientific and technological capabilities and trained man power, can still catch the opportunity.

Plants, like human beings, are attacked by fungi, microbes and viruses. They are also exposed to external stress such as high temperature, freezing conditions, salinity, flood, storm etc. Further, they have to defend themselves against feeding insects, birds and animals. In order to protect themselves from invading organisms and external stress factors, plants synthesize a variety of compounds known as secondary metabolites in small quantities and these are stored in various organs such as roots, stem, leaves, bark or seeds.

Some of these molecules may find application in the prevention and treatment of human ailments including diseases such as AIDS and cancer. In the search for bioactive molecules from plants, one may choose a plant for detailed investigation based on any one of the following criteria.

Random Selection

Investigators may pick up a plant at random for drug prospecting from a biodiversity rich area. A perusal of the reported results of such studies show that usually the investigations lead to the discovery of molecules with known or new structural features, but seldom such studies result in the discovery of useful bioactive compounds. However, there are exceptions such as the discovery of taxol, a potent anticancer drug from *Taxus brevifolia*.

Chemotaxonomy Based Selection

Chemotaxonomy is another criteria applied by the investigators for selection of plants or plant parts for detailed studies. Here, the selection is carried out with prior knowledge on the chemistry as well as the therapeutic properties of the constituents of a close relative belonging to the same genus or family of the target plant. Such studies may lead to the isolation and characterization of compounds which are chemically identical to the known ones or compounds with close structural features having similar therapeutic properties.

Ecological Considerations

One may choose a plant for investigation based on ecological, environmental and edaphic factors. Mycorrhizal, microbial, fungal and mineral associations are also known to induce synthesis of certain secondary metabolites in plants which may find use as therapeutic agents. Also some plants produce compounds which may act as deterrents to herbivorous animals, birds, insects etc. These compounds also may find use as therapeutic agents to humans. Hence any one of these criteria may be chosen for selection of a plant for detailed investigations.

Ethnomedical Considerations

The traditional knowledge base in every culture includes the knowledge on the biodiversity of the particular region. Ethnomedical information consists of the intimate knowledge on the properties, uses, and mode of application of products derived from plants, animals and minerals acquired by successive generations of humans through experiments and observations for the prevention and treatment of diseases and promotion of health. Ethnomedical leads have helped in the discovery of a number of bioactive molecules in the recent past and in this article the advantage of basing ethnomedical leads for selection of plants for investigations will be highlighted.

Indigenous Communities

According to the International Labour Organisation there are about 5,000 indigenous or tribal communities living in seventy countries. The total population of indigenous communities is estimated to be about 300 million. All definitions of the concept of 'indigenous' regards self identification as a fundamental criterion for determining the groups to which the term indigenous should be applied. With in the UN family the International Labour Organisation (ILO) Convention 169 defines indigenous and tribal peoples as follows:

Tribal people in independent countries whose social, cultural and economic conditions distinguish them from other sections of the national community and whose status is regulated wholly or partially by their own customs or traditions or by special laws of regulations.

People in independent countries who are regarded as indigenous on account of their dissent from the populations which inhabited the country, or geographic regions to which the country belongs, at the time of conquest or colonization or establishment of present state boundaries and who irrespective of their legal status retains some or all of their own social, economic, cultural and political institutions.

The Indian sub continent is inhabited by over 53 million tribes belonging to over 550 tribal communities that come under 227 linguistic groups. They inhabit varied geographic and climatic zones of the country. Their vocation ranges from hunting-gathering, cave dwelling, nomadic to societies with settled culture living in complete harmony with nature. There are about 106 different languages, 227 subsidiary dialects spoken by the tribes of India (1).

Indigenous Knowledge

Indigenous knowledge is a community based functional knowledge system, developed, preserved and refined by generations of people through continuous interaction, observation and experimentation with their surrounding environment. It is a dynamic system, ever changing, adapting and adjusting to the local situations and has close links with the culture, civilization and religious practices of the communities. Indigenous knowledge covers all spheres of human activity such as art, literature, health, education, agriculture, environment etc. Indigenous knowledge related to traditional medicine in India can be broadly classified into two streams *viz.* classical health traditions and oral health traditions. Classical health traditions have conceptual and theoretical foundations and philosophical explanations. Classical health traditions are codified in the ancient Vedic texts such as 'Rig Veda', 'Adharva Veda' etc. and Samhithas such as 'Charaka Samhita', 'Susrutha Samhitha', 'Ashtanga Hridaya' and numerous text books in Sanskrit and later Indian languages. Oral health traditions are transmitted to successive generations by word of mouth and are practiced by indigenous and tribal communities. The practitioners of oral health traditions are folk healers, village physicians, bone setters, dais, specialists in treating poisonous bites, jaundice, mental disorders etc., tribal physicians and elderly men and women of tribal communities. During a survey covering a period of more than a decade under the All India Coordinated Research Programme on Ethnobiology (AICRPE), indigenous knowledge on about 10,000 wild plant species were documented. The survey revealed that about 8,000 plants are used by tribal communities for medicinal purposes, about 3,500 plants for edible purposes, 550 species for fibre, 425 species for dyes, resins and gums, 325 species for pesticides and 1,000 species for other purposes. We have utilized this database for validation of the ethnomedical claims on some of these plants on specific disease conditions. The plants were chosen based on their reported antihypertensive/anticancer/antimalarial properties.

Screening of Plants at TBGRI for Drug Discovery: A Case Study

Random Selection

During the period 1995-1998, five hundred species of plants belonging to 130 families were collected. Different plant parts from the same species were studied separately. Thus a total of 1,000 extracts from these plants were prepared using 70 per cent aqueous alcohol. The extracts were subjected to *in vitro* throughput analysis using different test models. The study resulted in the identification of eight extracts with potentials for further studies for drug development. The positive hit rate in this case was 0.008 (2).

Ethnomedical Lead Based Selection

Search for Antihypertensive Drugs Based on Ethnomedical Leads

The plants for this investigation were selected based on the ethnomedical data obtained from the tribal communities. We have chosen plants which the tribes use to cure symptoms that can be compared to hypertension. The symptoms reported are:

1. Redness of skin, eye and fullness of veins.
2. Severe pain between muscle and bone, body ache, burning sensation, oedema, generalized skin eruption.
3. Headache, sleeplessness, vomiting, chest pain, heaviness around neck and ears, dyspepsia, giddiness, fits, strokes, diminished vision, hyper perspiration, anxiety, aversion to food, and attitude of anger.
4. Coughing sound in chest
5. Numbness resulting from bleeding of the nose, ear and mouth, excessive thirst, complaints with the blood vessels of the legs, heaviness and numbness of legs, pain and heaviness below neck, hip and hands, depression, giddiness, blurred vision, and scanty urine.

Thus plants traditionally used for the above symptoms and those used for diuretics and against poisonous bites were collected for this study during the period

1993-1997. A total of 273 plants were selected. Different plant parts from the same species were extracted with acetone, ethanol and water and these extracts were screened using an HPLC technique involving inhibition of angiotensin converting enzyme (ACE). The studies have resulted in the identification of 47 plants with potential ACE inhibition activity which showed that 17.2 per cent of the plants studied were active (3,4,5)

Search for Antiplasmodial Extracts from Plants Traditionally Used for Fever or Malaria

The problems of resistant lines of *Plasmodium* are on the increase. Laboratory studies have revealed development of resistance to almost every antiplasmodial drug known today. Hence there is an urgent need of new antimalarial drugs. New drugs of herbal origin such as artemisinin discovered through ethnopharmacological studies have shown interesting results. Plants on which ethnomedical leads were available in our database were selected for this study. The plants were selected based on their reported use in fever, intermittent fever with shivering and malaria. 47 plants were selected for this study. Eighty ethanol extracts were prepared from different parts of 47 plants. The plants were assayed for antiplasmodic activity as under:

Into each well of 96-well micro titer plates, 50 µL of parasitized erythrocytes (3 per cent) at a concentration of 5 x 10^8 cells/mL and 50 µL of medium containing the extracts at four different concentrations were added. The cultures were incubated at 37°C for 48 h in an atmosphere of 2 per cent O_2, 5 per cent CO_2 and 93 per cent N_2. Twenty four hours before the termination of incubation, 20µL of L-[2,3,4,5,6-3H]phenylalanine (37µl/mL) was added into each well. The effect of the extracts in the cultures was monitored by the measurement of L-[2,3,4,5,6-3H]phenylalanine incorporation into the parasite nucleic acids. The assay was performed in triplicates. The IC_{50} value of chloroquine-diphosphate has been determined to approximately 30 ng/ml.

Of eighty analyzed ethanol extracts from 47 species examined significant effects were found for 31 extracts. This represents 23 different sp. from 20 families. Of the active species, 20 were tested against *Plasmodium falciparum* for the first time. Among the active species *Casearia elliptica, Holarrhena pubescens, Pongamia pinnata, Plumbago zeylanica* and *Soymida febrifuga* were the most active. Plant extracts with an inhibiting effect on *P. falciparum* of more than 80 and 50 per cent at 100 µg/ml and 50µg/ml respectively were considered active (6).

In this study, we tested different parts of the same plant species such as root, stem, bark and leaf. The study revealed that the activity clearly depended on the plant part tested. This is in accordance with the traditional medicinal use where very often a particular part of the plant species is used as drug. The high rate of positive hits may be explained by the ethnomedical approach adopted in this study.

Anticancer Activity

On the basis of ethnomedical leads we have selected 31 plants for studying their anticancer properties. The plants were selected on the basis of their reported use in treatment of cancer like afflictions, ulcers, wounds etc. The plants were collected from different parts of Kerala. 30 per cent aqueous alcoholic extracts of the plants were prepared as per the protocol recommended by the National Institute of Health, USA. The extracts were screened for anticancer activity using different cell lines such as Louse Lymphocytic Leukemia (L1210), Human Adeno Carcenoma (COLO320DM) and by DNA scission. The study had led to the identification of six plants with potential anticancer activity. Only those plants which showed 100 per cent inhibition were selected. The number of positive hits obtained in this study is 19.3. The high positive hit rate clearly shows that selection of plants based on ethnomedical leads is definitely advantageous.

Conclusion

The drug discovery programme from plants begins with the selection of plants. As has been explained there can be several criteria in selecting a plant for drug discovery. In this article, we have presented the data of the screening carried out in our laboratory during the last decade. It is seen that plants with a history of use in traditional medicine give a substantially higher positive hit rate as compared to plants selected on other criteria such as random selection etc. The results which are presented are based on preliminary *in vitro* assays. To generate preliminary data on the biological activity of a plant, the investigator has to follow several steps, such as selection of plant, literature search, collection and taxonomic identification of the plant, documentation and preparation of voucher specimens, processing of the plant material involving drying, powdering or wet grinding, extraction with suitable solvents, concentration of the extracts using appropriate methods (distillation, evaporation, lyophilisation) and finally *in vitro* bioactivity assay using different enzymatic models. These activities in Indian laboratories may cost a minimum of Rs. Twenty thousand per plant. Thus if we base our search for bioactive molecules on random selection, in order to obtain a single positive hit about Rs. Twenty lakhs have to be spent (Assuming 1 per cent positive hit). On the other hand, investigations based on ethnomedical leads would bring down the cost to Rs. 1.4 lakhs (Assuming 15 per cent positive hit). Thus the study reveals that selection of plants on ethnomedical leads for drug discovery helps to save considerable time and money and it always provides a very high positive hit rate.

References

1. Anonymous: *Ethnobiology in India: A status report*. Ministry of Environment and Forest, New Delhi 1994.

2. Pushpangadan P, George V, Sathish Kumar C: Sustainable utilisation of lesser known forest products of Kerala–Final scientific and technical report. TBGRI, Trivandrum 1998.

3. Somanadhan B, Smitt UW, George V, Pushpangadan P, Rajasekharan S, Duus JO, Nyman U, Olsen CE Jaroszewski JW: Angiotensin converting enzyme (ACE) inhibitors from *Jasminum azoricum* and *Jasminum grandiflorum*. *Planta Med*, 1998, 64, 246-250.

4. Nyman U, Joshi P, Madsen LB, Pedersen TB, Pinstrup M, Rajasekharan S, George V, Pushpangadan P: Ethnomedical information and *in vitro* screening for

angiotensin converting enzyme inhibition of plants utilized as traditional medicines in Gujarat, Rajasthan and Kerala (India). *J Ethnopharmacol* 1998, 60, 247-263.

5. Somanadhan B, George V, Pushpangadan P, Rajasekharan S, Gudiksen L, Smitt UW, Nyman U: An ethnopharmacological survey for potential angiotensin converting enzyme inhibitors from Indian medicinal plants. *J Ethnopharmacol* 1999, 65, 103-111.

6. Simonsen HT, Nordskjold JB, Smitt UW, Nyman U, Pushpangadan P, Joshi P, George V: *In vitro* screening of Indian medicinal plants for antiplasmodial activity. *J Ethnopharmacol* 2001, 74, 195-204.

Chapter 10

Quality of Natural Health Products through Marker Profiling: Promotion and International Coordination

Pulok K. Mukherjee[1,2] *, V. Kumar[1], Peter J. Houghton[2]

[1]*School of Natural Product Studies, Department of Pharmaceutical Technology, Jadavpur University, Kolkata – 700 032, India*

[2]*Department of Pharmacy, Pharmacognosy Research Laboratories, King's College London, Franklin-Wilkins Building, 150 Stamford Street, London SE1 9NH, UK*

**E-mail: pknatprod@yahoo.co.in*

ABSTRACT

Renewed interest in Natural Health Products [NHP] globally has opened new areas of exploration and debate. NHP are not only a part of primary health care in developing countries but also the developed countries are taking interest due to possibilities of exploring the new chemical entities for medicinal purposes. NHP including functional food, health food and nutraceuticals is a part of health care globally. Safety and efficacy of the NHP is always a cause of concern to promote and rationalize their use. Quality control of botanicals, validated processes of manufacturing, customer awareness and post marketing surveillance are the key points which could ensure the safety and efficacy of NHP. Identification and quality evaluation of crude drugs is a fundamental requirement of industry and other organizations dealing with NHP. Marker analysis based on chemo profiling and development of characteristic fingerprints for individual plants could help to develop uniform standardization tool for their promotion through international co-ordination. Implementation of GMP guidelines and product information to customers through awareness program could be helpful in monitoring the manufacturing and use of NHP. Development of NHP so much so their regulations and promotional aspects vary country to country and this makes it difficult to maintain uniform standards for NHP.

In order to rationalize the use of herbal products in different forms more particularly the extracts in therapy as is being used nowadays, a need-based and novel concept of marker analysis is getting momentum. Marker is the chemical entity in the plant material that serves as a characteristic fingerprint for that plant which helps to develop the analytical techniques to ascertain the limits of the phyto-constituents in an herbal preparation. This technique helps to develop quality control profile of herbals based on their chemo profile, which can dictate the quality of phyto-constituents present in individual herb. Standardized manufacture procedures and suitable analytical tools required to establish the necessary framework for quality control in herbals which can best be performed through chemo profiling of the NHP through marker analysis. The assessment/ evaluation of phytomedicine, in what ever form it is being documented, the objective to be met are generally stated in terms of what is to be achieved in several areas of manufacture and control, which is the basis for quality drug development from natural resources so much so their promotion through international co-ordination.

Introduction

The beneficial role of plant derived products in therapeutic treatment is an important breakthrough in the history of mankind. Since ancient time medicinal plants have proved their efficacy and safety in therapeutics. The evidences for the therapeutic actions of herbal drugs are documented in Indian, Chinese, European and African systems of medicine. Ayurveda is an ancient Indian system of medicine and is in therapeutic practice since thousands of years. Ayurveda provides us information about various diseases, their symptoms and specific natural remedy for curing the diseases [1]. In the last few decades pharmaceutical companies have given keen stress on research and development of plant and plant derived drugs. The modern approaches involve isolation, characterization and pharmacological studies of plants with the help of sophisticated instruments. The outcome of such research work was the generation of new drugs, which are found to be active in specific diseases. Natural Products has become an integral part of human health care system. The popularity of these products is due to its efficacy and low toxicity. Most of the world population depends on the traditional medicine. World Health Organization (WHO) has formulated remedies of traditional medicine to study their potential usefulness, safety and efficacy. The global herbal product market is worth USD 14.2 billion and is growing at a rate of about 9-15 per cent annually [2].

Medicinal herbs yielding desired relief or results were remembered for future reference. Thus this natural way of healing was transferred from person to person and place to place. Persons acting as physicians or guide were much respected. As time passed, search for new herbs was intensified and numerous groups at different places were formed. Accordingly, different branches dealing in particular system of treatment came into existence in China (Chinese Medicine), Egypt (Egyptian Medicine), Iran (Iranian Medicine), Italy (Roman Medicine), and India (Ayurveda). One such system of medicine was also formed in Greece (Unani). Alternative medicines had never been static. Its practitioners had been innovative and dynamic in the therapeutic practice and carried out clinical trials out of the local flora. In fact, on study of literature, one comes across several references of permitting the use of a substitute drug when the classical drug is not available. However, during the last 100 years, crude drug supplying agencies came up and commercial manufacture of

Alternative medicines in factories started [3, 4]. The new economic set up was such that the practitioner generally could no longer process and prepare his own medicines but had to purchase his drugs from those sources with no means to ascertain authenticity of the medicines and formulations [5].

There are several government control parameters being implemented through various agencies on the manufacturer to ensure the quality of the medicines marketed, prescribed and administered to patients.

Surprisingly this regulation and control varies from countries to countries, which lack uniformity in the quality evaluation and also for their safety and toxicity assessment criteria. While very less efforts are made to investigate the efficacy and potency of these drugs, there are also very few systematic policy to encourage such moves to develop these systems of medicine. Some time even these systems are projected as out-dated and unscientific native systems. It is under these circumstances that some of the rationalists, scientists, scholars and protagonists of alternative medicines dedicated themselves for the development of these alternative systems for drug development from natural resources, which required to be harmonized through international coordination [3, 4].

Recently rules from the US FDA on the 'guidelines for the botanical drug industry' have come up. German investigators have published 410 monographs dealing with 324 different plants and plant substances used as medicinal. They represent a cogent, rational system of blending historical traditional use with modern scientific information. The council is publishing these monographs in English. Various guidelines on the quality on herbal drugs are coming up from different organizations, associations like EMEA, ESCOP, AESGP etc. which are even available in the internet web pages which will definitely help to make the rules and regulations of the herbals for different countries which are getting momentum to a large extent these days [6, 7]. In India separate Department or the Indian System of Medicine and Homeopathy (ISM and H) has been made who are specially dealing with the rules and regulations for the herbals along with the Drugs and Cosmetic act and rules which has come up with the rules for the implementation of GMP in herbals, which will not only help to make quality herbal products but also to safeguard the adverse effects of the herbals too. To establish the quality and standardization parameters of botanicals different approaches on phyto-markers as well as biomarker profiling of herbals need to be established through various chemo profiling techniques with the lead from therapeutically potent medicinal plants [8].

Traditional Use to Scientific Validation and Industrial Utilization of Natural Products from Indian System of Medicine (ISM)

Majority of the rural people in developing countries use plant based traditional medicines for health care. These are still produced using age old methods which can affect their quality, stability and efficacy. Resurgence of interest in green products in the industrialized countries has created an expanding market for plant based products that could be produced by developing countries to be competitive provided the quality and safety specifications could be satisfied. The possibilities for value addition, processing, product improvement and technical assistance are required to be strengthened for the industrial utilization of medicinal plants [9, 10]. The promotion and development of plant based products have been given a fresh impetus due to certain ground realities as under:

1. Green consumerism and the current resurgence of interest in the use of "Naturals" throughout the globe.
2. Free market economy bringing in more openness and expanding markets and demand for new resource materials and products.
3. A growing acceptability of the social responsibility of minimizing socio-economic inequalities in favor of rural people resulting in creating additional jobs and income opportunities for poor people.
4. Increasing awareness regarding biodiversity conservation and the sustainable and protective use of plant resources.
5. Search for new phytopharmaceuticals for the prevention and cure of deadly disease such as cancer and AIDS.

The chemistry of medicinal plants assumes great significance these days. When one wants to elevate the complementary alternative medicine (CAM) to the level of tested, proved Western medicine, the most important single component coming to force is the active principle. The knowledge of active components, their chemical nature, mode of action, limitation etc. will reveal the properties of the drugs and elevate CAM to a legitimate branch of science [9, 10]. Every part of plant exhibits one or more medicinal properties same or different from the action of other parts of the same plant. But the data available may only be of a single part of the plant, may be of the root, leaves or fruits, while for certain plants, nothing is known about their chemical constituents.

General Concepts of Evaluation and Quality Control of Herbal Drugs in Traditional Medicine

Herbal medicines are prepared from a variety of plant materials–leaves, stems, roots, bark and so on. They usually contain many biologically active ingredients and are used primarily for treating mild or chronic ailments. Herbs can be prepared at home in many ways, using either fresh or dried ingredients. Herbal teas and infusions can be steeped to varying strengths. Roots, bark or other plant parts can be boiled into strong solutions called decoctions. Honey or sugar can be added to infusions and decoctions to make syrups. Herbal remedies can also be purchased in the form of pills, capsules or powders, or in more concentrated liquid forms called extracts and tinctures. They can be applied topically in creams or ointments, soaked into clothes and used as compresses, or applied directly to the skin as poultices.

Herbal drug preparations are also diverse in character ranging from simple, comminuted plant material to extracts, tinctures, oils and resins. A comprehensive specification must be developed for each herbal drug preparation based on recent scientific data. Herbal medicinal products are now available in different dosage forms [11]. The following tests and acceptance criteria are considered generally applicable to all herbal medicinal products:

Description

A qualitative description of the dosage form should be provided (*e.g.*, size, shape, colour). If any of the characteristics change during manufacture or storage, this change should be investigated and appropriate action is to be taken. The acceptance criteria should include the final acceptable appearance. If colour changes during storage, a quantitative procedure may be appropriate.

Identification

Identification testing should establish the identity of the herbal drug preparation(s) in the herbal medicinal product and should be able to discriminate between closely related preparations which are likely to be present. Identity tests should be specific for the herbal drug preparation. Identification solely by chromatographic retention time, for example, is not regarded as being specific, however, a combination of chromatographic tests (*e.g.* HPLC and TLC-densitometry) or a combination of tests into a single procedure, such as HPLC/UV-diode array, HPLC/MS, or GC/MS may be acceptable.

Qualitative Statement

Qualitative statement about the characteristic organoleptic character of the herbal drug preparation is important. If any of these characteristics change during storage, this change should be investigated and appropriate action is to be taken.

Following test parameters are usually considered for the quality control of herbal drug preparation:

Residual Solvents

Refer to the European Pharmacopoeia Monograph *Residual solvents* for detailed information.

Water Content

This test is important where the herbal drug preparations are known to be hygroscopic. The acceptance criteria may be justified with data on the effects of hydration or moisture absorption. A Loss on Drying procedure may be adequate; however, in some cases (essential-oil containing preparations), a detection procedure that is specific for water is required.

Microbial Limits

There may be a need to specify the total count of aerobic microorganisms, the total count of yeasts and mould, and the absence of specific objectionable bacteria. These limits should comply with the European Pharmacopoeia.

Mycotoxins

The potential for mycotoxins contamination should be fully considered. Where necessary, suitable validated methods should be used to control potential mycotoxins and the acceptance criteria should be justified.

Pesticides, Fumigation Agents, etc.

The potential for residues of pesticides, fumigation agents etc. should be fully considered. Where necessary, suitable validated methods should be used to control potential residues and the acceptance criteria should be justified. In the case of pesticide residues the method, acceptance criteria and guidance on the methodology of the European Pharmacopoeia should be applied unless fully justified.

Assay

In the case of herbal drug preparation with constituents of known therapeutic activity, assays of their content are required with details of the analytical procedure. Where possible, a specific, stability-indicating procedure should be included to determine the content of the herbal drug in the herbal drug preparation. In cases where use of a non-specific assay is justified, other supporting analytical procedures should be used to achieve overall specificity. For example, where a UV/Visible spectrophotometric assay is used *e.g.* with anthraquinone glycosides a combination of the assay and a suitable test for identification (*e.g.* fingerprint chromatography) can be used. In the case of herbal drug preparations where the constituents responsible for the therapeutic activity are unknown, assays of marker substances or other justified determinations are required. The appropriateness of the choice of marker substance should be justified.

Impurities

Organic and inorganic impurities and residual solvents are included in this category. The need for inclusion of tests and acceptance criteria for inorganic impurities should be studied during development and based on knowledge of the plant species, its cultivation and the manufacturing process. The potential for manufacturing process to concentrate toxic residues should be fully addressed. Where justified, procedures and acceptance criteria for sulfated ash/residue on ignition should follow pharmacopoeial procedures; other inorganic impurities may be determined by other appropriate procedures, *e.g.* atomic absorption spectroscopy etc. In this context for individual preparation the ICH Guidelines on Impurities in New Drug Products and other official documents plays a major role which can be further explained by the following points.

1. Impurities arising from the herbal drug preparation *e.g.* contaminants such as pesticide/fumigant residues, heavy metals, are normally controlled during the testing of the herbal drug preparation and it is not necessary to test for these in the herbal medicinal product.
2. Similarly, residual solvent arising from the manufacture of the herbal drug preparation (*e.g.* an extract) need not be controlled in the finished herbal medicinal product provided it is appropriately controlled in the extract specification. However, solvents used for example in tablet coating will need to be controlled in the dosage form.
3. Major impurities arising from degradation of the herbal drug preparation should be monitored in the herbal medicinal product. Acceptance limits should be stated for individual specified degradation products, which may

include both identified and unidentified degradation products as appropriate and total degradation products.

4. When it has been conclusively demonstrated via appropriate analytical methodology with a significant body of data, that the herbal drug preparation (herbal drug) does not degrade in the specific formulation and under the specific storage conditions proposed in the marketing authorization, degradation product testing may be reduced or eliminated upon approval by the regulatory authorities.

Herbal medicines should be free not only from botanical contaminants, but also from residual pesticides or fumigation agents and from pathogenic microorganisms or microbial toxins. There is evidence, for instance, that medicinal plant materials from India and Sri Lanka can be contaminated with toxigenic fungi (*Aspergillus, Fusarium*). Since aflatoxin B (I) has sometimes been recovered from such materials in potentially unsafe amounts, it would certainly be prudent to improve their storage conditions of great practical concern is the presence, intentionally or by accident, of toxic metals (such as lead and arsenic) or conventional pharmaceuticals (such as corticosteroids and non-steroidal anti-inflammatory drugs) in certain herbal medicines of Asian origin [12, 13]. Although these hazards have been denounced for more than two decades now, they continue to pose an occasional threat to public health [14, 15]. The contamination of herbal medicines with pharmaceuticals is not necessarily limited to products of Oriental origin but also to products from other countries because of the not too stringent rules and regulations governing the quality of the herbals in different countries [16].

Many conventional drugs or their precursors are derived from plants, but there is a fundamental difference between administering a pure chemical and the same chemical in a plant matrix. It is this issue of the advantage of chemical complexity, which is both rejected by orthodoxy as having no basis in fact and avoided by most researchers as introducing too many variables for comfortable research. Herein lies the fundamental difference between the phytotherapist, who prefers not just to prescribe chemically complex remedies but often to administer them in complex formulations. Synergy is an important concept in herbal pharmacology. In the context of chemical complexity, it applies if the action of a chemical mixture is greater than the arithmetical sum of the actions of the mixture's components: the whole is greater than the sum of the individual parts. A well-known example of synergy is exploited in the use of insecticidal pyrethrins. A synergist known as piperonyl butoxide, which has little insecticidal activity of its own, interfaces with the insect's ability to break down the pyrethrins, thereby substantially increasing their toxicity. This example emphasizes what is probably an important mechanism behind the synergy observed for medicinal plant components: increased or prolonged levels of key components at the active site. In other words, components of plants which are not active themselves can act to improve the stability, solubility, bioavailability or half-life of the active components (17, 18). Hence a particular chemical in pure form might have only a fraction of the pharmacological activity that it has in its plant matrix. This important example of synergy therefore has a pharmacokinetic basis. Synergy can also have a

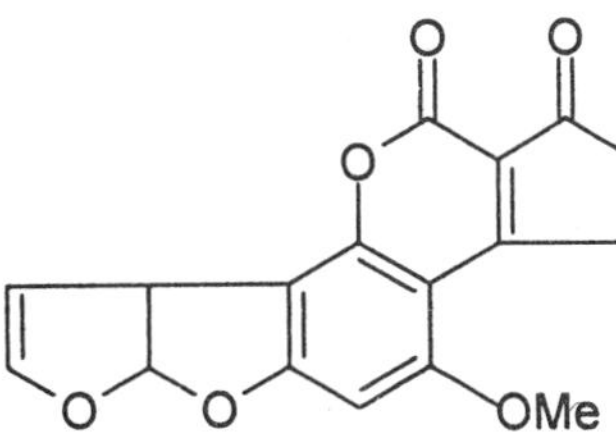

Aflatoxin B (I)

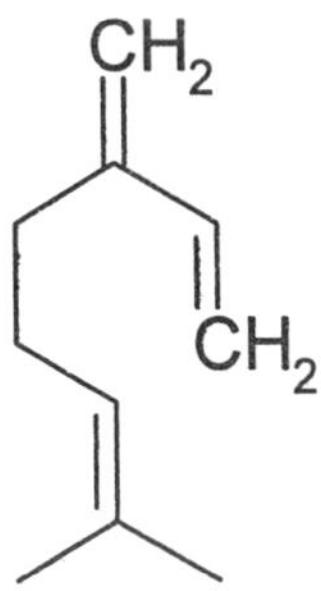

Myrcene (II)

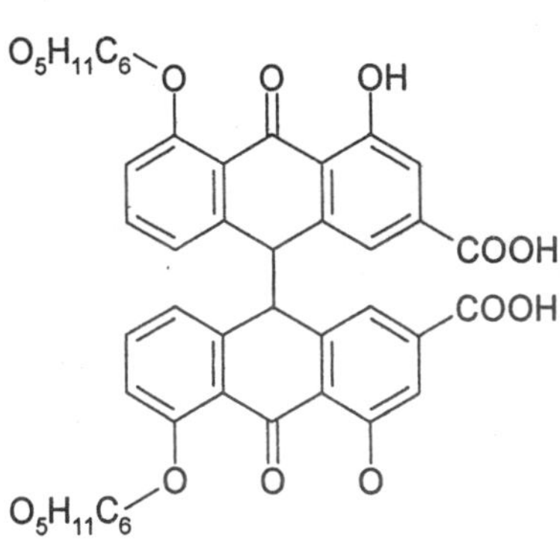

Sennoside A (III)

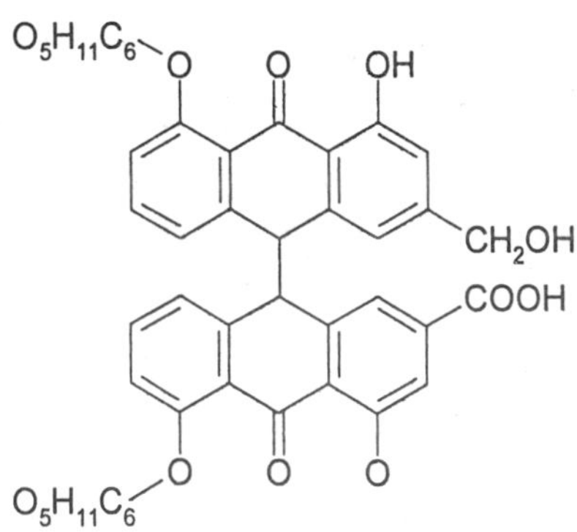

Sennoside C (IV)

pharmacodynamic basis. One example is the antibacterial activity of major components of lemongrass essential oil. While geranial and neral individually elicit antibacterial action, the third main component myrcene do not show any activity. However, myrcene (II) enhances the activities when mixed with either of the other two main components (19). Sennoside A (III) and sennoside C (IV) from senna have similar laxative activities in mice, however, a mixture of these compounds in the ratio 7:3 (which somewhat reflects the relative levels found in senna leaf) has almost double the laxative activity (20). Thus chemical complexity leading to enhanced solubility or bioavailability of key components has been the theme of a number of scientific studies.

Marker Analysis: Tool for Quality Evaluation of Botanicals

In the herbal boom world wide it is estimated that high quality phyto-medicinals will provide safe and effective medication. For the development of the quality and standardization parameters of botanicals and thereby to assist the herbal drug manufacturers engaged in production of medicinal plants, the special quality problems they pose, and the corresponding needs for international guidance on reliable methods of quality control and development of standardization parameters is of great importance. Highlights are being made on various approaches of biomarker profiling of herbals to establish the quality control approaches with chemo profiling techniques with the lead from some therapeutically potent medicinal plants [11]. It is an accepted fact that qualitative and quantitative analysis of major bioactive chemical components (marker) of plant material constitute an important and reliable part of quality control protocol as any change in quality of the plant material directly affects the constituents. If a marker itself is a biologically active principle of the plant, qualitative and quantitative analysis of these biomarker not only helps to control the quality of herbal material used, but also can be used to estimate the quantity of biologically active chemical entities required to produce specific pharmacological activity, provided the marker assay is validated as a reliable estimate of the quantities of other constituents, under specified conditions of growing, harvesting, storage and production. This can be used to estimate the dose required [21].

Markers can be defined as a chemical entity present in the plant material. The markers are chemically defined and of interest for quality control purposes. Markers are generally employed when constituents of known therapeutic activity are not found or are uncertain. Through various analytical techniques like TLC and HPLC, markers can be visualized. Analysis of such chemical entities may be used to calculate the quantity of plant material or preparation in the finished product. The biomarkers on the other hand are a group or chemical compounds which are in addition to being unique for that plant material also correlative with biological efficacy. Biomarker profiling of a maximum number of medicinal plants being used in therapy required to be established to highlight the quality control development based on this new emerging techniques which is being utilized by the people through out the globe for drug development from natural resources.

Quality evaluation of crude drugs and herbal preparations is a fundamental requirement of industry and other organizations dealing with Ayurvedic and herbal products. Unfortunately this requirement is often not possible to meet with usual Pharmacognostical tests such as macro and microscopical evolution, ash value, extractive value etc. Directives on the analytical control of crude drugs must take account of the fact that the material to be examined has a complex and inconsistent composition, therefore the analytical limits are not as precise as for the single chemical entity based on chemoprofiling through marker analysis [11, 22]. The use of indicative substances for development of quality control profiles has been considered as the thrust area for standardization of botanicals globally. They can be selected among the constituent substances of the plant, irrespective of whether these are active or accompanying substances. They should however be characteristic of the drug plant under investigation and easily demonstrable. Analytical data other than those obtained by thin layer chromatography can also be used for identification and quality assurance [23, 24].

Based on experience attempts have been made at the School of Natural Product Studies for development of marker profile for several medicinal plants. For example the marker profile of *Phyllanthus amarus* has been reported [25]. Phyllanthin (V) and Hypophyllanthin (VI) are phytomarkers of *Phyllanthus amarus.* In India the plant is often used in traditional system of medicine for a variety of ailments including flu, dropsy, asthma, bronchial infections, and diseases of the liver. In Ayurvedic system of medicine it is used in problems of stomach, genito-urinary system, liver and kidney. Apart from the major bio active lignan constituents of the plants Phyllanthin (V) and Hypophyllanthin(VI), the plant is reported to contain, geraniin (VII), corilagin (VIII), rutin (IX) and quercetin (X) [10, 26]. To make standardization profile for *Phyllanthus amarus*, various parameters prescribed in Indian Herbal Pharmacopoeia (IHP) were considered. The macroscopical characteristics like color, appearance, odor and taste were studied and noted as per requirement of Indian Herbal Pharmacopoeia. Parameters like tests for extraneous material and physio-chemical analysis were carried out on the basis of protocol prescribed by WHO [27, 28]. Successive extractive values, quantitative analysis of extract for the presence of Phyllanthin and Hypophyllanthin were carried out by HPLC. Phyllanthin and Hypophyllanthin were used as standards for HPTLC finger printing and to analyze the extract qualitatively. Marker profile based on HPTLC finger printing based on 6-gingerol (XI) in ginger (*Zingiber officinale*) and other plants has been reported from our laboratory [29]. Marker testing is in no way a substitute for other tests like Physico-chemical, chemical, macro and microscopical characterization etc. Nevertheless, it is an efficient procedure to ensure the identity and purity of herbal drugs. There are several constraints in adapting this technique for regular testing of the herbs and herbal formulations in the traditional system of medicine as follow:

1. Non availability of library of marker compounds isolated from herbs in their pure form
2. Lack of proper communication and the willingness of quality assurance department to undertake tedious testing procedures
3. Non availability of a system where standard or properly identified herbs are available for the industry.
4. High cost involved in procurement of costly instruments and also its validation and proper maintenance.

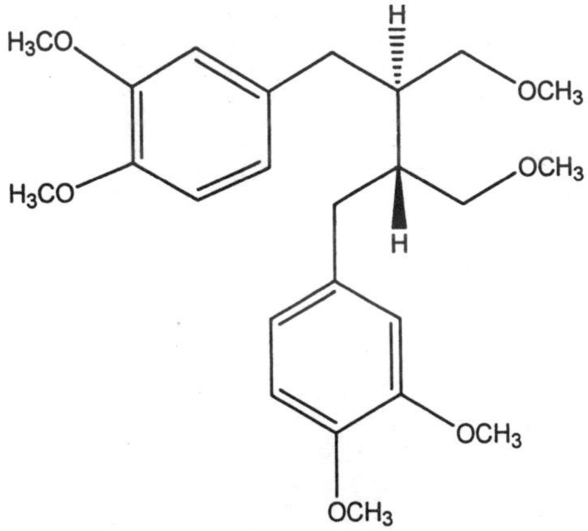

Phyllanthin (V)

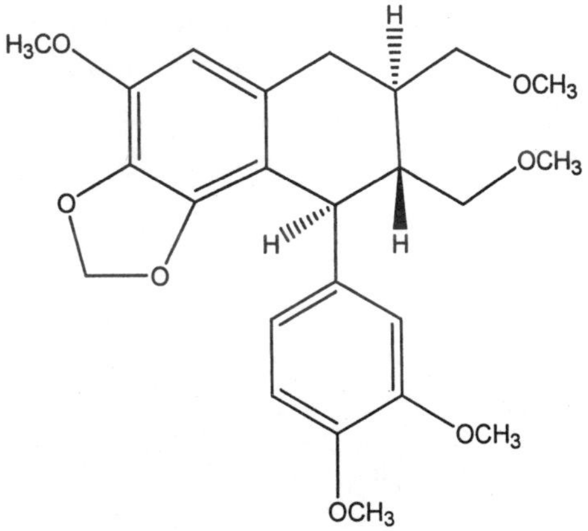

Hypophyllanthin(VI)

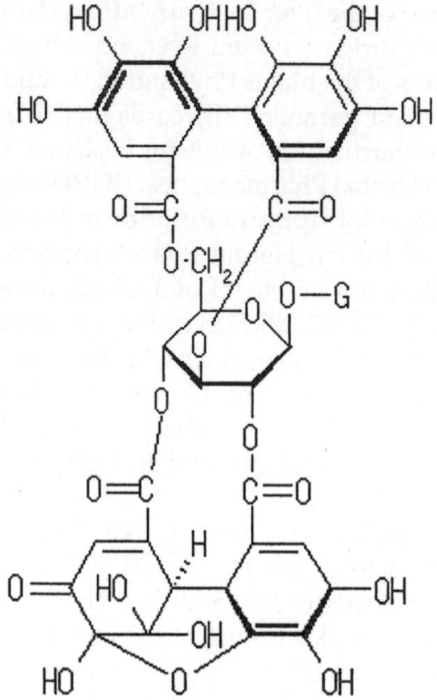

Geraniin (VII)

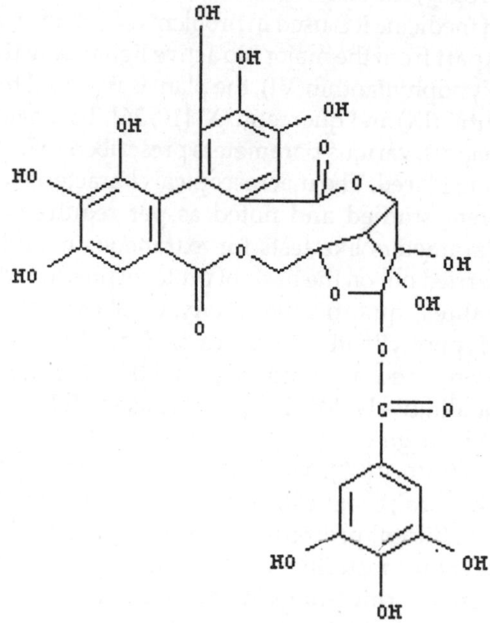

Corilagin (VIII)

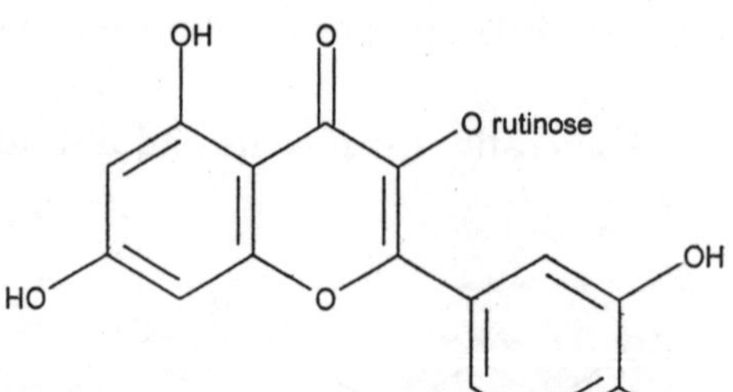

Rutin (IX)

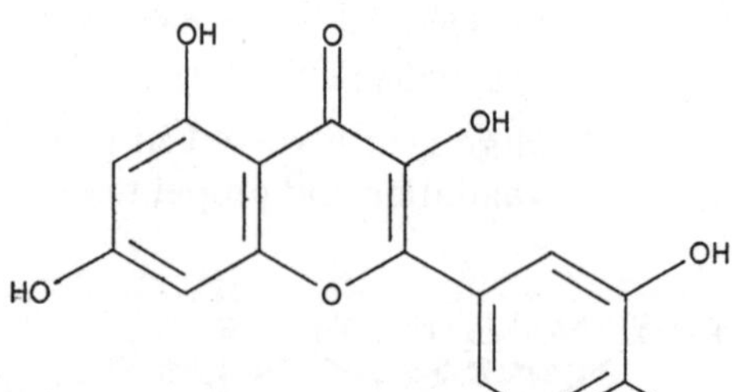

Quercetin (X)

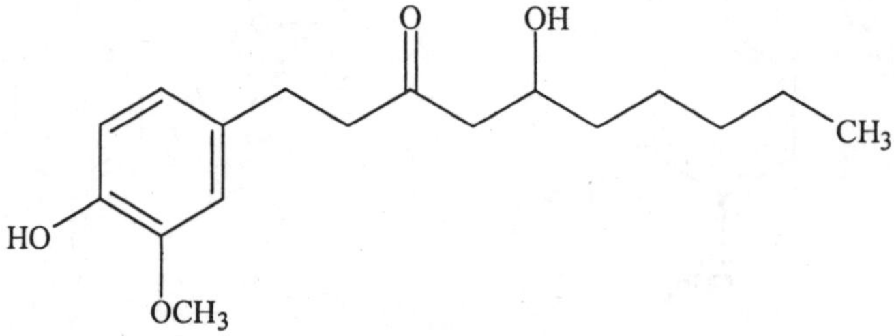

6-Gingerol (XI)

Conclusion

Nobody deserves a remedy, which is worse than his disease, and herbal markets should be actively improved by banning unsafe remedies and by discouraging unsafe practices. Unfortunately, the introduction of herbal medicine-like products into the market is not adequately monitored in various countries. This unsatisfactory situation could be greatly improved by the creation of a special licensing system for herbal medicines in particular, besides the laws for the Ayurvedic and Siddha medicines that already exist in the Indian Drugs and Cosmetics Act (1940). Such a system would not only help to keep out preparations from herbs with known toxicity but it would also provide a valuable tool to improve herbal product quality. This is of particular importance as herbal health problems are too often due to contaminants rather than to declared ingredients. Not only the quality of a finished herbal product is important, but also the quality of the consumer information about that product. Understandable warnings in the package insert can certainly help to reduce the risk of inappropriate uses and adverse reaction instances, the German health authorities have limited the indication of herbal anthranoid laxatives to constipation that has not responded to bulk-forming therapy. In addition, they have imposed restrictions to the laxative use of most anthranoid containing herbs, that is, not to be used for more than 1 to 2 weeks without medical advice, not to be used in children under 12 years of age, and not to be used during pregnancy and lactation. This example illustrates that herbal health risks do not always require a full ban of specific herbal ingredients but can sometimes be pushed back by appropriate warnings in the product information. This example also makes it clear that the quality assurance of herbal prescriptions is an important issue that should not be overlooked. The same can be said, of course, about the quality of crude herbal materials also.

The botanicals are evaluated and marketed by different countries based on the regulations of their own. Exploring botanicals with international coordination in the context of modern development is the need of the day and was mostly discussed through the international conferences. Formulation of important guidelines in defining the extent and type of our participation is important while discussing the acceptance of the role of traditional systems of medicine and their practitioners in the primary health care. Therefore, to establish the potentiality of traditional medicine, research needs to be simultaneously conducted on important aspects of these disciplines to meet the requirement of the society were they have to serve. Safety and efficacy of the Natural Health Products (NHP) is always a cause of concern to promote and rationalize their use. Quality control of botanicals, validated processes of manufacturing, customer awareness and post marketing surveillance are the key points which could ensure the safety and efficacy of NHP. Currently there is an urgent need for international collaboration in the development and promotion of operational methodologies that should include a variety of standard operating procedures addressing the nomenclature, quality, safety, and efficacy of these products, when used as phytomedicines. International coordination on botanical's development in the context of modern drug development will broaden the use of these products in both developing and industrialized nations. So there is a need for coordination and harmonization of regulations related to research and development of natural products as both pharmaceuticals and food supplements.

Acknowledgements

The authors wish to express their gratitude to the Commonwealth Scholarship Commission, Association of Commonwealth Universities, UK, for the Commonwealth Academic Staff Fellowship Award to Dr. Pulok K. Mukherjee through the University Grants Commission (UGC), India.

References

1. Mukherjee PK, Wahile A: Integrated Approaches towards Drug Development from Ayurveda and other Indian System of Medicines. *J Ethnopharmacol,* 2006, 103, 25–35.
2. Mukherjee PK: Promotion and development of botanicals with international coordination. *In: Promotion and development of botanicals with international coordination* [ed. Mukherjee PK], Allied Book Agency, Kolkata, India, 2005, 1-9.
3. Mukherjee PK: Exploring green resources for drug development through Ethnobotany. *In: Chemistry for green environment* (ed. Srivastava MM, Sanghi R), Narosa Publishing House, New Delhi, India, 2005, 287-301.
4. Mukherjee PK, Mukherjee K: Evaluation of botanical-perspectives of quality safety and efficacy. In *Advances in medicinal plants* (ed. Prajapati ND, Prajapati, Sushma JS), Asian Medicinal Plants, 2005, 87-110.
5. Mukherjee PK, Maiti K, Mukherjee K, Houghton PJ: Better herbal therapy with phospholipid based drug delivery systems of botanicals. *J Pharm Pharmacol,* 2006 [in press].
6. Farnsworth NR: The role of medicinal plants in drug development. In *Natural Products and Drug Development* (ed. Krogsgaard-Larsen P, Christensen SB, Kolod H) Munksgaard, Copenhagen, 1984, 17-28.
7. Mukherjee PK: Exploring botanicals in Indian systems of medicine–regulatory perspectives. *Clinical Res Reg Affairs,* 2003, 20, 249-264.
8. Mukherjee PK, Wahile A: Perspectives of safety for natural health products. In *Herbal drugs–a twenty first century perspectives* (ed. Sharma RK, Arora R), Jaypee Brothers Medicinal Publishers Ltd., New Delhi, 2006, 50-59.
9. Mukherjee PK: Problems and prospects for the GMP in herbal drugs in Indian systems of medicine. *Drug Inf J,* 2002, 63, 635-644.
10. Mukherjee PK, Maiti K, Mukherjee K, Houghton PJ: Leads from Indian medicinal plants with hypoglycemic potentials. *J Ethnopharmacol,* 2006, 106, 1-28.
11. Mukherjee PK: *Quality Control of Herbal Drugs–An approach for Evaluation of Botanicals,* Business Horizons Ltd, New Delhi, 2002.
12. Marwick C: Trials reveal no benefit, possible harm of beta carotene and vitamin A for lung cancer prevention. *JAMA,* 1996, 275, 422-423.

13. Abeywickrama K, Bean GA: Toxigenic *Aspergillus flavus* and aflatoxins in Sri Lankan medicinal plant material. *Mycopathologia*, 1991,113, 187-90.

14. De Smet PAGM, D'Arcy PF: Drug interactions with herbal and other non-orthodox drugs. In *Drug interactions* (ed. Wellington PJ, D'Arcy PF), Springer Verlag, Heidelberg, 1996, 327-352.

15. Shaw D, House I, Kolev S, Murray V: Should herbal medicines be licensed? *BMJ*, 1995, 311, 451-452.

16. Gertmner E, Marshall PS, Filandrinos D, Potek AS, Smith TM: Complications resulting from the use of Chinese herbal medications containing undeclared prescription drugs. *Arthritis Rheum*, 1995, 38, 614-617.

17. Mukherjee PK: Plant products with hypocholesterolemic potentials. In *Advances in food and nutrition research*, (ed.Taylor SL), Elsevier Science, USA, 2003, 277-338.

18. Mukherjee PK: Evaluation of Indian traditional medicine. *Drug Inf J*, 2001, 35, 623-632.

19. Onawunmi GO, Yisak W, Ogunlana EO: Antibacterial constituents in the essential oil of *Cymbopogon citratus* (DC). Stapf. *J Ethnopharmacol*, 1984, 12, 279-286.

20. Kisa K, Sasaki K, Yamuchi K, Kuwano S: Potentiating effect of sennoside C on purgative activity of sennoside A in mice. *Planta Med*, 1981, 42, 302-312.

21. Anonymous: GMP for Ayurveda, Siddha, Unani (ASU) Medicines. *IDMA Bulletin*, 2000, 31, 612-620.

22. Mukherjee PK, Manoranjan S, Suresh B: Indian herbal medicines. *The Eastern Pharmacist*, 1998, 42, 21-24.

23. De Smet PAGM, Smeets OSNM: Potential risks of health food products containing yohimbe extracts. *BMJ*, 1994, 309, 958

24. Mukherjee PK: GMP in Indian system of medicine. In *GMP for Botanicals–Regulatory and Quality Issues on Phytomedicine* (ed. Mukherjee PK, Verpoorte R), Business Horizons, New Delhi, India, 2003, 99-112.

25. Mukherjee PK, Wahile A, Kumar V, Rai S, Mukherjee K: Marker profiling for a few botanicals used for hepatoprotection in Indian System of Medicine". *Drug Inf J*, 2006, 40,131–139.

26. Maiti K, Gantait A, Mukherjee K, Saha BP, Mukherjee PK, Therapeutic potentials of andrographolide from *Andrographis paniculata*: A review. *J Natural Remedies*, 2006, 6, 1-13.

27. World Health Organization, Quality Control Methods for Medicinal Plant Materials, Geneva, 1998, 4-21.

28. World Health Organization, Regulatory Situation of Herbal Medicine, World Wide Review. 1998, 1-5.

29. Rai S, Mukherjee K, Mal M, Wahile A, Saha BP, Mukherjee PK: Determination of 6-gingerol in ginger (*Zingiber officinale*) using high-performance thin-layer chromatography. *J Separation Science*, 2006, 29 [in press].

Chapter 11

Potential Use of Some Natural Compounds as Radioprotectors

C.K.K. *Nair*

Department of Radiation Biology, Amala Cancer Research Centre, Trichur – 680 555, Kerala, India

E-mail: ckknair@yahoo.com

ABSTRACT

Radioprotective agents are classified into three broad groups–adaptogens–agents which act as stimulants of radioresistance; absorbents–which protect the organism against internal radionuclide and radioprotectors–which include sulphydryl compounds, antioxidants etc. Several compounds having antioxidant properties exhibit radioprotective ability and these include several nutraceuticals such as vitamin A, E, C etc, cytoprotective agents, drugs such as captopryl, MESNA, hormones like melatonin and phytochemicals such as curcumin, ferulic acid, epicatechin, vanillin, orientin, vicinin, glycyrrhizic acid etc. Also, the crude extracts of a number of plants have been reported to exhibit radioprotective ability. Several of these protect cells, membranes and biomolecules such as DNA and proteins *in vitro* However many of these though present promising results in laboratory studies are of limited application due to several factors such as toxicity, difficulties in administering required amounts, lack of preference for normal tissues, limited availability etc. A water soluble derivative of vitamin E, called Tocopherol monoglucoside (TMG) is of particular relevance in this context because of its nontoxic nature and antioxidant and radioprotective properties *in vitro* and *in vivo* in animal studies. The phytoceuticals epicatechin and ferulic acid are also effective in protecting DNA and membranes in biological systems exposed to ionizing radiation under *in vitro* as well as *in vivo* conditions. Radiation induced damages in vital cellular targets such as DNA and membrane are mainly due to radiation induced oxidative free radicals and the these antioxidant compounds scavenge the free radicals and thereby prevent deleterious effects of the radiation. TMG and ferulic acid have also been found to enhance cellular DNA repair in animal studies. This study will present an overview of some of the recent work on protection of biological systems against ionizing radiation induced damages by natural compounds and discuss the data from studies on epicatechin, ferulic acid and TMG.

Introduction

Ionizing radiation is being used in a large number of therapeutic, industrial and other applications apart from nuclear power generation development of new varieties of high-yielding crops, sterilization of materials for surgical and medical use and enhancing storage-period of food materials. In many instances where radiation is used for power generation, industrial/ medical purposes or agricultural uses and food preservation personnel manning the radiation sources may be subjected to low-level exposures. High exposures to radiation may occur due to accidents or during 'nuclear war'. Besides, radiation poses a major, currently un-resolvable risk for astronauts, especially for long-duration space flights. Cancer is one of the leading causes of morbidity and mortality in several populations of the world and radiotherapy is a dominant and effective mode of cancer treatment. Radiation injury to normal tissues surrounding the tumour is one of the major problems limiting the success of radiotherapy and there is a need to protect normal tissues from deleterious effects of radiation during radiotherapy. Understanding the mechanisms of radiation damage to humans is necessary for its possible prevention by drugs such as 'radioprotectors'. Several compounds, developed for this purpose which have been found very effective in the laboratory studies, have failed in human applications due to toxicity problems or lack of significant protective effects at radioprotective doses (1-3).

Many natural and synthetic chemicals have been investigated in the recent past for their efficacy to protect against radiation-induced damage in biological systems (3-5). However, the inherent toxicity of some of the synthetic agents at the effective radioprotective concentration warranted further search for safer and more effective radioprotectors. In fact, no radioprotective agent is now available, either alone or in combination to meet all the requisites of an ideal radioprotector (6). Amifostine is the only compound that is currently in use having good radioprotection to normal tissues during radiotherapy, even though there are reports about contra-indications in some cases (7). Though a large number of compounds have been shown to be promising as radioprotectors in laboratory studies, few could pass the transition from bench to bed-side. Most of them failed even before reaching the preclinical stage due to toxicity and side effects. For clinical application of any compound as a radioprotector, it would require absolute certainty about its relative protection factors for tumor and normal tissues accompanied by minimum toxicity to avoid unacceptable clinical risk.

Classification of Radioprotective Agents

Radioprotective agents can be classified as: (i) chemical radioprotectors, (ii) adaptogens and (iii) absorbents (3). The first group constitutes mainly sulfhydryl compounds and other antioxidants. Adaptogens act as stimulators of radioresistance.

These are natural protectors that offer chemical protection under low levels of ionizing radiations. They are generally extracted from the cells of plants and animals and have least toxicity. They can influence the regulatory system of exposed organisms, mobilize the endogenous background of radioresistance, immunity, and intensify the overall nonspecific resistance of an organism. Absorbents protect organisms from internal radiation and chemicals. These include drugs which prevent the incorporation of radioiodine by the thyroid gland and the absorption of radionuclides like ^{137}Cs, ^{90}Sr and ^{239}Pu.

Post-irradiation radioprotectors are important when an accidental exposure occurs during operation of equipments with radiation source or intentional exposures during war and such unnatural calamities. This area of radiation biology is a very slowly developing area since it is rather difficult to get such effective protectors.

Mechanisms Underlying Radioprotection

Radiation causes damage by direct and indirect mechanisms. The radioprotectors can elicit their action by various mechanisms such as: (*i*) suppressing the formation of free radicals, (*ii*) detoxifying the radiation induced reactive species, (*iii*) inducing the cellular radioprotectors such as superoxide dismutase (SOD), glutathione, prostaglandins and interleukin-1, (*iv*) enhancing the DNA repair by triggering one or more cellular DNA repair pathways, and (*v*) delaying cell division and inducing hypoxia in tissues (3). Scheme 1 gives an outline of the general strategies for protection, repair and regeneration following radiation exposure.

Importance of Free Radicals in Radiation Damage and Protection

Most of the cellular alterations induced by ionizing radiation is indirect and is mediated by the generation of free radicals and related reactive species, mainly derived from oxygen. Free radicals can be defined as atoms or a group of atoms having an unpaired electron. Because of the presence of unpaired electron, free radicals are highly reactive and are capable of altering all biological molecules including lipids, DNA and protein. In biological systems radiolysis of water gives rise to a large number of free radicals and related reactive species collectively known as 'reactive oxygen species' (ROS). These include hydrated electron e_{aq}^-, hydrogen radical.H, hydroxyl radical.$^{\bullet}$OH, H_2O_2, peroxyl radical ROO·, $O_2^{\cdot-}$, singlet oxygen $^1O_2$ etc. Radiolysis of aqueous solutions such as those forming cellular constituents results in the following reactions (8).

DNA and Membrane: The Major Targets of Radiation Inactivation

DNA forms the primary cellular target of radiation damage and membrane the alterative target. Mainly two types of changes are observed in DNA at the molecular level namely altered bases and strand breaks. Both types of changes, if not repaired affect the cell structure and function. Among the DNA bases, $^{\bullet}$OH is non selective in its reaction while $^1O_2$ reacts mainly with guanosines. Membrane protein and lipids can be damaged by radiation. In proteins it can lead to formation of protein carbonyls and loss of protein thiols besides loss of activity of membrane bound enzymes. Membrane lipids are highly susceptible for radiation damage mainly due to the presence of polyunsaturated fatty acids. The resulting damage results in lipid peroxidation. Unchecked peroxidative decomposition of membrane lipids has severe consequences for the cell and the organism. Since many cellular reactions are membrane based they are affected by lipid peroxidation. The products formed during this phenomenon also have effects at other targets away from the site of generation.

Tocopherolmonoglucoside (TMG) as Radioprotector

Vitamin E is a known radioprotector (3), possessing antioxidant property, effective in scavenging peroxyl radicals and other active oxygen species like superoxide anion, singlet molecular oxygen and hydroxyl radical (9-10). Vitamin E is only soluble in non polar solvents such as lipids and insoluble in aqueous medium. Due to its long hydrophobic phytyl side chain, the mobility of vitamin E, and hence, its radical scavenging activity, are restricted to the biological lipid membrane (9). Tocopherol monoglucoside (TMG) is a water soluble derivative of vitamin E–Scheme II (11). It has high solubility in water 100 per cent w/v and it also retains a high η-Octanol: H2O partition co-efficient of 3.5 (12). TMG inhibited γ-radiation induced conversion of thymine to thymine glycol (Rajagopalan *et al.* (13). TMG also inhibited the formation of γ-radiation induced single strand breaks SSBs in plasmid pBR322 DNA in a concentration dependent manner; at 500μM TMG there was complete protection of the DNA from radiation damage. The protective effect of TMG was found higher than that of Trolox, another structural analog of alpha Tocopherol (13).

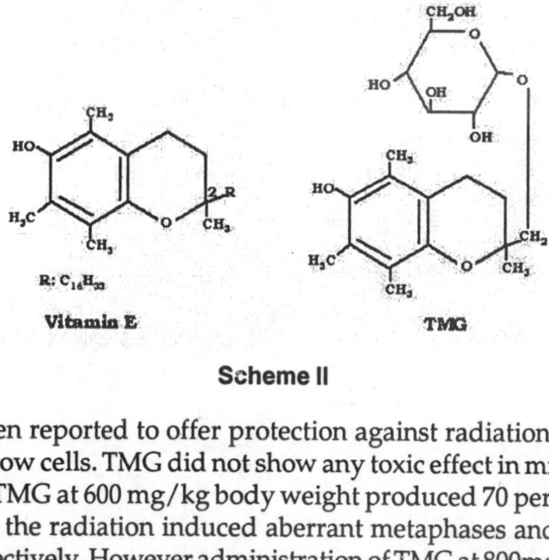

Scheme II

TMG has been reported to offer protection against radiation clastogenicity in mouse bone marrow cells. TMG did not show any toxic effect in mice up to 600 mg/kg body weight. TMG at 600 mg/kg body weight produced 70 per cent and >60 per cent reduction in the radiation induced aberrant metaphases and micronucleated erythrocytes respectively. However administration of TMG at 800mg/kg body weight showed some genotoxicity as revealed by increase in percentage of aberrant metaphase cells in mice. The LD_{50} of TMG administered i.p. for 24 hours and 30 days were found to be 1120 mg/kg body weight and 1000 mg/kg body weight respectively. Thus the maximum tolerated single dose of TMG is about 60 per cent of its LD_{50} for i.p. administration (12). Post irradiation administration of 600mg/kg body weight TMG within 10 min of lethal irradiation increased survival, giving a dose modification factor DMF of 1.09. DMFs of 1.22 and 1.48 for percentage aberrant metaphases and 1.6 and 1.98 for micronuclei were obtained for 400mg/kg body weight and 600mg/

kg body weight TMG respectively (12). Studies with yeast indicate that TMG confers radio-resistance *S. cerevisiae* possibly by two mechanisms *viz.* (*i*) by eliminating radiation-induced reactive free radicals when irradiation is carried out in the presence of TMG and (*ii*) by activating an error prone repair process involving RAD52 gene, when the cells are grown in medium containing TMG (14).

The effect of TMG administration on ionizing radiation-induced damage to membrane and DNA in mice under *in vivo* conditions has been investigated. The damages to cellular DNA were monitored by alkaline single cell gel electrophoresis comet assay (15,16), and the damages to membrane were studied by measuring peroxidation of membrane lipids. The membrane damage was measured in terms TBARS (17). The alteration in the lipid peroxidation values from different tissues are presented in Figure 11.1. It was observed that administration of TMG 400mg/kg alone could lower the basal level of lipid peroxidation in the cells of liver and intestinal crypt considerably. Exposure of mice to whole body gamma-radiation resulted in elevated levels of TBARS in tissues such as liver, spleen and intestinal crypt. Administration of TMG prior to radiation exposure could inhibit this peroxidative

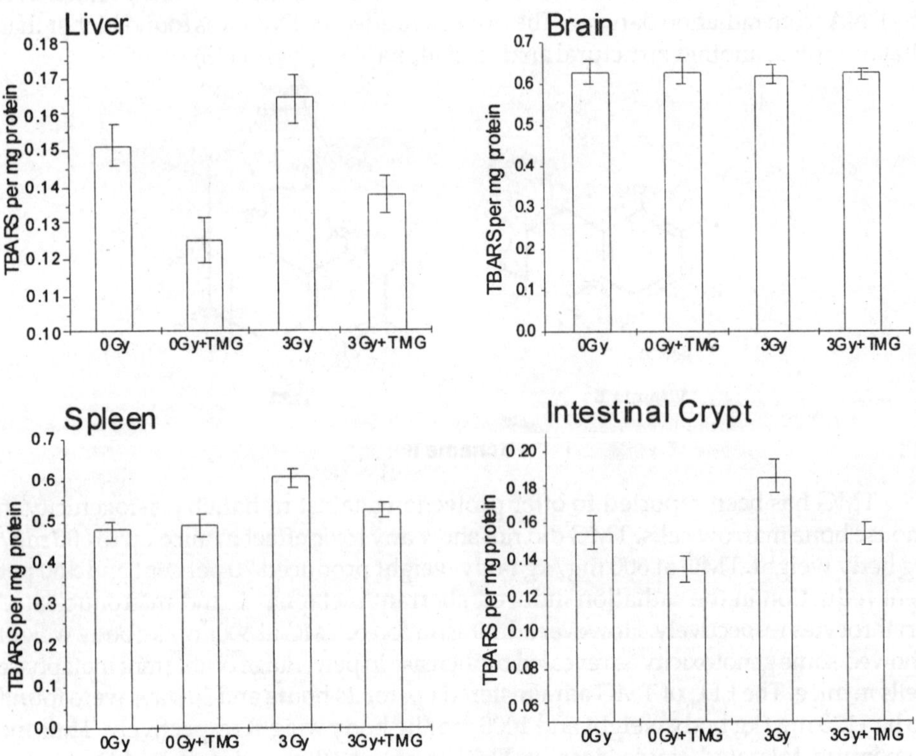

Figure 11.1: Protection of Membrane by TMG in Different Tissues of Whole-body Irradiated Mice Against Gamma-radiation Induced Lipid Peroxidation. Each point represents the mean ± SEM.

damage at different levels in these tissues as can be evidenced from the data presented in Figure 11.1.

DNA Damage and its Modification by TMG

Exposure to whole body gamma irradiation resulted in damage to cellular DNA in normal and tumor cells. The damage was manifested as increase in different comet parameters such as tail length TL, tail moment TM and percent DNA in tail of all the tissues. Administration of TMG after irradiation reduced this increase in the cells of normal tissues to a great extent. Figure 11.2 presents typical comet images of mouse blood leucocytes after different treatments.

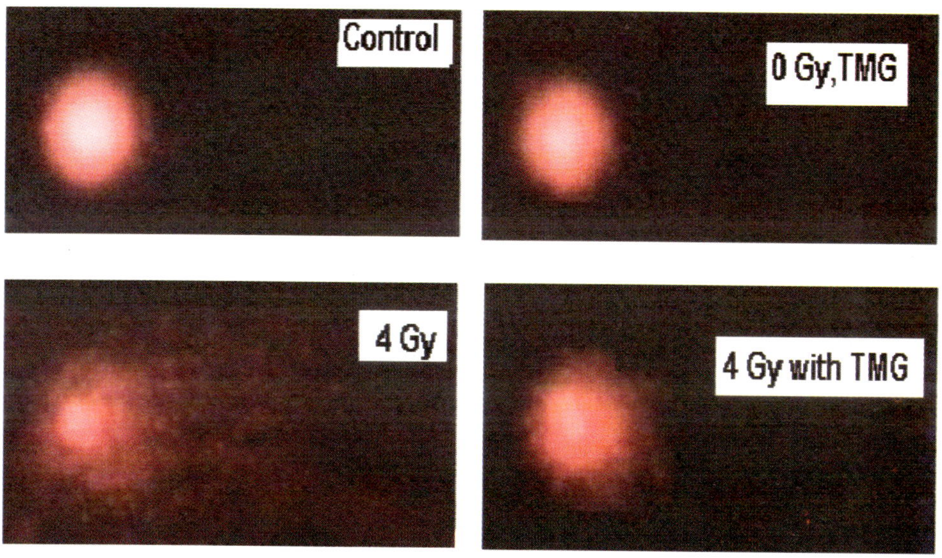

Figure 11.2: Protection of Cellular DNA by TMG in Peripheral Blood Leucocytes of Tumor Bearing Mice; Typical Comet Images of Mouse Blood Leucocytes After Different Treatments

The effect of TMG administration on cellular DNA damage in various tissues and tumor after whole-body gamma-irradiation can be inferred from Figure 11.3. The decrease in the parameters was more pronounced in the comets obtained from liver cells. The biodistribution of TMG in various tissues could be different, and the low tissue availability could result in lower protection in tissues other than liver. The comet parameter 'tail moment' has been regarded as one of the best indices of induced radiation damage among other parameters calculated by computerized image analysis (18), the DNA damage is quantified by measuring the tail moment TM which is calculated as the product of the tail length and percent DNA in tail. The protection of gamma-radiation induced single strand breaks in murine tissue by TMG was calculated using the formula,

$$TM_{4Gy} - TM_{4Gy,TMG} / TM_{4Gy} - TM_{0Gy} \times 100$$

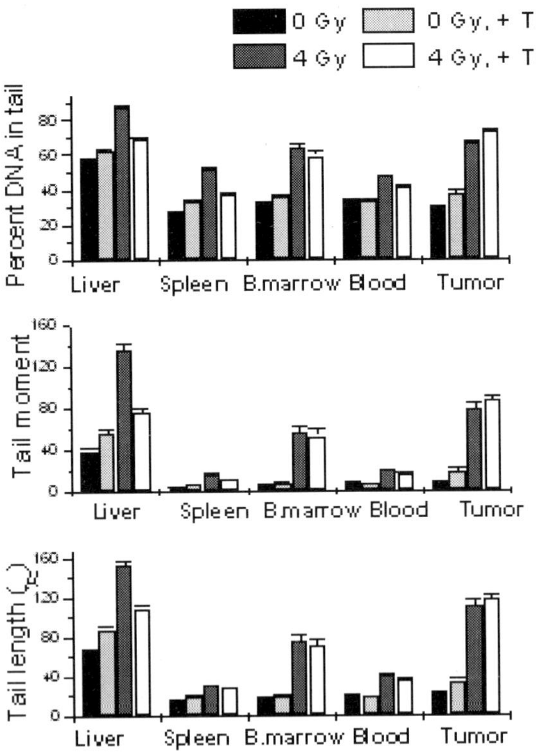

Figure 11.3: Protection of Different Tissues of Mice Against Gamma-radiation Induced DNA Strand Breaks Measured by Alkaline Comet Assay. Each figure represents the mean ± SEM.

It was found that TMG protected normal tissues selectively against gamma-irradiation and did not show any protection of tumor cells (12). Maximum protection was seen in cells of liver 60 per cent, followed by spleen 48 per cent, blood 34 per cent and bone marrow 7 per cent, while in tumor cells there was no protection observed.

Studies on Repair of Radiation-induced Single Strand Breaks in Cellular DNA in Blood Leucocytes of Whole Body Irradiated Mice

Figure 11.4 presents the data on the effect of post-irradiation administration of TMG 400mg/kg, on repair of DNA strand breaks in peripheral blood leucocytes of mice exposed to 4 Gy whole body gamma-radiation, in terms of comet parameters such as Percent DNA in tail, Tail length, Tail moment and Olive tail moment (OTM). The comet parameters of the blood leucocytes of the irradiated mice were found to decrease with increase in post-irradiation time of blood-withdrawal indicating repair of radiation induced damages in DNA of these cells. In irradiated mice administered with TMG this decrease of comet parameters was much faster than in mice irradiated but without TMG administration as can be evident in Figure 11.3. This would suggest that administration of TMG enhanced DNA repair. As the decrease in Olive tail

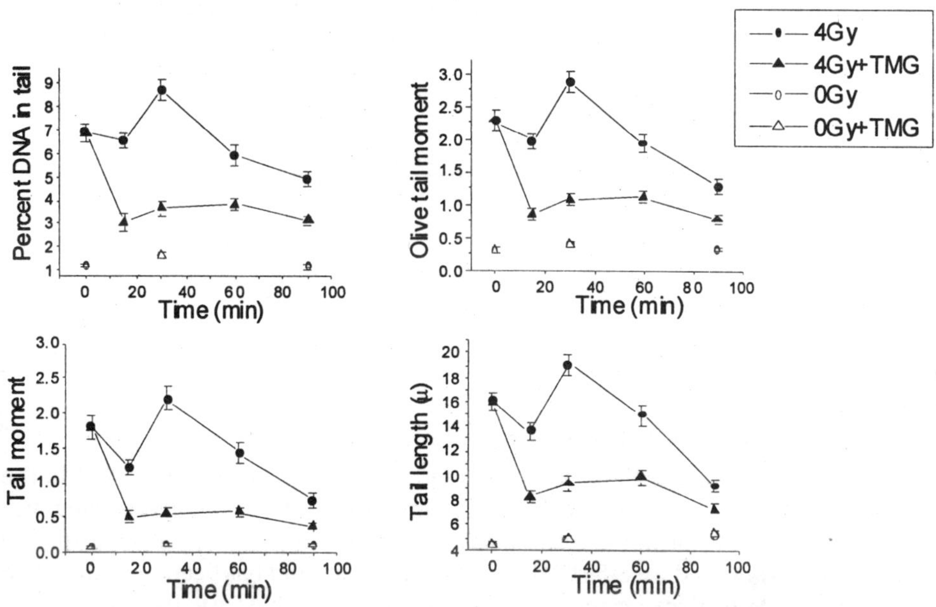

Figure 11.4: Effect of Post-irradiation Administration of TMG on DNA Repair in Peripheral Blood Leucocytes of Whole Body Irradiated Mice 4Gy *in vivo*. Each point represents the mean ± SEM standard error of mean.

moment can be considered as an index of DNA repair it was thought befitting to compare the DNA repair status in blood leucocytes from irradiated mice with and without TMG administration.

DNA repair index was measured as per cent decrease of Olive tail moment initial value of OTM immediately after irradiation taken as 100 per cent. It can be seen in Table 11.1, that the OTM of the blood leucocytes decreased by 15 per cent at 15 min post-irradiation but subsequently increased by about 30 per cent $p \leq 0.0001$at 30 min post irradiation and further decreased at the initial rate and reached to 56 per cent $p \leq 0.001$at 90 min post irradiation. When TMG was administered to the mice following irradiation, the OTM of the blood leucocytes decreased by 64 per cent $p \leq 0.0001$ in the first 15 min post irradiation. This would suggest that TMG or its metabolites accelerated the DNA repair process in these cells. At 30 min post irradiation there was a slight increase in OTM by 12 per cent, this increase remained constant till 60 min post irradiation and at 90 min post irradiation it was found that the OTM decreased by 66 per cent $p \leq 0.05$. The increase in the comet parameter such as OTM following 15 min post irradiation might be due to an increase in the DNA strand breaks characteristic of DNA repair corresponding to excision step at damaged sites (19,20). This would imply that TMG or its metabolite may be involved in DNA repair enhancement or TMG may be eliciting some biochemical pathway in the animal system *in vivo* to enhance the DNA repair process.

Table 11.1: DNA Repair Index Measured as Per cent Decrease of Olive Tail Moment (OTM) in Blood Leukocytes of Mice Following Exposure to Gamma-radiation and TMG Administration

Post Irradiation Time (min)	*% Olive Tail Moment*	
	Control irradiated	*Irradiated+TMG*
0	100	100
15	85	36
30	126	48
60	86	51
90	56	34

Epicatechin as a Radioprotector

Epicatechin–Scheme III–is one of the most potent antioxidants present in the human diet. Particularly high levels of this compound are found in tea, apples, and chocolate (21). Epicatechin is among the major constituents responsible for the protective and antioxidant effect exhibited by green tea and has been proved to be a very good free radical scavenger (22). It has been reported that tea extracts and/or its constituents have antibacterial (23) antiviral (24) antioxidative (25,26), antitumor and antimutagenic activities (27). Also it was shown that green tea extract can scavenge NO and O_2^- very effectively (28).

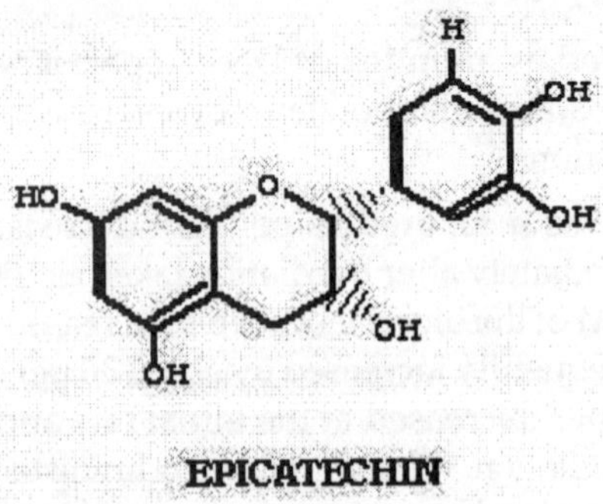

EPICATECHIN

Scheme III

It has been shown that EC has the capacity to quench OH$^\bullet$ radical almost 100 times more effectively than mannitol, a typical OH$^\bullet$ radical scavenger. It was demonstrated that EC possess DPPH free radical scavenging activity IC_{50}-1.5 μg, good hydrogen peroxide IC_{50}-11.18 μg and superoxide anion scavenging IC_{50}-1.64 μg activities (22). Various workers have documented the anti-lipid peroxidation activity of EC. Also it was shown that EC protected phospholipid bilayers against AAPH {2,2' -azobis2-amidinopropane, a water-soluble radical initiator} induced lipid peroxidation (29). Protection of membranes in isolated rat hepatocytes by EC against oxidative damage induced by *tert*-butylhydroperoxide was studied by Valls-Bellés *et al.* (30). EC reduced cell membrane damage by lowering lipid peroxidation. In addition, the activity of antioxidant enzymes such as superoxide dismutase and catalase were also shown to be restored (30). In the present report, protection of DNA by EC under *in vitro* conditions of irradiation was estimated in plasmid pBR322 DNA using plasmid relaxation assay. *In vivo* protection of cellular DNA was analyzed in peripheral blood leucocytes of whole body irradiated mice following prior administration of EC, using alkaline comet assay.

Effect of Epicatechin Gamma-radiation Induced Strand Breaks

Exposure to gamma-radiation lead to DNA strand breaks resulting into relaxation of plasmid DNA from super coiled ccc form to open circle oc form. It was seen that EC reduced ionizing radiation-induced disappearance of ccc form of the plasmid DNA significantly. Figure 11.5 presents the effect of 0.2 mM EC on formation of strand breaks in plasmid pBR 322 DNA by different doses of gamma-radiation 0-75 Gy. It was evident that at dose of 50 Gy and 75 Gy, 100 per cent of the plasmid DNA got converted into open circle form Figure 11.10, lane 7, 8. Presence of 0.2 mM EC inhibited this conversion from supercoiled form to open circle form almost to 40-60 per cent at different doses of gamma-radiation. Percent of ccc form of plasmid DNA remaining after exposure to various doses of gamma-radiation, with and without 0.2 mM EC was plotted against the radiation dose in Figure 11.6. The dose modifying factor D.M.F. was calculated at 50 per cent protection values from this figure as 6. Hence it was evident that EC could offer protection to DNA against gamma-radiation induced damage *in vitro* by reducing the formation of strand breaks significantly.

Effect of Epicatechin Administration on Gamma-Radiation-Induced DNA Strand Breaks in Peripheral Blood Leucocytes of Whole Body Irradiated Mice

Exposure to 4 Gy whole body gamma-radiation induced strand breaks in the DNA of peripheral blood leucocytes of mice. Figure 11.7 presents the comet parameters from blood leucocytes of mice exposed to 4 Gy whole body radiation, after EC administration, at 0 min post-irradiation. As depicted in Figure 11.7, all the comet parameters percent DNA in tail, tail length, tail moment and Olive tail moment increased from blood cells of animals subjected to radiation alone, implying formation of DNA strand breaks due to radiation exposure. The parameter, Olive tail moment was 4.247 ± 0.406 in mice administered with D/W and then exposed to gamma-

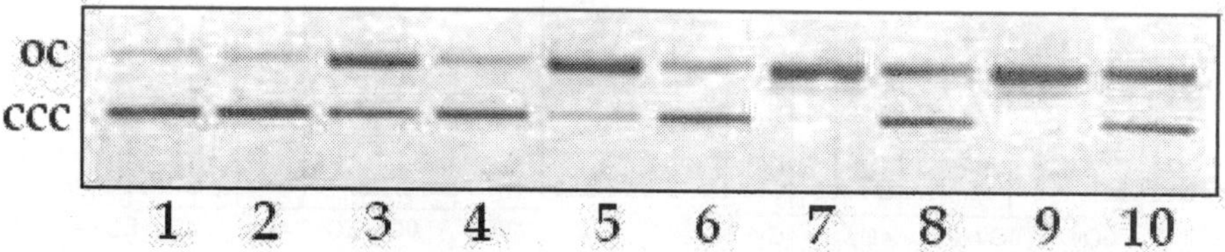

Figure 11.5: Protection of Plasmid DNA by 0.2mM EC, Against Different Doses of Gamma-radiation 0-75 Gy. Lane 1: 0 Gy, Lane 2: 0 Gy, EC, Lane 3: 10 Gy, Lane 4: 10 Gy, EC, Lane 5: 25 Gy, Lane 6: 25 Gy, EC, Lane 7: 50 Gy, Lane 8: 50 Gy, EC, Lane 9: 75 Gy, Lane 10: 75 Gy, EC

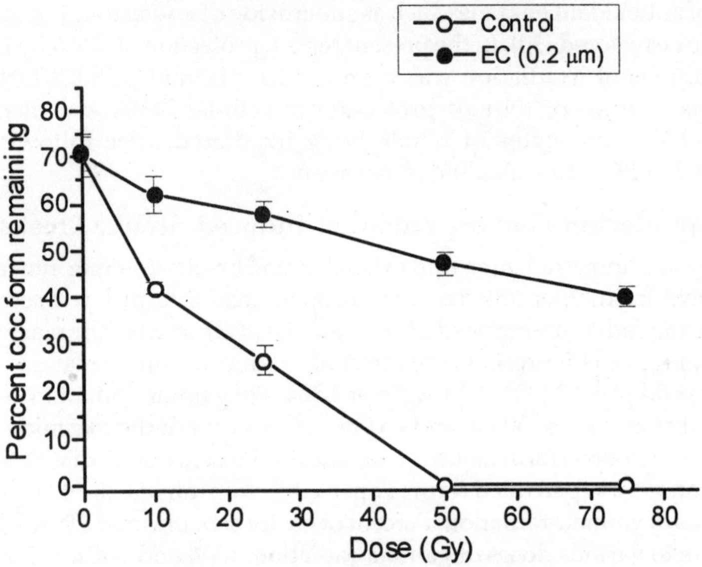

Figure 11.6: Protection of Plasmid DNA by 0.2mM EC, Against Different Doses of Gamma-radiation 0-75 Gy.
Each point represents the mean ± SEM from 3 individual experiments.

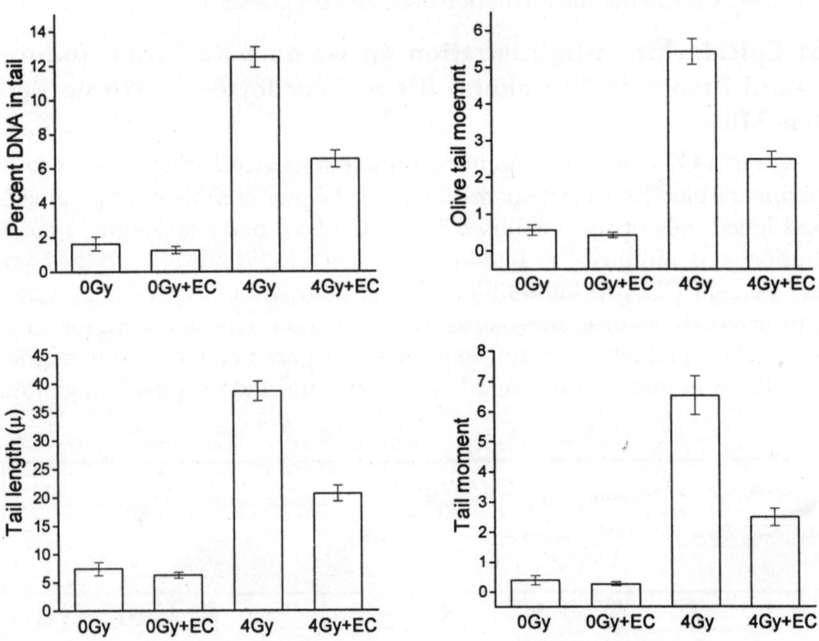

Figure 11.7: Comet Parameters Presenting the Effect of EC 40 mg/kg Body Weight Administration on Gamma-radiation-induced DNA Strand Breaks in Peripheral Blood Leucocytes of Whole Body Irradiated Mice, at 0 min Post-irradiation.
Each point represents the mean ± SEM.

radiation, and in mice administered with EC 40 mg/kg body weight it was found to be 3.042 ± 0.312 showing almost 37 per cent reduction in the formation of DNA lesions in EC administered group. This would imply that under *in vivo* condition of radiation exposure it was found that EC protected cellular DNA in peripheral blood leucocytes of mice against gamma-radiation induced strand breaks. Thus the studies indicate that EC has the capacity to protect DNA against radiation-induced damage under both, *in vitro* as well as *in vivo* conditions of gamma-irradiation. As EC is a dietary ingredient and has been used by man from time immemorial, this compound could be non toxic and safe. The present study denotes its usefulness as a radioprotector for planned radiation exposures. Studies on toxicity and pharmacokinetics and dynamics of EC are necessary before applying this drug in human subjects. Also the mechanism of radioprotection by this compound and its effect on DNA repair process are to be elucidated.

Ferulic Acid as Radioprotector

Ferulic acid (FA) is a monophenolic phenylpropanoid, Scheme IV, occurring in plant products such as rice bran, green tea and coffee beans. It has ability to act as an antioxidant against peroxyl radical induced oxidation in neuronal culture and synaptosomal membranes. It scavenges the reactive oxygen species such as hydroxyl radical.OH, hypochlorous acid HOCl and peroxyl radical RO_2 (25) and stable free radical 1,1-diphenyl-2-picrylhydrazyl (DPPH). The pulse radiolysis studies showed that the rate constant of ferulic acid for nitrogen dioxide radicals.NO_2 is 7.4×10^8 $dm^3mole^{-1}s^{-1}$ (31) and for trichloromethyl peroxyl radical Cl_3COO. is $\sim 2 \times 10^7$ dm^3 $mole^{-1}s^{-1}$ (32). It significantly reduces the NO production by lipopolysaccharide LPS-stimulated mouse macrophage like cells Raw 264.7 cells and is useful in preventing cell damage caused by O^{2-}, OH and NO in living systems (33).

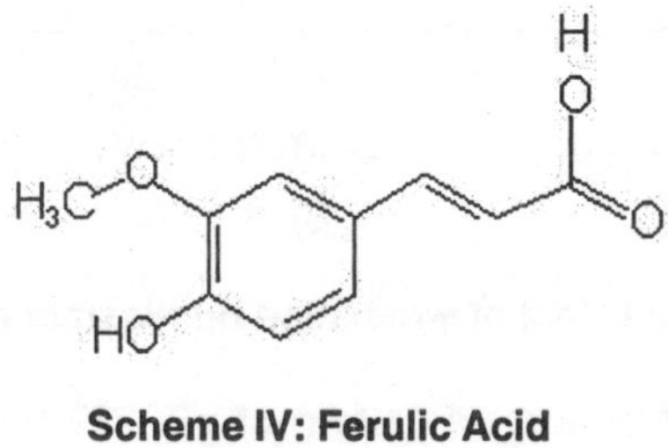

Scheme IV: Ferulic Acid

Effect of Ferulic Acid on Gamma-radiation Induced Strand Breaks in Plasmid pBR322 DNA

Figures 11.8 a and b present the data on the effect of 0.5mM ferulic acid on production of strand breaks in plasmid pBR322 DNA exposed to different doses of gamma-radiation (0-75 Gy). It can be seen from the figure that presence of 0.5 mM FA significantly inhibited the disappearance of super-coiled ccc form of plasmid pBR322, with a dose modifying factor DMF of 2.0 as can be evidenced from Figure 11.8b. This would imply that FA at 0.5mM effectively protected DNA *in vitro* against gamma-radiation induced strand breaks.

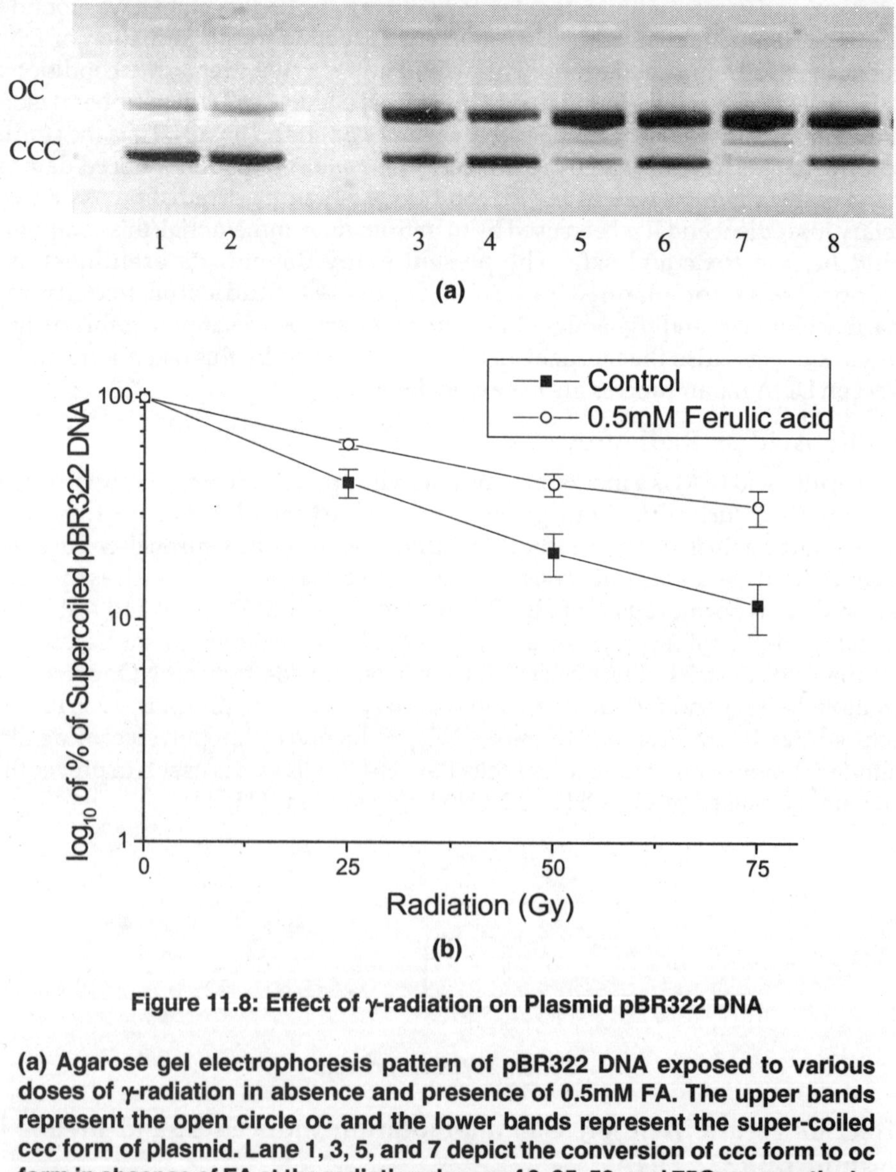

Figure 11.8: Effect of γ-radiation on Plasmid pBR322 DNA

(a) Agarose gel electrophoresis pattern of pBR322 DNA exposed to various doses of γ-radiation in absence and presence of 0.5mM FA. The upper bands represent the open circle oc and the lower bands represent the super-coiled ccc form of plasmid. Lane 1, 3, 5, and 7 depict the conversion of ccc form to oc form in absence of FA at the radiation doses of 0, 25, 50, and 75Gy respectively, where as lane 2, 4, 6, and 8 represent in presence of 0.5mM FA. (b) Presentation of log of per cent of ccc form of pBR322 DNA against various doses of γ-radiation.

Effect of FA on Gamma-radiation Induced Cellular DNA Damage in Whole Body Irradiated Mice

Whole body exposure of mice to 4 Gy gamma-radiation resulted in increase in comet parameters of peripheral blood leukocytes as can be evidenced in Figure 11.9.

Administration of FA 50 mg/ kg body weight i.p one hour prior or immediately after gamma-radiation exposure resulted in reduction of the comet parameters as can be seen in Figure 11.9.

When the animals were exposed to radiation, 4Gy, per cent DNA in tail was increased from 0.69 ± 0.08 to 2.87 ± 0.24, tail length was increased from 3.39 ± 0.09 to 8.04 ± 0.44, tail moment was increased from 0.034 ± 0.006 to 0.45 ± 0.06 and Olive tail moment was increased from 0.15 ± 0.02 to 0.84 ± 0.08 in blood leukocytes. But i.p administration of FA 1 hour prior to irradiation brought down these parameter to a level of 1.64 ± 0.14, 5.8 ± 0.27, 0.16 ± 0.02 and 0.44 ± 0.04 respectively in the irradiated group as can be seen in Figure 11.9. It was also found that administration of FA immediately after completion of irradiation also protected cellular DNA in peripheral blood and bone marrow cells of mice but the level of protection was less than the pre-administration of FA (Maurya D.K. and Nair C.K.K. unpublished results).

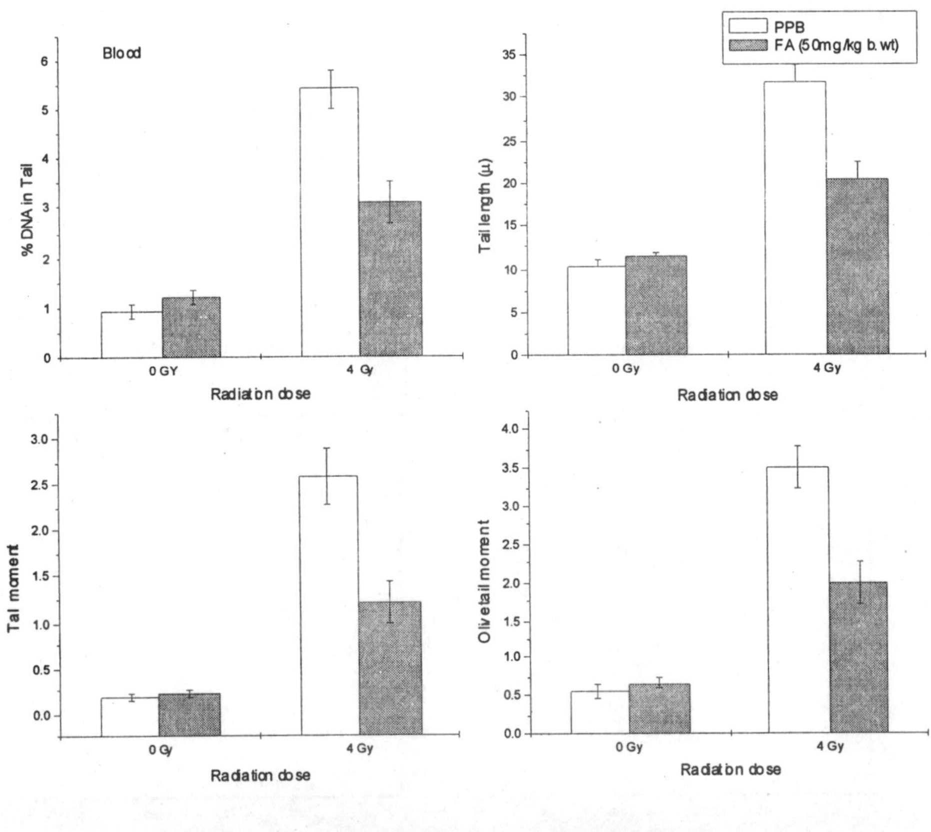

Figure 11.9: Effect of FA on DNA Damage in Murine Blood Leucocytes Assayed by Comet Assay. Mean comet parameters–per cent DNA in tail, Tail length, Tail moment and Olive tail moment of single cells of blood leukocytes subjected to alkaline single cell gel electrophoresis after administration of 50 mg/kg body weight FA immediately after radiation exposure are presented with ± SEM. N=4, ** p<0.001, * p<0.01.

Effect of FA Administration on Repair of Radiation Induced Damage to Cellular DNA of Peripheral Blood Leukocytes in Mice

The effect of FA on DNA repair was ascertained by examining the comet parameters of the peripheral blood leucocytes from whole-body irradiated mice at different post-radiation intervals after post-irradiation administration of 50 mg/kg body weight of FA. The comet assay parameters of the peripheral blood leucocytes are presented in Figure 11.10. In the FA treated animals the decrease of the comet parameters were found more than that of untreated animals. From Figure 11.10 it is clear that during initial 30 min the repair of most of DNA damages were completed. It can be understood from the figure that at 10 min post-irradiation most of the repair is completed. It can be seen that there was fast rejoining of DNA strand breaks in the first 10 min post-irradiation in mice exposed to gamma-radiation and treated with FA. Thus it is clear that the repair of DNA takes place at a faster rate in FA treated mice than in untreated ones. In irradiated group there is a peak at 20 min which is absence in the FA treated group. After 30 min the comet parameters started increasing this may be because of the commencement of excision repair process (20). This would

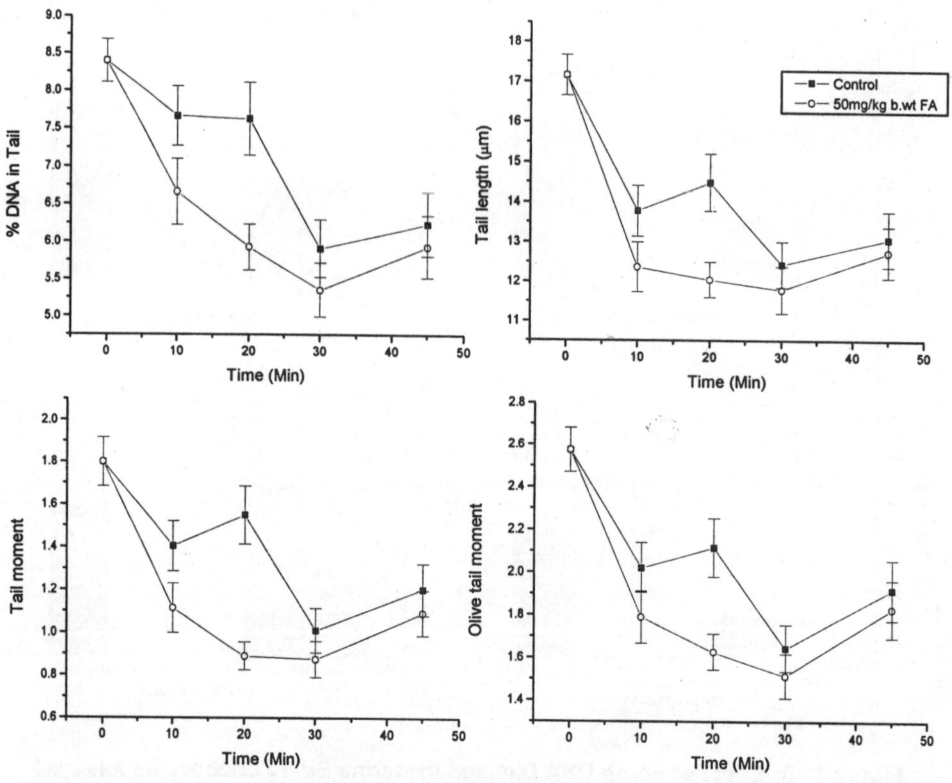

Figure 11.10: Effect of FA 50 mg/ kg Body Weight on Murine Blood Leucocytes DNA Strands Breaks at Different Time Interval After Exposure of 4Gy γ-radiation in Term of Decrease in Comet Parameters–per cent DNA in Tail, Tail Length, Tail Moment and Olive Tail Moment. N= 3

indicate that apart from offering protection to cellular DNA against radiation, FA also enhances repair of DNA in these cells.

Conclusions and Future Prospects

The effects of radiation exposure on human health have been well documented from the epidemiological studies on the survivors of the Hiroshima and Nagasaki atom bombing. There has been extensive research on radioprotective or anti-radical compounds since World War II on account of the relevance of these compounds in military, clinical and industrial application. Radiation protection is also relevant in these days as there is a global increase in attacks by terrorist groups and there is a possible threat of nuclear terrorism. Radioprotectors could reduce the cancer risk to population exposed to radiation directly or indirectly through industrial and military application. Radioprotectors are required to reduce normal tissue injury during radiotherapy of cancer. There is also a greater awareness on deleterious effects of radiation exposure due to medical X-rays and CT scans done for routine diagnostic purposes (34,35). In space travel, risk due to ionizing radiations is one of the medical adversities other than physical and mental effects of zero gravity (36). In these scenarios, the present study reveals that TMG, EC and FA have great potential to be used either alone or in combination as effective radioprotector for human application as these compounds are non toxic and some of them are constituents of human diet.

Acknowledgements

The author is thankful to Ms. Veena P.Salvi and Mr.D.K Maurya, Radiation Biology and Health Sciences Division, Bhabha Atomic Research Cenre for their participation in the experimental work and the data presented here.

References

1. Bump EA, Malaker K: Radioprotectors: chemical, biological and clinical perspective. CRC Press, Boca Raton, Fl., USA, 1998.
2. Weiss JF, Landauer MR: Protection against ionizing radiation by antioxidants and phytochemicals. *Toxicol*, 2003, 189, 1-20.
3. Nair CKK, Parida DK, Nomura T: Radioprotectors in radiotherapy. *J Radiat Res*, 2001, 42, 21-37.
4. Arora R, Gupta D, Chawla R, Sagar R, Sharma A, Kumar R, Prasad J, Singh S, Samanta N, Sharma RK: Radioprotection by plant products: present status and future prospects. *Phytother Res*, 2005, 19, 1-22.
5. Maurya DK, Devasagayam TPA, Nair CKK: Some novel approaches for radioprotection and the beneficial effects of natural products. *Ind J Experimental Biol*, 2006, 44, 93-114.
6. Maisin JR Bacq, and Alexander award lecture–chemical radioprotection: past present and future. *Int. J.Radiat.Biol.*, 1998, 73, 443-450.
7. Tannehill SP, Mehta MP: Amifostine and radiation therapy: past, present and future. Semin. *Oncol.*,1996, 23, 69-77.

8. Swallow AJ: Radiation chemistry, an introduction, Longman, London, 1996.

9. Murase H, Yamauchi R, Kato K, Kuneida T, Yoshikawa T, Terao J: Antioxidant activity of a novel vitamin E derivative, 2 (alpha-D-glucopyranosyl) methyl-2,5,7,8-tetramethylchroman-6-ol. *Free Radical Bio Med*, 1998, 24, 217-225.

10. Chow CK: Vitamin E and oxidative stress. *Free Radical Bio Med*, 1991 11, 215-32.

11. Murase H, Yamauchi R, Kato K, Kuneida T, Terao J: Synthesis of a novel vitamin E derivative, 2(alpha-D-glucopyranosyl)methyl-2,5,7,8-tetramethylchroman-6-ol by alpha-galactosidase–catalyses transglycosylation. *Lipids*, 1997, 32, 73-78.

12. Nair CKK, Umadevi P, Shimanskaya R, Kunugita N, Murase H, Gu YH, Kagiya TV: Water soluble vitamin E (TMG) as a radioprotector. *Ind J Experimental Biol*, 2003, 41, 1365-1371.

13. Rajagopalan R, Wani K, Huilgol NG, Kagiya VT, Nair CKK: Inhibition of gamma-radiation induced DNA damage in plasmid pBR $_{322}$ by TMG, a water soluble derivative of vitamin E. *J Radiat Res*, 2002, 43, 153-159.

14. Singh RK, Verma NC, Kagiya VT: Effect of water soluble derivative of alpha-tocopherol on radiation response of *Saccharomyces cerivisiae*. *Ind J Bichem Biophys*, 2001, 38, 399-405.

15. Gandhi NM, Nair CKK: Protection of DNA and membrane from gamma-radiation induced damage by gallic acid. *Molec Cell Biochem*, 2005, 278, 111-117.

16. Maurya DK, Balakrishnan S, Salvi VP, Nair CKK: Protection of cellular DNA from gamma-radiation induced damages and enhancement in DNA repair by troxerutin. *Molec Cell Biochem*, 2005, 280, 57-68.

17. Gandhi NM, Nair CKK: Radiation protection by *Terminalia chebula*: some mechanistic aspects. *Cell Biochem*, 2005, 277, 43-48.

18. Hellman B, Vaghef H, Bostrom B: The concepts of tail moment and tail inertia in single cell gel electrophoresis assay. *Mutat Res*, 1995, 336, 123-131.

19. Bowden RD, Buckwalter MR, McBride JF, Johnson DA, Murray BK, O'Neil KL: Tail profile: a more accurate system for analyzing DNA damage using comet assay, *Mutat Res*, 2003, 537, 1-9.

20. Mendiola-Cruz MT, Morales –Ramirez P: Repair kinetics of gamma-ray induced DNA damage determined by single cell gel electrophoresis assay in murine leukocytes in vivo. *Mutat Res*, 1999, 433, 45-52.

21. Natsume M, Osakabe N, Oyama M, Sasaki M, Baba S, Nakamura Y, Osawa T, Terao J: Structures of epicatechin glucuronide identified from plasma and urine after oral ingestion of epicatechin: differences between human and rat. *Free Radical Biol Med*, 2003, 34, 840-849.

22. Geetha T, Garg A, Chopra K, Kaur IP: Delineation of antimutgenic activity of catechin, epicatechin and green tea extract. *Muta Res*, 2004, 556, 65-74.

23. Edwards-Jones V, Buck R, Shawcross SG, Dawson MM, Dunn K: The effect of essential oils on methicillin resistant *Staphylococcus aureus* using a dressing model. *Burns*, 2004, 30, 772-774.

24. Yamaguchi K, Honda M, Ikigai H, Hara Y, Shimamura T: Inhibitory effects of epigallocatechin gallate on the life cycle of human immunodeficiency virus type I (HIV-I). *Antiviral Res,* 2002, 53-1, 19-34.

25. Scott BC, Butler J, Halliwell D, Aruoma OI: Evaluation of the antioxidant action of ferulic acid and catechins. *Free Radical Res Commun,* 1993, 19, 241-253.

26. Choi YB, Kim YI, Lee KS, Kim BS, Kim DJ: Protective effect of epigallocatechin gallate on brain damage after transient middle cerebral artery occlusion in rats. *Brain Res,* 2004, 1019, 47-54.

27. Zhu A, Wang H, Guo Z: Study of tea polyphenol as a reversal agent for carcinoma cell lines' multidrug resistance (study of TP as a MDR reversal agent). *Nucl Med Biol,* 2001, 26, 735-740.

28. Nakagawa T, Yokozawa T: Direct scavenging of nitric oxide and superoxide by green tea. *Food Chem Toxicol,* 2002, 40, 1745-1750.

29. Terao J, Piskulaand M, Yao Q: Protective effect of epicatechin, epicatechin gallate and quercetin on lipid peroxidation in phospholipids bilayers. *Archives Biochem Biophys,* 1994, 308, 278-284.

30. Valls-Bellés V, Gonzalez P, Muniz P: Epicatechin effect on oxidative damage induced by tert-BOOH in isolated hepatocytes of fasted rats. *Process Biochem,* 2004, 39, 1525-1531.

31. Zhouen Z, Side Y, Weizhen L, Wenfeng W, Yizun J, Nianyun L: Mechanism of reaction nitrogen dioxide radical with hydrocinnamic acid derivatives: a pulse radiolysis study. Free *Radical Res,* 1998, 29, 13-16.

32. Pan JX, Wang WF, Lin WZ, Lu CY, Han ZH, Yao SD, Lin NY: Interaction of hydroxyl cinnamic acid derivatives with the Cl_3COO radical: a pulse radiolysis study. *Free Radical Res,* 1990, 30, 241-245.

33. Ogiwara T, Satoh K, Kadoma Y, Murakami Y, Unten S, Atsumi T, Sakagami H, Fugisawa S: Radical scavenging activity and cytotoxicity of ferulic acid. *Anticancer Res,* 2002, 22, 2711-2717.

34. De Gonzalez AB, Darby S: Risk of cancer from diagnostic X-rays: estimates for UK and 14 other countries. *Lancet,* 2004, 363, 345-351.

35. Brenner DJ, Ellision CD: Estimated radiation risks potentially associated with full body CT scanning. *Radiology,* 2004, 232, 735-738.

36. Simonsen LC, Wilson JW, Kim MH, Cucinotta FA: Radiation exposure for human Mars exploration. *Health Phys,* 2000, 79, 515-525.

Chapter 12

Resveratrol Miracle: From Chemoprevention to Cardioprotection

Samarjit Das and Dipak K. Das*

Cardiovascular Research Center, University of Connecticut School of Medicine, Farmington, Connecticut, 6030 1110, USA

E-mail: ddas@neuron.uchc.edu

ABSTRACT

A mild-to-moderate wine drinking habit attenuates cardiovascular, cerebrovascular and peripheral vascular risk due to reduced platelet and monocyte adhesion, and attenuates the risk of prostate as well as a variety of cancers including pancreatic, gastric and thyroid cancer. Although epidemiological evidence strongly supports a beneficial role for wine, the experimental basis for these beneficial actions is not fully understood. Since all wines contain varying amounts of alcohol and more importantly, polyphenolic antioxidants, it seems that the protective effects of wine are due to both these constituents. Among approximately 500 different antioxidants, recent studies revealed that resveratrol and proanthocyanidins are the two most important polyphenolic antioxidants present in wine that attenuate various health problems. Resveratrol is mainly found in the grape seeds and skins while proanthocyanidins are found in seeds only; both are mainly found in red wine. Resveratrol, a polyphenol phytoalexin, possesses diverse biochemical and physiological properties including estrogenic, antiplatelet and anti-inflammatory actions. Several recent studies revealed resveratrol mediated protections from a wide variety of degenerative diseases. Cancer and Heart problem are the two major causes of death throughout the world. Resveratrol promises to be a better alternative against both the diseases. The most important point about resveratrol is that at a lower concentration, it inhibits apoptotic cell death, thereby providing protection from various diseases including myocardial ischemic reperfusion injury, artherosclerosis and ventricular arrhythmias. Both in acute and in chronic models, resveratrol-mediated cardioprotection is achieved through the preconditioning effect (the state-of-the-art technique of cardioprotection), rather than direct effect as found in conventional medicine. The same resveratrol when used in higher doses facilitates apoptotic cell death and also behaves as a chemo-preventive alternative. Resveratrol likely fulfills the definition of a pharmacological preconditioning compound and gives hope for the therapeutic promise of alternative medicine. The purpose of this review is to provide evidence in favor of resveratrol to be used as a preventive medicine for the maintenance of healthy lifestyle.

Keywords: *Alcohol, Polyphenolics, Resveratrol, Proanthocyanidins, Red wine, Antioxidant.*

Introduction

The beneficial effects of wine can be traced back to the dawn of human civilization. It is a global socio-religious symbol associated with a multitude of therapeutic benefits including medicinal as well as magical powers. The current popular propositions about the benefits of 'moderate wine drinking,' in fact, date back through history and were first proposed by the father of medicine, Hippocrates of Kos in Greece. The first scientific evidence, however, for the cardiovascular benefits of red wine was put forward by Renaud and associates in 1992. In this study, popularly known as 'French Paradox', the researchers found that there had been a low mortality rate from, and incidence of, coronary heart disease among the French men aged above 40 years compared to men in the UK and USA, despite their high consumption of saturated fats and the prevalence of other risk factors such as smoking (45). This was attributed to their so-called 'Mediterranean diet', which includes a moderate intake of wine. In 1997, a Dutch epidemiological study (23) showed that coronary heart disease in elderly males was inversely proportional to their intake of flavonoid polyphenolics.

Alcohol and polyphenolic antioxidants are the two components of wine attributed for the protective action and it seems that such protection may come from both these constituents. There is evidence from different research groups showing that oxidative stress disturbs the normal balance between the pro-oxidants (oxygen free radicals) and antioxidants either by increasing the formation of free radicals or by decreasing the amount of antioxidants in the cells and tissues. This oxidative stress plays a major role in the various diseases of the human body. Several studies highlight the role of free radicals in various diseases (8, 30). These studies indicate that the antioxidant reserve and antioxidant enzymes are significantly reduced during ischemia reperfusion injury or other injury caused by the free radicals. During ischemia and/or reperfusion injury, there is a loss of antioxidant enzymes and antioxidants, and thus the overall antioxidant reserve of the tissue is reduced. That is the reason why the antioxidant part of red wine gets more attention than the alcoholic part.

There are numerous polyphenolic antioxidants present in wine among which 3,4',5-trihydroxy-*trans*-stilbene (resveratrol) and the proanthocyanidins are believed to be the major compounds responsible for the protective effects of wine against various diseases. Recent studies revealed that resveratrol, a phenolic phytoalexin, present in grape skins and seeds is the most important wine-derived compound, exerting a wide range of health benefits, as shown in Figure 12.1.

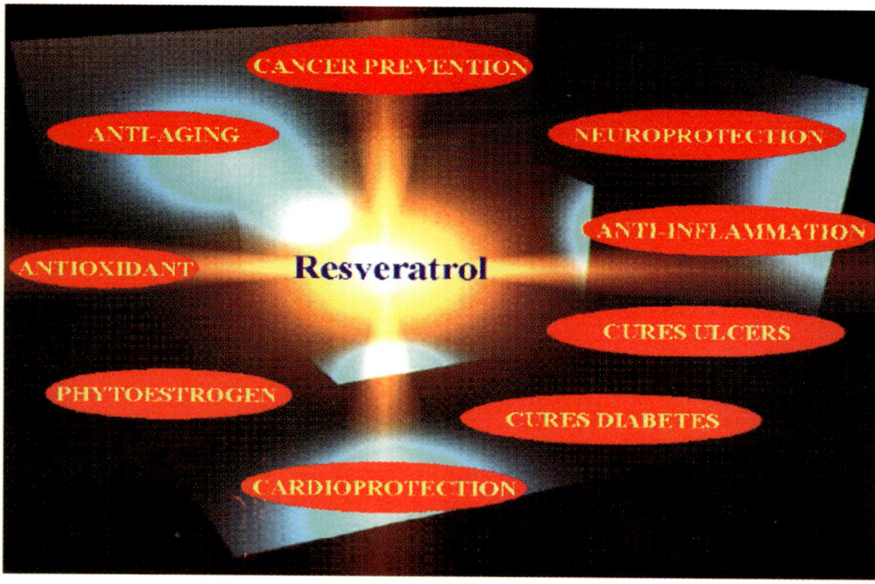

Figure 12.1: Health Benefits of Resveratrol.
Resveratrol has been implicated as a therapeutic in a number of major diseases.

Sources of Resveratrol

Resveratrol belongs to the stilbene class of compounds, which can modulate its production in grapes by protecting them from external stimuli such as fungal attack and UV-radiation. These external stimuli activate the stilbene synthase (STS) genes in the grapes to produce resveratrol in order to adequately protect the grapes from those stimuli (39). This STS gene is also found in peanut root, strawberry, blue berry, mulberry, grapes etc and other plants like eucalyptus, spruce, and lily. *Vitis vinifera*, labrusca, and muscadine types of grapes contain maximum concentration of resveratrol. The skins and seeds of these types of grapes contain 50–100 µg/gm of resveratrol. These varieties of grapes are particularly suitable for making red wine. Thus, grapes and red wines are considered as the major sources of resveratrol. In addition to grapes, a large variety of fruits including mulberry, bilberry, lingonberry, sparkle-berry, deerberry, partridgeberry, cranberry, blueberry and jackfruit, peanut, and a wide variety of flowers and leaves including gnetum, white hellebore, corn lily, butterfly orchid tree, eucalyptus, spruce, poaceae, scots pine and rheum also contain resveratrol

Resveratrol: A Polyphenolic Antioxidant

Resveratrol is capable of scavenging several intracellular reactive oxygen species (ROS). Although it possesses antioxidant properties, reseveratrol does not function as a strong antioxidant in vitro (61). Resveratrol can scavenge hydroxyl radicals with a reaction rate constant of $9.45 \times 10^{8} M^{-1} sec^{-1}$, which is much slower than the potent scavenging demonstrated by ascorbic acid (58). Depending on the biological system, resveratrol can also scavenge the superoxide anion (O_2^-) (46, 47, 58).

Although resveratrol behaves as a poor in vitro scavenger of ROS, it functions as a potent antioxidant in vivo. The in vivo antioxidant property of resveratrol probably arises from its ability to increase nitric oxide (NO) synthesis, which in turn functions as an in vivo antioxidant, scavenging superoxide radicals. In the ischemic reperfused heart, brain or kidney, resveratrol induces NO synthesis and lowers oxidative stress (20, 22). Having an unpaired electron, NO behaves as a potent antioxidant in vivo, rapidly reacting near the diffusion-limited rate ($6.7 \times 10^9 M^{-1}sec^{-1}$) with O_2 that is presumably formed in the ischemic reperfused myocardium. The affinity of NO for O_2^- is far greater than the affinity of superoxide dismutase (SOD) for O_2^-. In fact, NO may compete with SOD for O_2^-, thereby removing O_2^- and sparing SOD for other scavenging duties. The effects of resveratrol have been tested in specific cell lines and differentiated cell types. For example, resveratrol inhibits 12-*o*-tetradecanoylphorbol-13-acetate (TPA)-induced free radical formation in cultured HL-60 cells (33). In DU 145 cells–a prostate cancer cell line–administration of resveratrol inhibited proliferation that had been accompanied by a reduction in NO production and inhibition of inducible nitric oxide synthase (iNOS) (61). Resveratrol also inhibited the formation of O_2^- and H_2O_2 produced by macrophages stimulated by lipopolysaccharide (LPS) or TPA (54). In a related study, resveratrol inhibited reactive oxygen intermediates and lipid peroxidation induced by tumor necrosis factor (TNF) in a wide variety of cells (61). Resveratrol also scavenges peroxyl and hydroxyl radicals in the postischemic reperfused myocardium, thereby lowering malonaldehyde formation, a presumptive marker of lipid peroxidation (44, 54).

Resveratrol can maintain the concentrations of intracellular antioxidants found in biological systems. For example, resveratrol maintained glutathione (GSH) amounts in oxidation-stressed peripheral blood mononuclear cells isolated from healthy humans (1). In another study, resveratrol increased GSH amounts in human lymphocytes that were activated by hydrogen peroxide (5). Similarly, resveratrol restored glutathione reductase in cells subjected to TPA-mediated oxidative stress (63). In human lymphocytes, resveratrol increased the amounts of several antioxidant enzymes, including glutathione peroxidase, glutathione-*S*-transferase and glutathione reductase (57).

Resveratrol: A Phytoestrogen

Resveratrol has been recognized as a phytoestrogen based on its structural similarities to diethylstilbesterol (DES). Resveratrol can bind to the estrogen receptor (ER), thereby activating transcription of estrogen-responsive reporter genes transfected into cells (24, 60, 62, 63). Resveratrol functions as a superagonist when combined with estradiol (E2) to induce the expression of estrogen-regulated genes (24); however, several other studies showed conflicting results. Using the same cell line, Ashby *et al.*, showed that resveratrol possessed antiestrogen activity, because it suppressed progesterone receptor expression induced by E2 (3). Another recent study showed that both isomers of resveratrol possessed superestrogenic activity only at moderate concentration (>10 ìM), whereas at lower concentrations (<1 ìM), antiestrogenic effects prevailed (51).

Most of the *in vivo* studies have failed to confirm the estrogenic potential of resveratrol. At physiologic concentrations, resveratrol does not appear to induce any changes in uterine weight, uterine epithelial cell height, or serum cholesterol (64). Only at very high concentrations does resveratrol interfere with the serum cholesterol-lowering activity of E2. Elsewhere, resveratrol given orally or subcutaneously did not affect uterus weight at any concentration (0.03 to 120 mg/kg/day) (3). In a related study, resveratrol reduced uterine weight and decreased the expression of ER-α mRNA and protein and progesterone receptor (PR) mRNA (64).

In contrast, resveratrol possesses estrogenic properties in stroke-prone spontaneously hypertensive rats (65). When ovariectomized rats were fed resveratrol at the concentration of 5 mg/kg/day, it attenuated an increase in systolic blood pressure. In concert, resveratrol enhanced endothelin-dependent vascular relaxation in response to acetylcholine and in a manner similar to estradiol, prevented ovariectomy-induced decreases in femoral bone strength. Resveratrol also acts as an estrogen receptor (ER) agonist in breast cancer cells stably transfected with ERα (66). Although more data accumulate on the estrogenic behavior of resveratrol, the controversy continues to persist.

Resveratrol in Cancer Prevention

Carcinogenesis is a multi-step process involving (*i*) initiation, a mutation, (*ii*) promotion, selective outgrowth of the mutated cell and subsequent mutation in a sub-population and (*iii*) progression, a few more cycles of mutations to an established neoplastic phenotype. There are many cellular processes involved to predispose cells for these changes or prevent the acquisition of the abnormal phenotype directly or indirectly regulating the process of carcinogenesis. These cellular processes regulate intracellular redox status, cell-cycle checkpoint genes, transcription factors, and cell survival and apoptosis pathways. Each of these factors or pathways therein provides logical targets for drug design or for evaluating the effect of a candidate compound on the process as a whole. Therefore, by implication, an effect on these critical mediators of cellular transformation could provide insight into the ability of a given compound to favorably or adversely affect the process of carcinogenesis.

Jang *et al.* (29) evidenced in their research that resveratrol was able to manifest anti-mutagenic activity in a bacterial mutagenesis model and was capable of inducing the Phase II enzyme, quinine reductase, to potentiate carcinogen detoxification metabolism in hepatoma cells and curb the initiation stage of carcinogenesis. Regarding the initiation of antagonism, a recent study has shown that resveratrol encumbers carcinogen activation using at least two mechanisms. In the first mechanism, resveratrol hinders induction of the carcinogen triggered cytochrome P-450 1A1 (CYP1A1) by meddling with the binding of the aryl hydrocarbon receptor (AHR) to the promoter of the CPY1A1 gene, and in the second mechanism, resveratrol directly inhibits the enzymatic activity of CYP1A1 (6, 55).

In cultured human prostate cancer cells, resveratrol treatment provoked differential inhibitory responses among protein kinase D (PKD) and various protein kinase C (PKC) isozymes. Resveratrol is known to possess anti-inflammatory properties, but anti-inflammatory vehicles are seen as a valuable chemopreventive modality against this phase of carcinogenesis (28, 55). Cyclooxygenase (COX) enzymes are possibly central targets to the cancer preventative activity of resveratrol because prostaglandins both suppress immune surveillance and stimulate cell growth (55, 56). Resveratrol also holds the potential, through its effects on the androgen receptor (AR), to forage incipient populations of androgen-dependent prostate cancer cells (26, 55).

Associated with cell-growth suppression and induction of apoptosis, Mitchell *et al.* (1999) showed that in the androgen-dependent human prostate cancer cell line LNCaP, the AR-specific co-activator ARA70 and other various AR-regulated genes, resveratrol has key antiandrogenic effects (38). The potential value of resveratrol lies in the evidence that it may have cancer preventative properties through its ability to scavenge androgen-dependent prostate cancer cells, and its ability to be used as an adjuvant therapeutic for hormone-dependent prostate cancer. There is undeniable evidence that resveratrol impedes the final phase of multi-stage carcinogenesis as well as further amplification of the malignant cancer phenotype. It has been shown that resveratrol suppressed Lewis lung carcinoma tumor cell growth and tumor angiogenesis and metastasis to the lung (32, 55). Resveratrol has the capacity to arrest cell growth at the G_1 phase, and also has the ability to endue apoptotic responses in tumor cells through P-53 dependent pathway, that is BCl-2 sensitive, reactive oxygen species (ROS) dependent and mitochondrial dependant (2, 27, 40, 59).

Anti-inflammatory Response of Resveratrol

Polyphenols, specifically resveratrol and quercetin, possess antiaggregability activity in human platelets (42). It has also been shown that aggregation in response to ADP and thrombin in human platelets is strongly inhibited by red wine (43). Quercetin has been demonstrated to decrease platelet activity by reducing platelet cytosolic calcium as a consequence of increased cGMP phosphodiesterase activity (42). In a human study, the subjects who had 375 mL/day of red wine for 2-4 weeks had decreased ADP-induced platelet aggregation (52). Red wine, administered intravenously or intragastrically at doses of 1.6 and 4.0 mL/kg in the stenos canine coronary arteries, reduced the cyclic blood flow caused by periodic formation of acute platelet mediated thrombi (13). The same effects were observed when high quantities of grape juice was given, unlike white wine, thus suggesting a role for red wine polyphenols in this attenuation of platelet aggregation (13). In a related study, resveratrol, through a nitric oxide (NO) producing mechanism, blocked pro-adhesive molecules such as I-CAM, V-CAM and e-SELECTIN generated in the myocardium during ischemia-reperfusion phase (10). This study provides further positive evidence of the anti-inflammatory effect of red wine.

Resveratrol in Neuroprotection

One of the common causes of death and disability at an early age (<45 years) in almost all industrialized countries is traumatic brain injury. That is why researchers are more and more attracted to do research on neuroprotection and coming up with new strategies as well as some new neuroprotective compounds. Despite the fact that the mechanism of action of a particular compound becomes known, it fails the clinical trials for brain, as that particular compound can not cross the blood-brain barrier.

The first evidence of resveratrol being able to cross blood-brain barrier was published a little over a decade ago by Virgil *et al.* (19). In the same study Virgil *et al.*, showed that in young adult rats the chronic administration of resveratrol protects the damage caused by the systemic injection of the excitotoxin kainic acid, in the olfactory cortex and the hippocampus (19). They also concluded that resveratrol needs more attention to get a pharmacological tool in neuroprotection as the same treatment, which worked in-vivo, is not significantly protective in ex-vivo model. In contrast, some of the recent studies found that resveratrol could effectively protect the brain from traumatic brain injury (48) and also significantly inhibit the excitatory synaptic transmission in rat hippocampus (49). In another related study Raval *et al.*, showed resveratrol to be able to precondition and protect from cerebral ischemic injury (53). In this *in-vitro* model, Raval *et al.*, also found that such neuroprotective effect of resveratrol was mediated by SIRT1 (53). A similar study showed the neuroprotective effect of resveratrol by inhibiting the voltage-activated potassium currents in hippocampal neurons (4). Kiziltepe *et al.* (67) showed resveratrol-mediated protection of spinal cord from ischemia-reperfusion injury. In a rabbit model, they concluded the antioxidative effect and NO stimulating effect of resveratrol played a major role in this spinal cord protection. In an *in-vitro* study, Zamin *et al.*, showed the involvement of PI-3-Kinase pathways in resveratrol protection against oxygen free radicals during glucose deprivation in organotypic hippocampal (68). The most recent advance technology in bio-medical science, proteomic profiling, well established the fact that resveratrol can act as one of the important psychoactive compounds (69). In this proteomic study Kim *et al.*, discovered a wide variety of protein profiles which may actively involve in neuroprotection and now it is the time to discover further the mechanistic pathways of action involved with those newly found proteins or genes, which are activated during resveratrol mediated neuroprotection.

Resveratrol in Gastric and Peptic Ulcer

Dr. Barry J. Marshall and Dr. J. Robin Warren were awarded jointly The Nobel Prize in Physiology or Medicine for 2005 for their discovery of "the bacterium *Helicobacter pylori* (*H. pylori*) and its role in gastritis and peptic ulcer disease". In 1982, when this bacterium was discovered by Marshall and Warren, stress and lifestyle were considered to be the major causes of peptic ulcer disease by rupturing the mucus membrane of the stomach.

In an *in vitro* study, Marimon *et al.* (1998) showed that wine could effectively reduce the growth of *H. pylori* propagation (37). A few other studies showed that red wine is more effective over white wine to inhibit the growth of *H. pylori* (7, 36). Mahady *et al.* (2003) showed in their study, resveratrol is the active component which causes the inhibitory effect on 15 different strains of *H. pylori* (36). This observation is also confirmed by another *in vitro* study (35) by the same group of researchers.

Resveratrol–*In vino* Vitalis

In many eukaryotic cells such as rodents, flies and nematode worms and even single-celled organisms such as baker's yeast, only SIR2 among many longevity regulatory genes has received significant attention from researchers (21). In human cells, the analogus gene of SIR2 is SIRT1, which can extend lifespan (25). In a recent study, Howitz *et al.* (2003) showed red wine derived resveratrol could increase the SIRT1 activity 13 fold by inhibiting apoptotic cell death through the deacetylation of p53 (25). In the same study they also showed that resveratrol extended the lifespan by 70 per cent by minimizing calorie restriction by stimulating SIR2 in the yeast cells and, thus, increased DNA stability. In another very recent study on calorie restriction experiments on monkey and other mammalian species, the conception of wine as 'fountain of youth' was re-confirmed (34).

Resveratrol in Cardioprotection

Since cardiovascular disease contributes in a major way to the morbidity and mortality, it is becoming a strain on the economy of many countries worldwide. Wine polyphenols can reduce LDL sensitivity to lipid peroxidation. In an epidemiological study (14), when subjects consumed 375 mL/day of red wine for 2 weeks, lipid peroxides decreased by 40 per cent. This study also suggested a pro-oxidant effect of white wine because there was a 21 per cent to 28 per cent increase in thiobarbituric acid reactive substances in the subjects who consumed white wine. Fermenting white wine along with the grape pulp and solids increased its ability to scavenge free radicals and inhibit LDL's copper ion-induced oxidation. Oxidation properties of the wine were inhibited by up to 87 per cent when the grape juice was allowed to ferment for an additional 18 hours resulting in a wine with 18 per cent alcohol. The increased inhibition is due to the increased polyphenolic content and is similar to the 94 per cent inhibition seen with red wines (16). In another study, the LDL oxidation property of wine mainly came from the polyphenolic components, as an alcohol-free powder of red wine phenolic extract was shown to have similar effects to red wine on LDL (41). Wine-derived polyphenols have been found to strongly inhibit this oxidation induced by copper than that induced by aqueous peroxyl radicals (1). Polyphenols have also been found to reduce macrophage oxidative stress through the inhibition of NADPH oxidase, 15-lipoxygenase, cytochrome p450 and myeloperoxidase (14). Red wine polyphenols are absorbed efficiently in human subjects and bind to LDL, thus protecting it from oxidation (14, 15, 41).

Generally, in wine the concentration of polyphenolic compounds is about 1,8003,000 mg/L (18). Numerous studies have established resveratrol as the most cardioprotective compound among all the polyphenols present in wine (Figure 12.2). Several experimental studies have demonstrated the cardioprotective effect of resveratrol from ischemia/reperfusion injury (11, 12, 44). Initially, the researchers found the NO-dependent mechanism of resveratrol induced preconditioning effect (9, 22). A recent study (9) has suggested that a coordinated up-regulation of iNOS–VEGF–KDR–eNOS, to be one of the resveratrol preconditioning mechanisms. Adenosine receptors are also involved in the pharmacologically preconditioning effect of resveratrol (11). It has been suggested that adenosine A_1, A_3, A_{2a} or A_{2b} receptors,

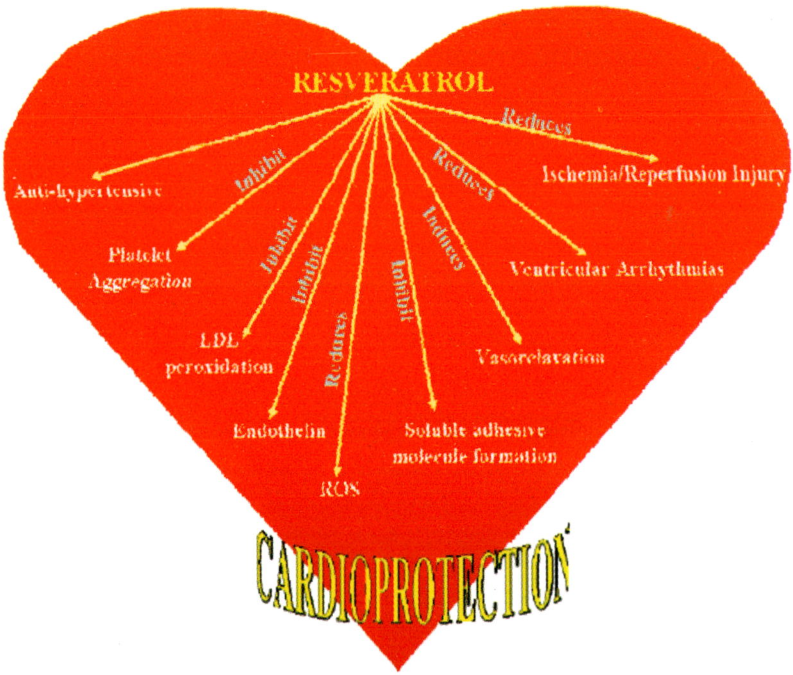

Figure 12.2: Cardioprotection with Resveratrol
The major contribution to health from resveratrol appears to be directed toward limiting progression of heart disease.

play a critical role in the pharmacological preconditioning by resveratrol. Resveratrol likely activates both adenosine A_1 and A_3 receptors that phosphorylate PI-3 Kinase, which then phosphorylates protein kinase B (Akt) and thus preconditions the heart by producing NO as well as by the activation of antioxidant BCl-2. Das *et al.* (12) showed that the activation of adenosine A_3 receptors could also precondition the heart by survival signal through the cAMP response element-binding protein (CREB) phosphorylation via PI-3 Kinase–Akt and via MEK (Mitogen-activated extracellular signal-regulated protein kinase)–CREB pathways. In another recent study, the activation of HO-1 and Trx-1 has been considered as an important cardioprotective factor of resveratrol-induced pharmacological preconditioning through the activation of VEGF under the angiogenesis point of view apart from the NO-dependent signaling mechanism (31). In this study, MAPK's signaling was found to be the only mechanistic pathway shown for the induction of HO-1 by the resveratrol-mediated cardioprotection. Resveratrol attenuates various soluble intercellular cytokines like I-CAM, V-CAM and e-Selectin through improvement in the endothelium function which reduces the infarct size of the ischemic myocardium (10). Apart from the REDOX signaling mechanism, resveratrol also protects the heart as a potent antioxidant by scavenging free radicals and inhibiting lipid peroxidation both *in vitro* and *in vivo* (50). Thus, resveratrol inhibits apoptotic cell death as well as release and/or generate inflammatory mediators.

For further exploring the molecular mechanisms of resveratrol mediated cardioprotection, Bezstarosti *et al.*, used the most promising bio-informatical technique, proteomic, and discovered a challenging list of proteins and genes profile (70). Some of these profile listed protein is already known to be cardioprotective and many of the proteins and genes will help the future cardiovascular researchers to find a link to make a concrete pathway for cardioprotective effect of resveratrol. In this study (70), Bezstarosti *et al.*, showed the listed proteins and genes are involved the cardioprotective effect of resveratrol from ischemia-reperfusion injury, but in the long run this list of protein will help us to find resveratrol as a therapeutic alternative against many cardiovascular diseases.

Resveratrol and Diabetes

Diabetes, a well known cardiovascular risk factor, is a disease when islets of Langerhans cells in the pancreas does not or poorly produce insulin or the body is not properly using the insulin present in the system. Insulin is the hormone which mobilizes sugar and starches to the blood stream to be converted into energy needed for the body for daily activity. What is the cause of diabetes is still a mystery to the research world. Although both genetics and environmental factors like obesity, food habit or lack of exercise in daily routine appear to play an important role, the underlying mechanism is still not very clear to the scientists.

According to the latest report of American Diabetes Association in 2006, there are at least 20.8 million children and adults in the United States, or 7 per cent of the population, who have diabetes. While an estimated 14.6 million have been diagnosed with diabetes, unfortunately, 6.2 million people (or nearly one-third) are unaware that they have the disease. That's why diabetes is also known as "Silent Killer". The rapid increase in the number of Silent Killer in the society catch the attention of the research world and recently almost double of the population are working in this area compared to the last decade.

A little over a year ago, a scientist from California, USA, hypothesized based on the evidences that IKK-β, a crucial catalyst of NFêB activation, is an obligate mediator of the disruption of insulin signaling induced by excessive exposure of tissues to free fatty acids, the inhibitors of IKK-β may have some important role against the type 2 diabetes. Indeed, resveratrol, a well known IKK-β inhibitor, reverses fat-induced insulin resistance (71). This observation provides more enthusiasm to the researchers to use resveratrol as an anti-diabetic agent. As an out come of this, the year 2006 brings quite a number of publications which short of pointed resveratrol possesses an insulin-like effect and can be used for the protection against diabetes. In a very recent study, Su *et al.*, showed that resveratrol significantly reduced the plasma glucose concentration as well as the dramatic reduction of triglyceride concentration in streptozotocin (STZ) induced diabetic mellitus rats in 14 days treatment (72). They concluded from this observation that resveratrol possesses hypoglycemic and hypolipidemic property. Baur *et al.*, add more value to this conclusion. As a part of an outstanding study, Baur *et al.*, showed that resveratrol increases insulin sensitivity by lowering the blood glucose level in a group of high calorie diet mice and they have pointed out reduced insulin-like growth factor-1 (IGF-I) levels and increased AMP-activated protein kinase (AMPK) probably playing a major role in it (73).

Some other related studies established that resveratrol can attenuate diabetic nephropathy in rats (74) and reduce thermal hyperalgesia and cold allodynia in streptozotocin-induced diabetic rats (75). This is just the beginning and there is lot to go with this Magic compound to reduce the number of Silent Killer from our society.

Summary and Conclusions

It is becoming increasingly clear that resveratrol has two faces. On one hand, it protects cells by potentiating a survival signal. On the other hand, it selectively kills cancer cells. It behaves as an antioxidant, yet it can induce redox signaling. It is an antiproliferative agent for cancer; it induces apoptosis in tumor cells and sensitizes cancer cells by inhibiting cell survival signal transduction and antiapoptotic pathways. In contrast, the same compound triggers a survival signal in the ischemic tissue by inducing antiapoptotic genes and blocks apoptosis in ischemic heart. At low doses, resveratrol stimulates angiogenesis, but at higher doses, it blocks angiogenic response. At low concentrations, resveratrol scavenges ROS, but at higher concentrations, it behaves like a prooxidant.

Probably this dual property of resveratrol gives a wide range of protection. There are very few compounds, both natural as well as synthetic, available which can provide protective journey from cancer to cardiovascular diseases like resveratrol does. Of course that's one of the major reasons of growing interest in the research world with resveratrol. More and more encouraging results establish resveratrol as a therapeutic alternative for the treatment of various diseases.

References

1. Losa GA: Resveratrol modulates apoptosis and oxidation in human blood mononuclear cells. *Eur J Clin Invest* 2003, 33, 818–823.
2. Ahmad N, Adhami VM, Afaq F, Feyes DK, Mukhtar H: Resveratrol causes WAF-1/p21-mediated G(1)-phase arrest of cell cycle and induction of apoptosis in human epidermoid carcinoma A431 cells. *Clin Cancer Res* 2001, 7, 1466-1473.
3. Ashby J, Tinwell H, Pennie W, Brooks AN, Lefevre PA, Beresford N, Sumpter JP: Partial and weak oestrogenicity of the red wine constituent resveratrol: Consideration of its superagonist activity in MCF-7 cells and its suggested cardiovascular protective effects. *J Appl Toxicol* 1999, 19, 39-45.
4. Gao ZB, Hu GY: Trans-resveratrol, a red wine ingredient, inhibits voltage-activated potassium currents in rat hippocampal neurons. *Brain Res* 2005, 1056, 68-75.
5. Olas B, Wachowicz B, Bald E, Glowacki R: The protective effects of resveratrol against changes in blood platelet thiols induced by platinum compounds. *J Physiol Pharmacol* 2004, 55, 467-476.
6. Ciolino HP, Yeh: Inhibition of aryl hydrocarbon-induced cytochrome P-450 1A1 enzyme activity and CYP1A1 expression by resveratrol. *Mol Pharmacol* **1999, 56,** 760-767.

7. Daroch F, Hoeneisen M, Gonzalez CL, Kawaguchi F, Salgado F, Solar H, Garcia A: In vitro antibacterial activity of Chilean red wines against *Helicobacter pylori*. *Microbios* 2001, 104, 79-85.

8. Das DK, Maulik N: Protection against free radical injury in the heart and cardiac performance. In: Sen CK, Packer L, Hanninen O (Eds.). *"Exercise and Oxygen Toxicity"*. Elsevier Science, Amsterdam, 1995, 359.

9. Das S, Alagappan VK, Bagchi D, Sharma HS, Maulik N, Das DK: Coordinated induction of iNOS-VEGF-KDR-eNOS after resveratrol consumption: a potential mechanism for resveratrol preconditioning of the heart. *Vascul Pharmacol* 2005, 42, 281-289.

10. Das S, Bertelli AA, Bertelli A, Maulik N, Das DK: Antiinflammatory action of resveratrol: a novel mechanism of action. *Drugs Exp Clin Res* (in press).

11. Das S, Cordis GA, Maulik N, Das DK: Pharmacological preconditioning with resveratrol: role of CREB-dependent Bcl-2 signaling via adenosine A3 receptor activation. *Am J Physiol Heart Circ Physiol* 2005, 288, 328-335.

12. Das S, Tosaki A, Bagchi D, Maulik N, Das DK: Resveratrol mediated activation of CREB through adenosine A3 receptor by Akt–dependent and–independent pathways. *J Pharmacol Exp Ther* 2005, 314, 762-769.

13. Demrow HS, Slane PR, Folts JD: Administration of wine and grape juice inhibits *in vivo* platelet activity and thrombosis in stenosed canine coronary arteries. *Circulation* 1995, 91, 1182-1188.

14. Fuhrman B, Aviram M: Flavonoids protect LDL from oxidation and attenuate atherosclerosis. *Curr Opin Lipidol* 2001, 12, 41-48.

15. Fuhrman B, Lavy A, Aviram M: Consumption of red wine meals reduces the susceptibility of human plasma and low-density lipoprotein to lipid peroxidation. *Am J Clin Nutr* 1995, 61, 549-554.

16. Fuhrman B, Volkova N, Suraski A, Aviram M: White wine with red wine-like properties increased extraction of grape skin polyphenols improve the antioxidant capacity of the derived white wine. *J Agric Food Chem* 2001, 49, 3164-3168.

17. Gaziano JM, Gaziano TA, Glynn RJ, Sesso HD, Ajani UA, Stampfer MJ, Manson JE, Hennekens CH, Buring JE: Light-to-moderate alcohol consumption and mortality in the Physicians' Health Study enrollment cohort. *J Am Coll Cardiol* 2000, 35, 96-105.

18. Goldberg DM, Tsang E, Karumanchiri A, Diamandis E, Soleas G, Ng E: Method to assay the concentrations of phenolic constituents of biological interest in wines. *Anal Chem* 1999, 68, 1688.

19. Virgili M, Contestabile A: Partial neuroprotection of *in vivo* excitotoxic brain damage by chronic administration of the red wine antioxidant agent, trans-resveratrol in rats. *Neurosci Lett* 2000, 281, 123-126.

20. Cadenas S, Barja G: Resveratrol, melatonin, vitamin E, and PBN protect against renal oxidative DNA damage induced by the kidney carcinogen KBrO3. *Free Radic Biol Med* 1999, 26, 1531-1537.

21. Hall SS: Longevity research. In vino vitalis? Compounds activate life-extending genes. *Science* 2003, 301, 1165.

22. Hattori R, Otani H, Maulik N, Das DK: Pharmacological preconditioning with resveratrol: role of nitric oxide. *Am J Physiol Heart Circ Physiol* 2002, 282, 1988-1995.

23. Hertog MGL, Feskens EJM, Kromhout D: Antioxidant flavonols and coronary heart disease risk. *Lancet* 1997, 349, 699.

24. Gehm BD, McAndrews JM, Chien P-Y, Jameson JL: Resveratrol, a polyphenolic compound found in grapes and wine, is an agonist for the estrogen receptor. *Proc Natl Acad Sci* U.S.A. 1997, 94, 14138-14143.

25. Howitz KT, Bitterman KJ, Cohen HY, Lamming DW, Lavu S, Wood JG, Zipkin RE, Chung P, Kisielewski A, Zhang LL, Scherer B, Sinclair DA: Small molecule activators of sirtuins extend *Saccharomyces cerevisiae lifespan. Nature* 2003, 425, 191-196.

26. Hsieh TC, Wu JM: Grape-derived chemopreventive agent resveratrol decreases prostate-specific antigen (PSA) expression in LNCaP cells by an androgen receptor (AR)-independent mechanism. *Anticancer Res* 2000, 20, 225-228.

27. Huang C, Ma WY, Goranson A, Dong Z: Resveratrol suppresses cell transformation and induces apoptosis through a p53-dependent pathway. *Carcinogenesis* 1999, 20, 237-242.

28. Hursting SD, Slaga TJ, Fischer SM, DiGiovanni J, Phang JM: Mechanism-based cancer prevention approaches: targets, examples, and the use of transgenic mice. *J Natl Cancer Inst* 1999, 91, 215-225.

29. Jang M, Cai L, Udeani GO, Slowing KV, Thomas CF, Beecher CW, Fong HH, Farnsworth NR, Kinghorn AD, Mehta, RG, Moon RC, Pezzuto JM: Cancer chemopreventive activity of resveratrol, a natural product derived from grapes. *Science* 1997, 275, 218-220.

30. Joshi G, Sultana R, Tangpong J, Cole MP, St Clair DK, Vore M, Estus S, Butterfield DA: Free radical mediated oxidative stress and toxic side effects in brain induced by the anti cancer drug adriamycin: insight into chemobrain. *Free Radic Res* 2005, 39, 1147-1154.

31. Kaga S, Zhan L, Matsumoto M, Maulik N: Resveratrol enhances neovascularization in the infarcted rat myocardium through the induction of thioredoxin-1, heme oxygenase-1 and vascular endothelial growth factor. *J Mol Cell Cardiol* 2005, 39, 813-822.

32. Kimura Y, Okuda H: Resveratrol isolated from *Polygonum cuspidatum* root prevents tumor growth and metastasis to lung and tumor-induced neovascularization in Lewis lung carcinoma-bearing mice. *J Nutr* 2001, 131, 1844-1849.

33. Lee SK, Mbwambo ZH, Chung H, Luyengi L, Gamez EJ, Mehta RG, Kinghorn AD, Pezzuto JM: Evaluation of the antioxidant potential of natural products. *Comb. Chem. High Throughput Screen.* 1998, 1, 35-46.
34. Kujoth GC, Hiona A, Pugh TD, Someya S, Panzer K, Wohlgemuth SE, Hofer T, Seo AY, Sullivan R, Jobling WA, Morrow JD, Van Remmen H, Sedivy JM, Yamasoba T, Tanokura M, Weindruch R, Leeuwenburgh C, Prolla TA: Mitochondrial DNA mutations, oxidative stress, and apoptosis in mammalian aging. *Science* 2005, 309, 481-484.
35. Mahady GB, Pendland SL: Resveratrol inhibits the growth of *Helicobacter pylori in vitro*. *Am J Gastroenterol* 2000, 95, 1849.
36. Mahady GB, Pendland SL, Chadwick LR: Resveratrol and red wine extracts inhibit the growth of CagA+ strains of *Helicobacter pylori in vitro*. *Am J Gastroenterol* 2003, 98, 1440-1441.
37. Marimon JM, Bujanda L, Gutierrez-Stampa MA, Cosme A, Arenas JI: *In vitro* bactericidal effect of wine against *Helicobacter pylori*. *Am J Gastroenterol* 1998, 93, 1392.
38. Mitchell SH, Zhu W, Young CY: Resveratrol inhibits the expression and function of the androgen receptor in LNCaP prostate cancer cells. *Cancer Res* 1999, 59, 5892-5895.
39. Morelli R, Das S, Bertelli A, Bollini R, Scalzo RL, Das DK, Falchi M: The introduction of the stilbene synthase gene enhances the natural antiradical activity of *Lycopersicon esculentum* mill. *Mol Cell Biochem* 2006, 282, 65-73.
40. Mouria M, Gukovskaya AS, Jung Y, Buechler P, Hines OJ, Reber HA, Pandol SJ: Food-derived polyphenols inhibit pancreatic cancer growth through mitochondrial cytochrome C release and apoptosis. *Int J Cancer* 2002, 98, 761-769.
41. Nigdikar SV, Williams NR, Griffin BA, Howard AN: Consumption of red wine polyphenols reduces the susceptibility of low-density lipoproteins to oxidation *in vivo*. *Am J Clin Nutr* 1998, 68, 258-265.
42. Pace-Asciak CR, Hahn S, Diamandis EP, Soleas G, Goldberg DM: The red wine phenolics trans-resveratrol and quercitin block human platelet aggregation and eicosanoid synthesis implications for protection against coronary heart disease. *Clin Chim Acta* 1995, 236, 207-219.
43. Pace-Asciak CR, Rounova O, Hahn SE, Diamandis EP, Goldberg DM: Wines and grape juices as modulators of platelet aggregation in healthy human subjects.
44. Ray PS, Maulik G, Cordis GA, Bertelli AAE, Bertelli A, Das DK: The red wine antioxidant resveratrol protects isolated rat hearts from ischemia reperfusion injury. *Free Radic Biol Med* 1999, 7, 160-169.
45. Renaud S, de Lorgeril: Wine, alcohol, platelets and the French paradox for coronary heart disease. *Lancet* 1992, 339, 1523-1526.

46. Orallo F, Alvarez E, Camina M, Leiro JM, Gomez E, and Fernandez, P: The possible implication of *trans*-resveratrol in the cardioprotective effects of long-term moderate wine consumption. *Mol Pharmacol* 2002, 61, 294-302.

47. Martinez J, Moreno JJ: Effect of resveratrol, a natural polyphenolic compound, on reactive oxygen species and prostaglandin production. *Biochem Pharmacol* 2000, 59, 865-870.

48. Ates O, Cayli S, Altinoz E, Gurses I, Yucel N, Sener M, Kocak, Yologlu S: Neuroprotection by resveratrol against traumatic brain injury in rats. *Mol Cell Biochem* (in press). 2006.

49. Gao ZB, Chen XQ, Hu GY: Inhibition of excitatory synaptic transmission by trans-resveratrol in rat hippocampus. *Brain Res* 2006, 1111, 41-47.

50. Sato M, Maulik N, Das DK: Cardioprotection with alcohol: role of both alcohol and polyphenolic antioxidants. *Ann N Y Acad Sci* 2002, 957, 122-135.

51. Basly JP, Marre-Fournier F, Le Bail JC, Habrioux G, Chulia AJ: Estrogenic/antiestrogenic and scavenging properties of (E)–and (Z)–resveratrol. *Life Sci* 2000, 66, 769-777.

52. Seigneur M, Bonnet J, Dorian B: Effect of the consumption of alcohol, white wine and red wine on the platelet function and serum lipids. *J Appl Cardiol* 1990, 5, 215.

53. Raval AP, Dave KR, Perez-Pinzon MA: Resveratrol mimics ischemic preconditioning in the brain. *J Cereb Blood Flow Metab* 2006, 26, 1141-1147.

54. Ray PS, Maulik G, Cordis GA. *et al.*: Myocardial protection by Protykin, a novel extract of *trans*-resveratrol and emodin. *Free Radic Res* 2000, 32, 135-144.

55. Stewart JR, Artime MC, O'rian CA: Resveratrol: A candidate nutritional substance for prostate cancer prevention. *Am Soc Nutr Sci* 2003, 22-3166, 2440S-2443S.

56. Subbaramaiah K, Chung WJ, Michaluart P, Telang N, Tanabe T, Inoue H, Jang M, Pezzuto JM, Dannenberg AJ: Resveratrol inhibits cyclooxygenase-2 transcription and activity in phorbol ester-treated human mammary epithelial cells. *J Biol Chem* 1998, 273, 21875-21882.

57. Yen GC, Duh PD, Lin CW: Effects of resveratrol and 4-hexylresorcicol on hydrogen peroxide-induced oxidative DNA damage in human lymphocytes. *Free Radic Res* 2003, 37, 509-514.

58. Leonard S, Xia C, Jiang BH, Stinefelt B, Klandorf H, Harris GK, Shi X: Resveratrol scavenges reactive oxygen species and effects radical-induced cellular responses. *Biochem Biophys Res Commun* 2003, 309, 1017-1026.

59. Tinhofer I, Bernhard D, Senfter M, Anether G, Loeffler M, Kroemer G, Kofler R, Csordas A, Greil R: Resveratrol, a tumor-suppressive compound from grapes, induces apoptosis via a novel mitochondrial pathway controlled by BCl-2. *FASEB J* 2001, 15, 1613-1615.

60. Lu R, Serrero G: Resveratrol, a natural product derived from grape, exhibits antiestrogenic activity and inhibits the growth of human breast cancer cells. *J Cell Physiol* 1999, 179, 297-304.

61. Manna SK, Mukhopadhyay A, Aggarwal BB: Resveratrol suppresses TNF-induced activation of nuclear transcription factors NF-κB, activator protein-1 and apoptosis: potential role of reactive oxygen intermediates and lipid peroxidation. *J Immunol* 2000, 164, 6509-6519.

62. Klinge CM, Risinger KE, Watts MB, Beck V, Eder R, Jungbauer A: Estrogenic activity in white and red wine extracts. *J Agri Food Chem* 2003, 51, 1850-1857.

63. Bowers JL, Tyulmenkov VV, Jernigan SC, Klinge CM: Resveratrol acts as a mixed agonist/antagonist for estrogen receptors alpha and beta. *Endocrinology* 2000, 141, 3657-3667.

64. Freyberger A, Hartmann E, Hildebrand H, Krotlinger F: Differential response of immature rat uterine tissue to ethinylestradiol and the red wine constituent resveratrol. *Arch Toxicol* 11, 709-715.

65. Mizutani K, Ikeda K, Kawai Y, Yamori Y: Resveratrol attenuates ovariectomy-induced hypertension and bone loss in stroke-prone spontaneously hypertensive rats. *J Nutr Sci Vitaminol* 2000, 46, 78-83.

66. Levenson AS, Gehm BD, Pearce ST, Horiguchi J, Simons LA, Ward JE III, Jameson JL, Jordan VC: Resveratrol acts as an estrogen receptor (ER) agonist in breast cancer cells stably tranfected with ERα. *Int J Cancer* 2003, 104, 587-596.

67. Kiziltepe U, Turan NN, Han U, Ulus AT, Akar F: Resveratrol, a red wine polyphenol, protects spinal cord from ischemia-reperfusion injury. *J Vasc Surg* 2004, 40, 138-145.

68. Zamin LL, Dillenburg-Pilla P, Argenta-Comiran R, Horn AP, Simao F, Nassif M, Gerhardt, D, Frozza RL, Salbego C: Protective effect of resveratrol against oxygen-glucose deprivation in organotypic hippocampal slice cultures: Involvement of PI3-K pathway. *Neurobiol Dis* 2006, 24, 170-182.

69. Kim H, Deshane J, Barnes S, Meleth S: Proteomics analysis of the actions of grape seed extract in rat brain: technological and biological implications for the study of the actions of psychoactive compounds. *Life Sci* 2006, 78, 2060-2065.

70. Bezstarosti K, Das S, Lamers JMJ, Das DK: Differential proteomic profiling to study the mechanism of cardiac pharmacological preconditioning by resveratrol. *J Cell Mol Med* 2006 (in press).

71. McCarty MF: Potential utility of natural polyphenols for reversing fat-induced insulin resistance. *Med Hypotheses* 2005, 64, 628-635.

72. Su HC, Hung LM, Chen JK: Resveratrol, a red wine antioxidant, possesses an insulin-like effect in streptozotocin-induced diabetic rats. *Am J Physiol Endocrinol Metab* 2006, 290, E1339-E1346.

73. Baur JA, Pearson KJ, Price NL, Jamieson HA, Lerin C, Kalra A, Prabhu VV, Allard JS, Lopez-Lluch, Lewis, K, Pistell PJ, Poosala S, Becker KG, Boss O, Gwinn D, Wang M, Ramaswamy S, Fishbein KW, Spencer RG, Lakatta EG, Le Couteur D, Shaw RJ, Navas P, Puigserver P, Ingram DK, de Cabo R, Sinclair DA: Resveratrol improves health and survival of mice on a high-calorie diet. *Nature* 2006 (in press)

74. Sharma S, Anjaneyulu M, Kulkarni SK, Chopra K: Resveratrol, a polyphenolic phytoalexin, attenuates diabetic nephropathy in rats. *Pharmacology* 2006, 76, 69-75.

75. Sharma S, Kulkarni SK, Chopra K: Resveratrol, a polyphenolic phytoalexin attenuates thermal hyperalgesia and cold allodynia in STZ-induced diabetic rats. *Ind J Exp Biol* 2006, 44, 566-569.

Chapter 13

Protective Effect of Phytochemicals in Cancer Chemoprevention, Wound Healing and Ischemia-Reperfusion Injury

Rajesh L. Thangapazham[1, 2], *Anuj Sharma*[1, 2] *and*
Radha K. Maheshwari[1*]
[1]*Department of Pathology, Uniformed Services University of the Health Sciences, 4301 Jones Bridge Road, Bethesda, MD 20814, USA*
[2]*Birla Institute of Technology and Science, Pilani – 333 031, India*
**E-mail: rmaheshwari@usuhs.mil*

ABSTRACT

There is increasing evidence of the health-protective benefits of numerous dietary components popularly known as phytochemicals, non-nutritive substances present in plants. Our laboratory is involved in research involving the elucidation of molecular targets and mechanism(s) of action of these phytochemicals which may provide health benefits like cancer chemoprevention and enhancement of wound healing. In this brief review we discuss the recent findings of our laboratory involving phytochemicals like curcumin, picroliv, shikonin and epigallocatechin gallate. A detailed understanding and importance of molecular targets and mechanism of action is pivotal to illustrate the use and development of non-toxic phytochemicals that regulate multiple pathways as therapeutics for the enhancement of wound healing, cancer chemoprevention and in ischemia-reperfusion injury.

Introduction

There is increasing number of research articles identifying the crucial role of numerous dietary components popularly known as phytochemicals, non-nutritive substances in plants possessing health-protective benefits [1]. Consuming a diet rich in vegetables and fruits containing antioxidants has been associated with protection from and/or treatment of conditions such as cancer, enhancement of wound healing and chemoprevention of various other diseases. The increasing popularity of phytochemicals has led to the development of a new branch of science coined nutrogenomics to understand how nutrients can interact with the human genome to alter the expression of genes. These studies on interaction between nutrients and genes may have great potential for exploring mechanisms and identifying susceptible individuals [2]. The important step in phytochemical research will be to identify molecular targets and mechanism of action by which they exert protective effects, which will enable further understanding of the molecular mechanism of disease. Such studies will help to develop preventive strategies beneficial to human health. This review specifically focuses on some of the beneficial effect and molecular targets of various phytochemicals like curcumin, picroliv, arnebin and epigallocatechin gallate (EGCG) in cancer chemoprevention, enhancement of wound healing and ameliorating ischemia-reperfusion injury.

Curcumin

Turmeric, *Curcuma longa* L. (Zingiberaceae family) rhizomes, has been widely used for centuries in indigenous medicine for the treatment of a variety of inflammatory conditions and other diseases. Its medicinal properties have been attributed mainly to the curcuminoids and the main component present in the rhizome includes curcumin (diferuloylmethane)-(1,7-bis(4-hydroxy-3-methoxyphenyl)-1,6-heptadiene-3,5-dione) (Figure 13.1).

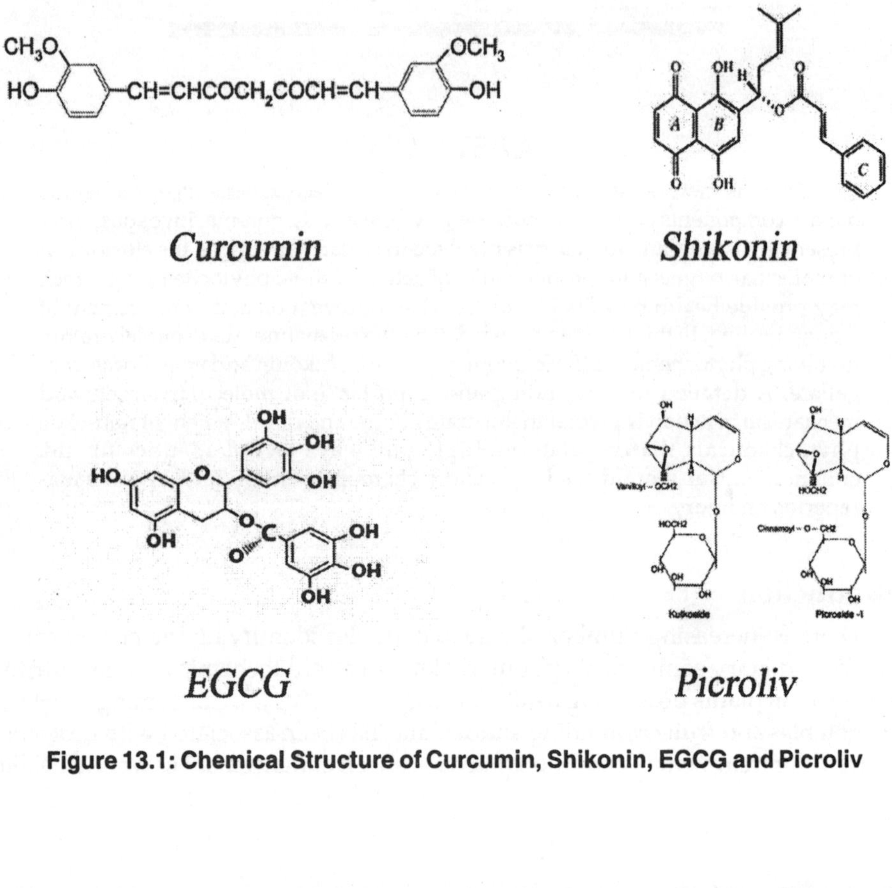

Figure 13.1: Chemical Structure of Curcumin, Shikonin, EGCG and Picroliv

Curcumin in Wound Healing

Every wound initiates bodily mechanisms that are intended to regenerate same or almost the same tissue as the original one. Wound healing proceeds in three interrelated dynamic phases with overlapping time courses irrespective of the wound type and degree of tissue damage [3]. According to morphological changes in the course of the healing process, three phases are clinically distinguished as (1) Inflammatory or exudative phase, for detachment of the deteriorated tissues and wound cleansing (2) Proliferative phase, for the development of granulation tissue and (3) Differentiation phase or a regeneration phase, for maturation, scar formation and epithelialization. In the normal healthy host, wound healing is usually uncomplicated and proceeds at a rapid rate. In contrast, most healing failures are associated with some form of host impairment, including diabetes, infection, immunosuppression, obesity or malnutrition. Impaired wound healing is a significant source of morbidity for the surgical patient and may result in complications such as wound-dehiscence, anastomotic breakdown and chronic non-healing ulcers.

Turmeric has been used since ancient times in India for the treatment of wounds. Multiple biological activities of curcumin and its beneficial effect in the enhancement of wound healing have been well described in recent reviews [4, 5]. Several studies have clearly substantiated the beneficial effects of topical application of curcumin in the acceleration of wound healing [6, 7]. In our work pertaining to curcumin in the field of wound healing we have shown that oral and topical administration of curcumin on punch biopsy wounds resulted in faster healing. Curcumin treatment resulted in faster re-epithelialization of the epidermis, increased migration of myofibroblasts, fibroblasts and macrophages in the wound bed, extensive neo-vascularization and greater collagen deposition [7]. This enhanced wound healing activity is attributed to increased expression of TGF*b*1 and collagen synthesis and modulation of levels of lipid peroxides, superoxide-dismutase, catalase and glutathione peroxidase in wounds by curcumin [6]. These studies show that curcumin can be effectively used in therapeutics for enhancing wound healing. We have also shown that curcumin enhances wound healing in dexamethasone and streptozotocin induced diabetes in rats and in genetically diabetic mice [8, 9]. These animals exhibit impaired healing without any treatment. Wounds of animals treated with curcumin showed earlier re-epithelialization, improved neovascularization, increased migration of dermal myofibroblasts, fibroblasts, and macrophages into the wound bed, and a higher collagen content. In these wounds curcumin treatment resulted in increased expression of transforming growth factor beta-1 [TGF-β1] and its receptor TGF-beta type I [tIrç] and type II [tIIrc] and induced nitric oxide species [iNOS] [9]. Apoptosis was also delayed in diabetic wounds as compared to curcumin treated wounds [8]. These studies show that curcumin has a positive impact on wound repair in diabetic impaired healing and could be developed as a pharmacological agent for treating diabetic wounds.

Curcumin in Ischemia-reperfusion

A great deal of effort has been directed, without much success, towards searching for compounds that can be used for better management of clinical consequences arising from renal ischemia–reperfusion. The pathophysiology of hemorrhagic shock is the result of ischemia/hypoxia, reperfusion, and subsequent inflammation. Sustained reduction in blood flow leads to diminished microcirculatory perfusion, which results in regional hypoxia. Resuscitation supplies oxygen to the ischemic region of the tissue, which in turn generates free radicals. These toxic oxygen and nitrogen species are central to cellular damage. They cause lipid peroxidation-related membrane damage and activate the cellular antioxidant defense, signal transduction, and gene expression. Studies in our laboratory have shown that pretreatment with curcumin resulted in significant restoration of the liver cytokines Interleukin-1α, IL-1β, IL-2, IL-6 and IL-10 to normal levels that were increased by hemorrhage/ resuscitation regimen in rats [10]. In fact, IL-1β levels were lower than sham levels. Nuclear factor kappa beta (NF-k β) and transcription factor AP-1 were differentially activated at 2 and 24 h post-hemorrhage and were inhibited by curcumin pretreatment. Serum aspartate transaminase estimates indicated decreased liver injury in curcumin-pretreated animals that were subjected to hemorrhage. These results suggested that protection by curcumin pretreatment against hemorrhage/resuscitation injury might have resulted from the down modulation of transcription factors involved and regulation of cytokines to beneficial levels [10].

Curcumin in Angiogenesis

Angiogenesis is a crucial step in the growth and metastasis of cancers. The migration, proliferation and differentiation of human umbilical vein endothelial cells (HUVEC) lead to angiogenesis, which facilitates tumor initiation and promotion. We have for the first time reported that curcumin inhibited the growth of HUVEC stimulated with fibroblast growth factor (FGF) and endothelial growth supplement (ECGS) and also resulted in an accumulation of around 46 per cent of the cells in early S-phase, as determined by the flow cytometry [12]. The studies have revealed a unique mode of action of curcumin whereby it effectively blocked the cell cycle progression of HUVEC during S-phase by inhibiting the activity of thymidine kinase enzyme [12]. Zymographs of curcumin-treated culture supernatants showed a decrease in the gelatinolytic activities of secreted 53 and 72-kDa metalloproteinase, MMP2 and 9 respectively [11]. Western and Northern analysis showed a dose-dependent decrease in the expression of protein transcript of 72 kDa, indicating that curcumin might be exerting its inhibitory effect at both the transcriptional and post-transcriptional level. These findings suggest that curcumin acts as an angiogenesis inhibitor by modulating protease activity during endothelial morphogenesis [11] and may be a useful compound in cancer chemoprevention. Recent studies in our laboratory have suggested a strong *in vitro* efficacy of curcumin to attenuate the expression and function of the androgen receptor (*AR*). In prostate cancer, ETS-related gene (*ERG*) is highly up regulated and *ERG* forms fusion with *TMPRSS2*. Microarray analysis have shown that TMPRSS2 is highly down regulated by curcumin (unpublished data) unveiling some of the mechanism(s) used by curcumin to inhibit LNCaP cell growth.

Picroliv

Iridiod glycosides Picroside I and Kutkoside are isolated from the roots and rhizomes of *Picrorhiza kurrooa*. A standardized fraction containing 1:1.5 mixture of Picroside I and Kutkoside has been named Picroliv (Figure 13.1).

Picroliv and Ischemia-reperfusion

Picroliv is known to have significant hepatoprotective, anti-inflammatory and antioxidant properties. As mentioned before lot of effort is aimed at developing of compounds that can be used for better management of clinical consequences arising from renal ischemia–reperfusion. Regional hypoxia, a pathophysiology of hemorrhagic shock results due to ischemia/hypoxia, reperfusion, and subsequent inflammation. Cellular adaptation to hypoxia involves regulation of specific genes such as vascular endothelial growth factor (VEGF), erythropoietin (EPO) and hypoxia inducible factor-1(HIF-1).

Picroliv treatment of HUVEC and Hep3B cells in vitro during normoxia and hypoxia resulted in increased expression of VEGF and HIF-1 subunits (HIF-1α /β), which upon re-oxygenation was significantly reduced [13]. In an in-vivo model of renal ischemia-reperfusion injury (IRI) in rats at a dose of 12 mg/kg orally for 7 days, picroliv pretreatment protects rat kidneys from IRI, perhaps by modulation of free radical damage and adhesion molecules as indicated by their lower lipid peroxidation, improved antioxidant status and reduced apoptosis [14]. In the same model picroliv ameliorated hepatic IRI by reducing oxidant induced cellular damage as measured by tissue malondialdehyde [MDA] levels, which was significantly less following picroliv pretreatment [15]. More over a reduction in neutrophil infiltration and an increased level of intracellular antioxidant enzyme superoxide dismutase was also found with picroliv pretreatment. Picroliv treatment resulted in reduction in tissue lipid peroxidation and inflammatory cytokines such as IL1α/β [15]. Picroliv significantly down-regulated the stress-sensitive transcription factor AP1 and decreased the level of c-fos mRNA as well as c-jun and c-fos proteins in liver tissue, indicating that its actions could be mediated through AP1 and associated signal transduction pathways [16]. In recent studies, insulin growth factor (IGF) has been implicated in tissue repair and regeneration after hypoxic-ischemic injury [17]. Significant reduction in the mRNA level of IGF-I, IGF-II and IGF-IR was observed in response to hypoxia in male Sprague-Dawley rats, placed in 10 per cent oxygen for 4 days [17]. Pretreatment with picroliv not only prevented such down regulation but more importantly resulted in increased levels of IGF-I and IGF-IR [17]. These studies suggest picroliv as a cost effective alternative for being developed as a therapeutic agent for the better management of ischemia–reperfusion injury [IRI].

Picroliv in Wound Healing and Angiogenesis

We have investigated the effect of Picroliv in an ex-vivo rat aorta ring model of angiogenesis and punch wound healing model in rat. Picroliv treatment resulted in improved re-epithelialization, neovascularization and migration of various cells such as endothelial, dermal myofibroblasts and fibroblasts into the wound bed after picroliv treatment [18]. Immunohistochemical localization showed an increased VEGF and alpha smooth muscle actin staining consistent with increased number of microvessels in granulation tissue. These findings suggest that picroliv could be developed as a therapeutic angiogenic agent for the restoration of the blood supply in diseases involving inadequate blood supply such as limb ischemia and ischemic myocardium and wound healing.

Arnebin and Shikonin Analogue 93/637 [SA]

Arnebin-1 (Figure 13.1) is a naphthaquinone characterized by the Central Drug Research Institute [CDRI], Lucknow, India and supplied to us.

Arnebin and Shikonin Analogue in Wound Healing

Arnebin has been shown to improve wound healing in both normal and hydrocortisone impaired wounds. Topical application of Arnebin-1 resulted in faster closure of full thickness punch wound model in rats [19]. Arnebin-1 promoted the wound healing by inducing the proliferation of cells, angiogenesis, and collagen synthesis. Fibronectin and TGFβ were also transcriptionally upregulated in wounds by arnebin-1 which may be responsible for the enhancement of wound healing [19].

The compound β,β-dimethyl acryloyl shikonin, an extract from the roots of plant Arnebia nobilis appear to have toxicity. Subsequently, several analogues of β,β-dimethyl acryloyl shikonin were synthesized and one of them shikonin analogue 93/637 [SA] was significantly less toxic compared to beta, beta-dimethyl acryloyl shikonin. In a wound healing study 0.1 per cent SA was applied topically daily as an ointment in polyethylene glycol base on wounds. The effect of shikonin was evaluated on normal and hydrocortisone-induced impaired healing in full thickness cutaneous punch wounds in rats [20]. SA treatment significantly accelerated healing of wounds, as measured by wound contraction in hydrocortisone induced diabetic animals. SA treatment promoted formation of granulation tissue including cell migration and neovascularization, collagenization and re-epithelialization [18]. The expression of basic fibroblast growth factor [bFGF] was higher as revealed by immunohistochemistry in SA treated wounds over untreated controls. However, the expression of TGF β-1 was not affected by SA treatment [20]. Since bFGF is known to accelerate wound healing, the increased expression of bFGF by SA may be partly responsible for the enhancement of wound healing.

Arnebin and Shikonin Analogue in Cancer Chemoprevention

Shikonin was found to have anti-cancer properties but its use was limited because of its toxicity. Less toxic analogue of shikonin, SA, showed slight inhibitory effect on the growth of prostate cancer cell lines, DU 145 and LNCaP cells at low doses ranging from 250 nM to 1 mM and has moderate inhibitory effect at concentrations 2.5 μM and above [21]. Decrease in mRNAs of *IGF-II* in DU 145, *IGF-I*, and *IGF-IR* in LNCaP, and *IGF-II* and *VEGF* in PC-3 cells and an increase in *IGFBP-3* in both DU 145 and PC-3 cells was found when the cells were treated with SA [21]. These results show inhibitory effect of SA on prostate cancer cell growth and *IGFs* cancer pathway suggesting a potential therapeutic use in treatment of prostate cancer.

Epigallocatechin gallate (EGCG)

Tea [*Camellia sinesis* (Theacacea)] is considered second only to water as the most popular beverage consumed worldwide. Consumption of tea has been associated with many health benefits and their role and mechanism in cancer chemoprevention has been studied recently. The biological activity of green tea is due to several catechins. Epigallocatechin gallate (EGCG) (Figure 13.1) is identified as the principal antioxidant present in tea.

Tea and Cancer Chemoprevention

Breast cancer cells when treated with green tea polyphenols (GTP) had lower proliferation potential with several proteins such as Cyclin D, Cyclin E, cyclin-dependent kinase 4 (CDK 4), CDK 1 and proliferating cell nuclear antigen (PCNA) down regulated [21]. GTP treatment of nude mice inoculated with human breast cancer MDA-MB-231 cells was effective in delaying the tumor incidence as well as reducing the tumor burden when compared to the water fed and similarly handled control. Both tumor incidence and mean tumor volume were significantly reduced by GTP and EGCG treatment. GTP and EGCG treatment were also found to induce apoptosis and inhibit the cell proliferation. TUNEL assay, to study apoptosis, revealed increased tumor cell death in-vivo in GTP (80±10 SEM cells/field) and EGCG (60±8 SEM cells/field) treatment as compared to untreated controls (23±5 SEM cells/field). PCNA staining in mice tumor xenograft showed decrease in the PCNA positive cells in EGCG (24±5.0 SEM cells/field) and GTP (33±4.3 SEM cells/field) as compared to controls (87±12 SEM cells/field), indicated the anti-proliferative effect of these polyphenols [21]. EGCG was also found to inhibit angiogenesis by modulating protease activity during endothelial morphogenesis [22]. In an *in-vivo* matrigel plug assay mouse model, plugs containing the growth supplement and EGCG (100–200 μg/ml) showed a dose-dependent decrease in the number of cells in the plugs compared to untreated control. This indicates that EGCG inhibited the migration of cells and vessel formation in matrigel plug model. However, such significant difference in the migration of cells was not observed at the lower concentrations of EGCG (40 μg/ml). Tube formation was inhibited by EGCG treatment both prior to plating and after plating endothelial cells on matrigel and was also found to stall migration of endothelial cells in matrigel plug model [22].

Conclusion

In conclusion, the approach of using phytochemicals for the prevention and treatment of certain diseases like cancer, enhancement of wound healing and ameliorating ischemia-reperfusion injury looks promising. The phytochemicals are known for their minimal acute or chronic toxicity and will be of great importance in condition requiring long term usage. Phytochemicals are also a cost effective treatment modality. Though epidemiological studies and preclinical and experimental studies, including all the work cited in this review, suggest the beneficial nature of these phytochemicals, we acknowledge that more structured work in transgenic animal models and human intervention trials will be the ultimate proof of the aforementioned protective nature of these phytochemicals. The beneficial effects of these phytochemicals are summarized in Figure 13.2.

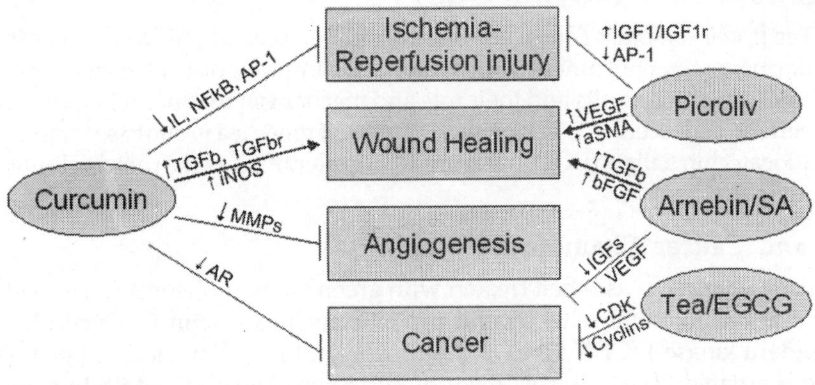

Figure 13.2: Schematic Representation of Molecular Targets of Phytochemicals in Cancer Chemoprevention, Wound Healing and Ischemia-Reperfusion Injury

Acknowledgements

Some of these studies were supported by a grant (G174KT) from the NCCAM, National Institute of Health, Bethesda and US-INDIA Foreign Currency Fund from US Department of State to USUHS. The opinions or assertions contained herein are the private views of the authors and should not be construed as official or necessarily reflecting the views of the Uniformed Services University of the Health Sciences or the Department of Defense, USA.

References

1. Craig W, Beck L: Phytochemicals: Health Protective Effects. *Can J Diet Pract Res*, 1999, 60, 78-84
2. Reszka E, Wasowicz W, Gromadzinska J: Genetic polymorphism of xenobiotic metabolising enzymes, diet and cancer susceptibility. *Br J Nutr*, 2006, 96, 609-19
3. Aukhil I: Biology of wound healing. *Periodontol*, 2000, 22, 44-50
4. Thangapazham RL, Sharma A, Maheshwari RK: Multiple molecular targets in cancer chemoprevention by curcumin. *Aaps J*, 2006, 8, E443-9
5. Maheshwari RK, Singh AK, Gaddipati J, Srimal RC: Multiple biological activities of curcumin: a short review. *Life Sci*, 2006, 78, 2081-2087
6. Panchatcharam M, Miriyala S, Gayathri VS, Suguna L: Curcumin improves wound healing by modulating collagen and decreasing reactive oxygen species. *Mol Cell Biochem*, 2006, 290, 87-96
7. Sidhu GS, Singh AK, Thaloor D, Banaudha KK, Patnaik GK, Srimal RC, Maheshwari RK: Enhancement of wound healing by curcumin in animals. *Wound Repair Regen*, 1998, 6, 167-77
8. Sidhu GS, Mani H, Gaddipati JP, Singh AK, Seth P, Banaudha KK, Patnaik GK, Maheshwari RK: Curcumin enhances wound healing in streptozotocin induced diabetic rats and genetically diabetic mice. *Wound Repair Regen*, 1999, 7, 362-374

9. Mani H, Sidhu GS, Kumari R, Gaddipati JP, Seth P, Maheshwari RK: Curcumin differentially regulates TGF-beta1, its receptors and nitric oxide synthase during impaired wound healing. *Biofactors*, 2002, 16, 29-43

10. Gaddipati JP, Sundar SV, Calemine J, Seth P, Sidhu, GS, Maheshwari RK: Differential regulation of cytokines and transcription factors in liver by curcumin following hemorrhage/resuscitation. *Shock*, 2003, 19, 150-156

11. Thaloor D, Singh AK, Sidhu GS, Prasad PV, Kleinman HK, Maheshwari RK: Inhibition of angiogenic differentiation of human umbilical vein endothelial cells by curcumin. *Cell Growth Differ*, 1998, 9, 305-12

12. Singh AK, Sidhu GS, Deepa T, Maheshwari RK: Curcumin inhibits the proliferation and cell cycle progression of human umbilical vein endothelial cell. *Cancer Lett*, 1996, 107, 109-115

13. Gaddipati JP, Madhavan S, Sidhu GS, Singh AK, Seth P, Maheshwari RK: Picroliv–a natural product protects cells and regulates the gene expression during hypoxia/reoxygenation. *Mol Cell Biochem*, 1999, 194, 271-281

14. Seth P, Kumari R, Madhavan S, Singh AK, Mani H, Banaudha KK, Sharma SC, Kulshreshtha DK, Maheshwari RK: Prevention of renal ischemia-reperfusion-induced injury in rats by picroliv. *Biochem Pharmacol*, 2000, 59, 1315-1322

15. Singh AK, Mani H, Seth P, Gaddipati JP, Kumari R, Banuadha KK, Sharma SC, Kulshreshtha, DK, Maheshwari RK: Picroliv preconditioning protects the rat liver against ischemia-reperfusion injury. *Eur J Pharmacol*, 2000, 395, 229-239

16. Seth P, Sundar SV, Seth RK, Sidhu GS, Sharma SC, Kulshreshtha DK, Maheshwari RK: Picroliv modulates antioxidant status and down-regulates AP1 transcription factor after hemorrhage and resuscitation. *Shock*, 2003, 19, 169-175

17. Gaddipati JP, Mani H, Banaudha KK, Sharma SK, Kulshreshtha DK, Maheshwari RK: Picroliv modulates the expression of insulin-like growth factor (IGF)-I, IGF-II and IGF-I receptor during hypoxia in rats. *Cell Mol Life Sci*, 1999, 56, 348-355

18. Singh AK, Sharma A, Warren J, Madhavan S, Steele K, Rajeshkumar NV, Thangapazham RL, Sharma SC, Kulshreshtha DK, Gaddipati JP, Maheshwari RK: Picroliv accelerates epithelialization and angiogenesis in rat wounds. *Planta Medica* (Accepted)

19. Sidhu GS, Singh AK, Banaudha KK, Gaddipati JP, Patnaik GK, Maheshwari RK: Arnebin-1 accelerates normal and hydrocortisone-induced impaired wound healing. *J Invest Dermatol*, 1999, 113, 773-781

20. Mani H, Sidhu GS, Singh AK, Gaddipati J, Banaudha KK, Raj K, Maheshwari RK: Enhancement of wound healing by shikonin analogue 93/637 in normal and impaired healing. *Skin Pharmacol Physiol*, 2004, 17, 49-56

21. Gaddipati JP, Mani H, Shefali, Raj K, Mathad VT, Bhaduri AP, Maheshwari RK: Inhibition of growth and regulation of IGFs and VEGF in human prostate cancer cell lines by shikonin analogue 93/637 (SA). *Anticancer Res*, 2000, 20, 2547-2552

22. Thangapazham RL, Singh AK, Sharma A, Warren J, Gaddipati JP, Maheshwari RK: Green tea polyphenols and its constituent epigallocatechin gallate inhibits proliferation of human breast cancer cells *in vitro* and *in vivo*. *Cancer Lett*, 2006, 3, (in press)
23. Singh AK, Seth P, Anthony P, Husain MM, Madhavan S, Mukhtar H, Maheshwari RK: Green tea constituent epigallocatechin-3-gallate inhibits angiogenic differentiation of human endothelial cells. *Arch Biochem Biophys*, 2002, 401, 29-37

Chapter 14

A Brief Review on Phytoconstituents with Potential Antidiabetic Activity

K. Rajendran and Annie Shirwaikar*

Department of Pharmacognosy, Manipal College of Pharmaceutical Sciences, Manipal – 576 104, Karnataka, India

** E-mail: annieshirwaikar@yahoo.com*

ABSTRACT

Pharmaceutical research conducted over the past three decades shows that natural products are a potential source of novel molecules for drug development. A wide array of plant-derived active principles, representing numerous classes of chemical compounds *viz.*, alkaloids, glycosides, peptidoglycans, steroids, carbohydrates, glycopeptides, terpenoids and amino acids have been found to demonstrate activity consistent with their possible use in the treatment of non-insulin dependent diabetes mellitus (NIDDM). The present paper is a review of the activity of some phytoconstituents used in the treatment of diabetes.

Introduction

Diabetes is recognised today as one of the leading causes of morbidity and mortality in the world. About 2.5-3 per cent of the world's population suffer from this disease, a proportion which, in some countries, can reach 7 per cent or more. In India, the prevalence rate of diabetes is estimated to be 1-5 per cent [1,2,3].

Historical accounts reveal that NIDDM was well known among the ancients and medicinal plants have been used for millennia to treat this disease. Studies on a medicinal plant, *Galega officinalis,* led to the discovery and synthesis of metform [4]. It may look a bit paradoxical (in spite of the remarkable advancements in synthetic medicaments) if one were to turn back to indigenous herbal drugs for a new antidiabetic remedy.

Since ancient times, plants have been an exemplary source of medicine. Ayurveda and other Indian literature mention the use of plants in the treatment of various human ailments. Research conducted in the last few decades on plants mentioned in ancient literature or used traditionally for diabetes has been encouraging and fruitful [5].

Given the likelihood that medicinal plants with a long history of human use will ultimately yield novel drug prototypes, a systematic and intensive research on plants for new drugs to treat Type 2 diabetes mellitus seems to be of great utility. The ethnomedicinal approach to plant drug discovery is practical, cost-effective, and logical. Till today about 1200 species of plants have been screened for antidiabetic activity on an ethnopharmacological or random basis [6,7]. A wide array of plant-derived active principles, representing numerous classes of chemical compounds *viz.*, alkaloids, glycosides, peptidoglycans, steroids, carbohydrates, glycopeptides, terpenoids and amino acids have been found to demonstrate activity consistent with their possible use in the treatment of NIDDM [8]. The present paper is a review of the activity of some phytoconstituents used in the treatment of diabetes.

Hypoglycin A and Hypoglycin B from *Blighia sapida*

Two extremely potent hypoglycaemic agents have been isolated from the unripe fruits of the *B. sapida* (Sapindaceae). They are cyclopropanoid amino acids known as hypoglycin A and hypoglycin B respectively. Hypoglycin A is found in both the aril and the seeds of the unripe fruit, hypoglycin B is present only in the seeds. The former constituent is almost twice as toxic as the latter. The mode of action of hypoglycins is quite different from that of insulin, in that they appear to act as antimetabolites capable of blocking the pathway of oxidation of fatty acids. This depletes liver glycogen and subsequently induces hypoglycaemia. Although the hypoglycins are too toxic to be used as a substitute for insulin, the fact that they do induce hypoglycaemia by oral administration makes them attractive models for the synthesis of non-toxic analogs [9].

Charantin, Momordin and Polypeptides from *Momordica charantia*

Charantin, a peptide resembling insulin isolated from *M. charantia* (Curcubitaceae) lowered fasting blood sugar in rabbits gradually beginning from the first and lasting till the fourth hour and slowly recovering to the initial level. Charantin (50 mg/kg) administered orally, lowered blood glucose by 42 per cent at the 4th h with a mean fall of 28 per cent during 5 h [10]. Another constituent polypeptide-p, isolated from fruit, seeds, and tissue of *M. charantia* showed potent hypoglycaemic effect when administered subcutaneously to gerbils, langurs, and humans [11]. Experiments in rats showed that 2 other important constituents of *M. charantia i.e.* oleanolic acid 3-*O*-glucuronide and momordin exert anti-hyperglycemic effect by inhibiting glucose transport at the brush border of the small intestine [12].

Gymnemosides and Gymnemic Acid from *Gymnema sylvestre*

Various hypoglycaemic principles of *G. sylvestre* isolated from the saponin fraction of the plant are referred as gymnemosides and gymnemic acid [13]. Its triterpene glycosides isolated from the plant inhibited glucose utilization in muscles [14]. However, triterpene glycosides exhibited little or no inhibitory activity against glucose absorption in oral glucose tolerance test (OGTT) conducted in rats. Gymnemic acid I and gymnema saponin V lacked anti-hyperglycemic effect [15].

Galegin from *Galega officinalis* L. (Leguminosae)

The active principle galegin, isolated from *G. officinalis,* has been reported as a hypoglycaemic agent by a number of workers [16].

Epicatechin, Marsupin and Pterostilbene from *Pterocarpus marsupium*

Epicatechin, a pure flavonoid isolated from the ethanol extract of *P. marsupium* bark has been shown to possess significant anti-diabetic effect. Epicatechin has been shown to enhance insulin release and conversion of proinsulin to insulin *in vitro* [17].

Phenolic constituents such as *marsupin* and *pterostilbene* significantly lowered blood glucose level in STZ diabetic rats and the effect was comparable to metformin [18]. *Pterostilbene* (a constituent derived from wood) caused hypoglycaemia in dogs (at the dose of 10 mg/kg i.v.). Higher dose (20, 30 and 50 mg/kg) caused initial hyperglycaemia followed by hypoglycaemia lasting for nearly 5 h [19]. Joglekar *et al.,* [20] associated its hypoglycaemic effect with the presence of tannins in the extract.

Leucopelargonidin, Leucocyanidin, Leucodelphinidin and Pelargonidin from *Ficus bengalenesis*: Indian Banyan tree

Oral administration of leucopelarogonidin derivative (100 mg/kg) isolated from bark of *F. bengalenesis* exerts significant hypoglycaemic activity in normal and moderately alloxanized diabetic dogs (60 mg/kg i.v. injection) [21]. Cherian and Augusti [22] proved the use of leucopelarogonidin derivative for significant hypoglycaemic, hypolipidemic and serum insulin raising effects in moderately diabetic rats.

A leucocyanidin derivative (100 mg/kg) isolated from the bark of *F. bengalenesis* was found to be hypoglycaemic in normal rats. Combination of single dose of this chemical and low dose of insulin controlled diabetes in alloxanized rats as effectively as that of a high dose of insulin. In addition, long term treatment with this combination showed equal response to double dose of insulin in respect to body weight, urine and blood sugar along with amelioration of serum cholesterol and triglyceride [23].

Leucodelphinidin (250 mg/kg) also showed hypoglycaemic action equal to that of glibenclamide (2 mg/kg) in normal and alloxan-diabetic rats. However, in OGTT, it was less effective as compared to glibenclamide (2 mg/kg) [24].

The glycoside, pelargonidin isolated from bark decreased fasting blood glucose by 19 per cent and improved glucose tolerance by 29 per cent in moderately diabetic rats at the dose of 250 mg/kg. In comparison, glibenclamide (2 mg/kg) showed 25 and 66 per cent reduction, respectively, versus controls [25]. Treatment with the same glycoside (100 mg/kg/day) for 1 month reduced the fasting blood glucose levels to almost half of the pretreatment levels. Glucose tolerance improved by 15 per cent in glycoside treated group versus 41 per cent in glibenclamide treated group (0.5 mg/kg/day). In addition, pelargonidin was more potent than leucocyanidin in stimulating *in vitro* insulin secretion by beta cells [25].

Pectin from *Coccinia indica*

Oral administration (2 g/kg/day) of pectin isolated from *C. indica* fruit showed a significant hypoglycaemic action in normal rats due to stimulation of glycogen synthetase activity and reduction of phosphorylase activity [26].

SMCS, SACS from *Allium cepa* and *A. sativum*

Sulfur containing amino acid, *S*-methyl cysteine sulphoxide (SMCS) isolated from *A. cepa* (200 mg/kg for 45 days) to alloxanized rats significantly controlled blood glucose and lipids in serum and tissues and normalized the activities of liver hexokinase, glucose 6-phosphatase and HMG CoA reductase. The effect was comparable to that of glibenclamide and insulin [27]. Sheela *et al.*, [28] showed beneficial effect of SMCS and *S*-allylcysteine sulfoxide (SACS) in alloxanized diabetic rats on glucose intolerance, weight loss and liver glycogen. It also decreased hyperglycaemic peak in subcutaneous glucose tolerance tests conducted in rabbits [29].

Administration of SACS, a sulfur containing amino acid and the precursor of allicin, isolated from *A. sativum* (200 mg/kg) significantly decreased the concentration of serum lipids, blood glucose and activities of serum enzymes like alkaline phosphatase, acid phosphatase and lactate dehydrogenase and liver glucose-6-phosphatase. It also significantly increased liver and intestinal HMG CoA reductase activity and liver hexokinase activity [30]. In another study, oral administration of SACS to alloxan-diabetic rats for 1 month ameliorated glucose intolerance, weight loss, depletion of liver glycogen in diabetic rats in comparison to glibenclamide and insulin [28]. SACS also controlled lipid peroxidation better than glibenclamide and insulin and ameliorated diabetic condition almost to the same extent as they did. Furthermore, SACS significantly stimulated *in vitro* insulin secretion from β-cells isolated from normal rats [31].

Beta Vulgarosides from *Beta vulgaris*: Garden Beet (English)

Beta vulgarosides II, III and IV are glycosides isolated from the root extract of *Beta vulgaris* and have been shown to increase glucose tolerance in OGTT experiments conducted in rats [32].

Mulinolic Acid, Azorellanol, and Mulin-11,13-dien-20-oic Acid from *Azorella compacta*

Antidiabetic activity of diterpenic compounds mulinolic acid, azorellanol, and mulin-11,13-dien-20-oic acid isolated from *Azorella compacta* were evaluated in streptozotocin diabetic rats. Blood glucose levels of animals treated with mulinolic acid and azorellanol decreased in a manner similar to chlorpropamide injection. Authors hypothesized that because of the similarity to the hypoglycemic medication chlorpropamide, azorellanol could be acting on the beta cells of pancreatic islets, while mulinolic acid may act upon glucose utilization or production in the liver [33].

Hydroxyisoleucine from *Trigonella foenum graecum*

4-hydroxyisoleucine, a novel amino acid has been extracted and purified from fenugreek seeds. It increased glucose-induced insulin release (ranging from 100 ìmol/l to 1 mmol/l) through a direct effect on the isolated islets of Langerhans in both rats and humans. This pattern of insulin secretion was biphasic, glucose dependent, occurred in the absence of any change in pancreatic alpha and delta cell activity and without interaction with other agonists of insulin secretion (such as leucine, arginine, tolbutamide, glyceraldehyde) [34].

Kotalanol and Salacinol from *Salacia reticulate* and *Salacia oblonga*

Potent natural α-glycosidase inhibitors such as kotalanol with thiosugar sulfonium sulfate structure and salacinol isolated from the roots and stems of *S. reticulata* exert potent inhibitory activity against sucrase [35].

Salacinol and kotalanol with nine other sugar related components were isolated from the water soluble portion while, a new triterpene, kotalagenin 16-acetate along with known diterpene and triterpenes isolated from the ethyl acetate portion of *S. oblonga* were found to be responsible components for the inhibitory activity on aldolase reductase [36].

Lepidine from *Lepidium ruderale* Linn

An active principle lepidine isolated from the aerial parts of *L. ruderale* had a dose dependant hypoglycaemic activity when given orally to rats having alloxan diabetes. Single or long-term administration of lepidine induced antihyperglycaemic effect in rats with induced mild chronic diabetes mellitus and an antihyperlipemic activity was also observed with the long-term administration of lepidine [37].

Pinitol from *Bougainvillea spectabilis*

Pinitol was isolated from the leaves of *B. spectabilis* (Nyctaginaceae) and evaluated for hypoglycaemic activity. Pinitol, which is readily soluble in water, induced significant hypoglycaemia when administered orally, at a dose of 0.01 g/kg in normal fasted albino mice, the maximum effect being at the end of two hours. In alloxan induced diabetic mice after treatment with pinitol for 72 h (5 doses), a significant fall in blood sugar level was observed [38].

Shamimin from *Bombax ceiba*: Red Silk Cotton Tree (English)

A C-flavonol glucoside isolated from *Bombax ceiba* leaves called as shamimin has been shown to exert significant hypoglycaemic activity at the dose of 500 mg/kg in rats [39].

Stilbene and anthraquinone derivatives from *Rheum undulatum*

Stilbene (a), desoxyrhapontigenin and anthraquinones, emodin and chrysophanol from *R. undulatum* (Polygonaceae) inhibited postprandial hyperglycemia by 35.8, 29.5, 42.3 per cent, respectively [40].

Swerchirin from *Swertia chirata*

In a study, Swerchirin (a xanthone isolated from hexane fraction of *S. chirata*) showed significant blood sugar lowering effect in fasted, glucose loaded and tolbutamide pre-treated albino rats. Oral ED50 of Swerchirin for 40 per cent blood sugar reduction in male albino rats is 23.1 mg/kg [41]. Force-feeding of Swerchirin (35 and 65 mg/kg i.v.) to STZ diabetic rats (50 mg/kg) showed significant anti-hyperglycemic effect at 0, 1, 3 and 7 h after the dose both in healthy as well as STZ rats (35 mg/kg) but not in the group treated with STZ (65 mg/kg) [42]. Single oral administration of Swerchirin (50 mg/kg) to rats caused a 60 per cent fall in blood glucose at 7 h post-treatment with marked depletion of aldehyde-fuchsin stained beta-granules and immunostained insulin in the pancreatic islets. *In vitro*, glucose uptake and glycogen synthesis by muscle (diaphragm) was significantly enhanced by the serum of Swerchirin-treated rat. Swerchirin at 100, 10 and 1 μM concentration greatly enhanced glucose (16.7 mM) stimulated insulin release from isolated islets [43].

Trihydroxyoctadecadiene acid from *Bryonia alba*

Effect of trihydroxyoctadecadiene acid from *B.alba* (Cucurbitaceae) on the activity of glycogen metabolizing enzymes has been studied and its phytoconstituent was found to directly exert effect on glycogen phosphorylase, phosphoprotein phosphatase and hexokinase in the liver and muscle tissues of alloxan induced diabetes white rats [44].

Ulopyranose from *Psacalium peltatum*

A new ulopyranose isolated from aqueous extract of roots and rhizomes of *P. peltatum* has been determined to have hypoglycaemic activity at doses of 100 mg/kg, comparable to that of tolbutamide and insulin in alloxan diabetic mice [45].

Phanoside from *Gynostemma pentaphyllum*

Phanoside is a dammarane-type saponin, and four stereoisomers differing in configurations at positions 21 and 23 were isolated from *G. pentaphyllum* (Cucurbitaceae). Each of these compounds was found to stimulate insulin release from isolated rat pancreatic islets. Dose-dependent insulin-releasing activities at 3.3 and 16.7 mM glucose levels were determined for the racemic mixture containing all four stereoisomers. Phanoside at 500 μM stimulates insulin release *in vitro* 10-fold at 3.3 mM glucose and potentiates the release almost 4-fold at 16.7 mM glucose. Interestingly, β-cell sensitivity to phanoside is higher at 16.7 mM than at 3.3 mM glucose, although insulin responses were significantly increased by phanoside below 125 μM only at high glucose levels. Also when given orally to rats, phanoside (40 and 80 mg/ml) improved glucose tolerance and enhanced plasma insulin levels at hyperglycemia [46].

3-Hydroxy-3-methylglutaric Acid from *Tillandsia usneoides*

3-Hydroxy-3-methylglutaric acid was isolated from the water soluble fraction of *T. usneoides* L. (Spanish Moss) (Bromeliaceae) and it has been shown to be hypoglycaemic in fasting healthy mice [47].

Bakuchiol from *Otholobium pubescens*

Oral administration of bakuchiol, a compound isolated from an extract of *O. pubescens* (Cupressaceae) reduced glycaemia in db/db mice in a dose-dependent fashion. In a new model of type 2 diabetes (fat-fed, streptozotocin treated rats) an oral dose of 150 mg/kg produced a strong reduction in blood glucose and triglycerides levels [48].

Kolaviron from *Garcinia kola*

Kolaviron, a mixture of C-3/C-8 linked biflavonoids obtained from *Garcinia kola* Heckel (Guttiferae) produced significant hypoglycaemic effects when administered intraperitoneally to healthy and alloxan diabetic rabbits at a dose of 100 mg/kg. The fasting blood glucose in normoglycaemic rabbits was reduced from 115 mg/100 ml to 65 mg/100 ml after 4 h. In alloxan-diabetic rabbits the blood sugar was lowered at 12 h [49].

Escins from *Aesculus hippocastanum*

Five triterpene oligologlycosides named escins-Ia, Ib, IIa, IIb and IIIa were isolated from the seeds of *A. hippocastanum* L. (Common Horse-Chestnut) plant (Hippocastanaceae). These compounds showed hypoglycaemic activity. Greater hypoglycaemic activities were obtained with escins IIa and IIb [50].

Fagomine, 4-O-β-D-glucopyranosylfagomine, 3-O-β-D-glucopyranosyl fagomine and 3-epifagomine from *Xanthocercis zambesiaca*

Four compounds, structurally related nitrogen-containing sugars (fagomine, 4-O-β-D-glucopyranosylfagomine, 3-O-β-D-glucopyranosylfagomine, and 3-epifagomine) were isolated from the aqueous methanolic extract of the leaves and root of *X. zambesiaca* (Leguminosae) and were evaluated for antihyperglycaemic effects in streptozotocin-induced diabetic mice. Glycaemia fell after i.p. injection of the extract (50 mg/kg). These four compounds reduced the blood glucose level after i.p. injection (150 μM/kg). Fagomine increased plasma insulin levels in diabetic mice and potentiated the 8.3-μM glucose-induced insulin release from the rat isolated-perfused pancreas. The fagomine induced potentiation of insulin release may contribute in part to its antihyperglycaemic action [51].

Masoprocol from *Larrea tridentote*

Masoprocol (nordihydroguaiaretic acid, a lipoxygenase inhibitor) is a pure compound isolated from *L. tridentata* (Creosote bush) (Zygophyllaceae). The oral administration of masoprocol produced a fall in the plasma glucose concentrations in two mouse models of type 2 diabetes;without any change in plasma insulin concentrations. In addition, oral glucose tolerance improved and the ability of insulin to lower plasma glucose concentrations was accentuated in masoprocol-treated db/db mice [51].

Leuropeoside from *Olea europea*

Leuropeoside isolated from *Olea europea* (Oleaceae) olive leaf, showed activity at a dose of 16 mg/kg. This compound also demonstrated antidiabetic activity in animals with alloxan induced diabetes. The hypoglycaemic activity of this compound may result from two mechanisms: (a) potentiation of glucose-induced insulin release, and (b) increased peripheral uptake of glucose [53].

Senegin-II, Senegasaponins and Desmethoxysenegin from *Polygala senega*

A triterpenoid glycoside named senegin II was isolated from *Polygala senega* (L.) var. *Latifolia* Torrey and Gray. Senega radix, (Polygalaceae) and identified as the active component for the hypoglycaemic effect of this plant [54].

E-senegasaponins a, b and c were isolated from the root of Senega radix. Their isomers include, Z-senegasaponins a, b, and c. The E and Z-senegasaponins a and b were found to be hypoglycaemic in the oral D-glucose tolerance test in rats [55].

Other bioactive saponins Z-senegasaponin c, were isolated from the roots of *P. senega* together with Z-senegins II, III and IV. The E and Z-senegasaponins c and E and Z-senegins II, III, and IV were also found to exhibit hypoglycaemic activity in the oral D-glucose tolerance test. E and Z-senegins II also showed an inhibitory effect on alcohol absorption in rats [56].

The effect of four triterpenoid glycosides isolated from the rhizomes of *P. senega*, senegins II-IV and desmethoxysenegin II were tested in healthy and KK-Ay mice. Senegins II and III reduced the blood glucose of healthy mice 4 h after intraperitoneal administration and also significantly lowered the glucose level of KK-Ay mice under similar conditions. Senegin IV and desmethoxysenegin II, as well as senegose A, an oligosaccharide ester, were inactive when tested in healthy mice [57].

Discussion and Conclusion

Diabetes is a metabolic disorder which can be considered as a major cause of high economic loss which can in turn impede the development of nations. Moreover, uncontrolled diabetes leads to many chronic complications such as blindness, heart failure and renal failure. In order to prevent this alarming health problem, the development of research into new hypoglycaemic and potentially antidiabetic agents is of great interest.

This review confirms the benefits of medicinal plants and their role in the management of diabetes mellitus. Numerous mechanisms of action have been proposed for these constituents. While, some hypotheses relate to the effect on the activity of pancreatic β cells (synthesis, release, cell regeneration/revitalization), or the increase in the protective/inhibitory effect against insulinase and the increase of the insulin sensitivity or the insulin-like activity, other mechanisms may involve improved glucose homeostasis (increase of peripheral utilization of glucose), increase of synthesis of hepatic glycogen and/or decrease of glycogenolysis acting on enzymes, inhibition of intestinal glucose absorption, reduction of glycaemic index of carbohydrates and the reduction of the effect of glutathione. All of these actions may be responsible for the reduction and or abolition of diabetic complications.

In conclusion, this paper has presented a list of anti-diabetic phytoconstituents used in the treatment of diabetes mellitus. Many new bioactive drugs isolated from plants showed antidiabetic activity equal to and sometimes even more potent than known oral hypoglycaemic agents such as daonil, tolbutamide and chlorpropamide. However, many other antidiabetic compounds obtained from plants have not been well characterized. Further investigations must be carried out to evaluate the mechanism of action of these constituents coupled with in-depth toxicity studies. Out of an estimated 250, 000 higher plants, less than 1 per cent have been screened pharmacologically and very few with regard to diabetes mellitus. The goal of medicine, no matter, to which group it belongs, remains the same *i.e.* the welfare of the patient. One can look forward to integrated medicine and hope that research in alternative medicine will help identify that which is safe and effective rather than marginalizing, unorthodox medical claims and findings.

References

1. Patel M, Jamrozik K, Allen O, Martin FI, Eng J, Dean B: A high prevalence of diabetes in a rural village in Papua New Guinea. *Diabetes Res Clin Pract,* 1986, **2,** 97-103.
2. Rao PV, Ushabala P, Seshiah V, Ahuja MM, Mather HM: The Eluru survey: prevalence of known diabetes in a rural Indian population. *Diabetes Res Clin Pract,* 1989, 5, 29-31.
3. Verma NP, Mehta SP, Madhu S, Mather HM, Keen H: Prevalence of known diabetes in an urban Indian environment: the Darya Ganj diabetes survey. *Br Med J,* 1986, **293,** 423-424.
4. Oubre AY, Carlson TJ, King SR, Reaven GM: From plant to patient: an ethnomedical approach to the identification of new drugs for the treatment of NIDDM. *Diabetologia,* 1997, **40,** 614-617.
5. Alarcon-Aguilara FJ, Roman-Ramos R, Perez-Gutierrez S, Aguilar-Contreras A, Contreras-Weber CC, Flores-Saenz JL, Study of the anti-hyperglycemic effect of plants used as antidiabetics. *J Ethnopharmacol,* 1998, **61,** 101–110.
6. Atta-Ur-Rahman, Zaman K: Medicinal plants with hypoglycemic activity. *J Ethnopharmacol,* 1989, **20,** 553-564.
7. Marles RJ, Farnsworth NR: Antidiabetic plants and their active constituents. *Phytomedicine,* 1995, 2, 137-189.
8. Bailey CJ, Day C, Turner SL, Leatherdale BA: Cerasee, a traditional treatment for diabetes. Studies in normal and streptozotocin diabetic mice. *Diabetes Res,* 1985, **2,** 81-84.
9. Hassall CH, Reyle K: Hypoglycin A and B, two biologically active polypeptides from *Blighia sapida, Biochem J* 1955, 60, 334-339.

10. Lolitkar MM, Rao MRR: Pharmacology of a hypoglycaemic principle isolated from the fruits of *Eugenia jambolana* Linn. *Ind J Pharm*, 1966, **28**, 129-133.

11. Khanna P, Jain SC, Panagariya A, Dixit VP: Hypoglycaemic activity of polypeptide-p from a plant source. *J Nat Prod* 1981, **44**, 648-655.

12. Matsuda H, Li Y, Murakami T, Matsumura N, Yamahara J, Yoshikawa M: Antidiabetic principles of natural medicines. III. Structure-related inhibitory activity and action mode of oleanolic acid glycosides on hypoglycemic activity. *Chem Pharm Bull (Tokyo)* 1998, **46**, 1399-1403.

13. Murakami N, Murakami T, Kadoya M, Matsuda H, Yamahara J, Yoshikawa M: New hypoglycemic constituents in gymnemic acid from *Gymnema sylvestre*. *Chem Pharm Bull (Tokyo)*, 1996, **44**, 469-471.

14. Shimizu K, Iino A, Nakajima J, Tanaka K, Nakajyo S, Urakawa N, Atsuchi M, Wada T, Yamashita C: Suppression of glucose absorption by some fractions extracted from *Gymnema sylvestre* leaves. *J Vet Med Sci* 1997, **59**, 245-251.

15. Yoshikawa M, Murakami T, Kadoya M, Li Y, Murakami N, Yamahara J, Matsuda H: Medicinal foodstuffs. IX. The inhibitors of glucose absorption from the leaves of *Gymnema sylvestre* R.BR. (Asclepiadaceae): structures of gymnemosides a and b. *Chem Pharm Bull (Tokyo)*, 1997, **45**, 1671-1676.

16. Petricic J, Kalodera Z: Galegin in the goats rue herb: its toxicity, antidiabetic activity and content determination. *Acta Pharm Jugosl* 1982, 32, 219-223.

17. Sheehan EW, Zemaitis MA, Slatkin DJ, Schiff PL: A constituent of *Pterocarpus marsupium*, (–)-epicatechin, as a potential antidiabetic agent. *J Nat Prod* 1983, **46**, 232-234.

18. Manickam M, Ramanathan M, Jahromi MA, Chansouria JP, Ray AB: Antihyperglycemic activity of phenolics from *Pterocarpus marsupium*. *J Nat Prod* 1997, **60**, 609-610.

19. Haranath PSRK, Haranath, RK, Anjaneyulu CR, Ramanathan JD: Studies on the hypoglycemic and pharmacological actions of some stilbenes. *Indian J Med Sci* 1958, **12**, 85-89.

20. Joglekar GV, Chaudhary NY, Aiaman R: Effect of Indian medicinal plants on glucose absorption in mice. *Indian J Physiol Pharmacol* 1959, **3**, 76-77.

21. Augusti KT, Daniel RS, Cherian S, Sheela CG, Nair CR: Effect of leucopelargonin derivative from *Ficus bengalenesis* Linn. on diabetic dogs. *Ind J Med Res* 1994, **99**, 82-86.

22. Cherian S, Augusti KT: Antidiabetic effects of a glycoside of leucopelargonidin isolated from *Ficus bengalenesis* Linn. *Indian J Exp Biol* 1993, **31**, 26-29.

23. Kumar RV, Augusti KT: Insulin sparing action of a leucocyanidin derivative isolated from *Ficus bengalenesis* Linn. *Indian J Biochem Biophys* 1994, **31**, 73-76.

24. Geetha BS, Mathew BC, Augusti KT: Hypoglycemic effects of leucodelphinidin derivative isolated from *Ficus bengalenesis* (Linn.) *Indian J Physiol Pharmacol* 1994, **38**, 220-222.

25. Cherian S, Kumar RV, Augusti KT, Kidwai JR: Antidiabetic effect of a glycoside of pelargonidin isolated from the bark of *Ficus bengalenesis* Linn. *Indian J Biochem Biophys* 1992, **29**, 380-382.

26. Kumar GP, Sudheesh S, Vijayalakshmi NR: Hypoglycaemic effect of *Coccinia indica*: mechanism of action. *Planta Med* 1993, **59**, 330-332.

27. Kumari K, Mathew BC, Augusti KT: Antidiabetic and hypolipidemic effects of *S*-methyl cysteine sulfoxide isolated from *Allium cepa* Linn. *Indian J Biochem Biophys* 1995, **32**, 49-54.

28. Sheela CG, Kumud K, Augusti KT: Anti-diabetic effects of onion and garlic sulfoxide amino acids in rats. *Planta Med* 1995, **61**, 356-357.

29. Roman-Ramos R, Flores-Saenz JL, Alarcon-Aguilar FJ: Anti-hyperglycaemic effect of some edible plants. *J Ethnopharmacol* 1995, **48**, 25-32.

30. Sheela CG, Augusti KT: Antidiabetic effects of *S*-allyl cysteine sulphoxide isolated from garlic *Allium sativum* Linn. *Indian J Exp Biol* 1992, **30**, 523-526.

31. Augusti KT, Sheela CG: Antiperoxide effect of *S*-allyl cysteine sulfoxide, an insulin secretagogue, in diabetic rats. *Experientia* 1996, **52**, 115-120.

32. Yoshikawa M, Murakami T, Kadoya M, Matsuda H, Muraoka O, Yamahara J, Murakami N: Medicinal foodstuff. III. Sugar beet. Hypoglycemic oleanolic acid oligoglycosides, betavulgarosides I, II, III, and IV, from the root of *Beta vulgaris* L. (Chenopodiaceae) *Chem Pharm. Bull (Tokyo)*, 1996, **44**, 1212-1217.

33. Fuentes NL, Sagua H, Morales G, Borquez J, San Martin A, Soto J, Loyola LA: Experimental antihyperglycemic effect of diterpenoids of *llareta Azorella compacta* (Umbelliferae) Phil in rats. *Phytother Res* 2005, 19, 713-716.

34. Sauvaire Y, Petit P, Broca C, Manteghetti M, Baissac Y, Fernandez-Alvarez J, Gross R, Roye M, Leconte A, Gomis R, Ribes G : 4-Hydroxyisoleucine: a novel amino acid potentiator of insulin secretion. *Diabetes* 1998, **47**, 206-210.

35. Yoshikawa M, Murakami T, Yashiro K, Matsuda H: Kotalanol, a potent alpha-glucosidase inhibitor with thiosugar sulfonium sulfate structure, from antidiabetic Ayurvedic medicine *Salacia reticulata*. *Chem Pharm Bull (Tokyo)*, 1998, **46**, 1339-1340.

36. Matsuda H, Murakami T, Yashiro K, Yamahara J, Yoshikawa M: Antidiabetic principles of natural medicines. IV. Aldose reductase and alpha-glucosidase inhibitors from the roots of *Salacia oblonga* Wall. (Celastraceae): structure of a new friedelane-type triterpene, kotalagenin 16-acetate. *Chem Pharm Bull (Tokyo)*, 1999, **47**, 1725-1729.

37. Raghunathan B, Sharma PV: Effect of *Tinospora cordifolia* Miers (*Guduchi*) on alloxan induced hyperglycaemia. *J Res Indian Med* 1969, 3, 203-209.

38. Narayanan CR, Joshi DD, Mudjumdar AM, Dhekne VV: Pinitol, a new anti-diabetic compound from the leaves of *Bougainvillea spectabilis*. *Curr Sci* 1987, 56, 139-141.

39. Saleem R, Ahmad M, Hussain SA, Qazi AM, Ahmad SI, Qazi MH, Ali M, Faizi S, Akhtar S, Hussein SN: Hypotensive, hypoglycemic and toxicological studies on the flavonol C-glycoside shamimin from *Bombax ceiba*. *Planta Med* 1999, **65**, 331-334.

40. Choi SZ, Lee So, Jang Ku, Chung Sh, Park Sh, Kang HC, Yang EY, Cho HJ, Lee KR: Antidiabetic stilbene and anthraquinone derivatives from *Rheum undulatum*. *Arch Pharm Res* 2005, 28, 1027-1030.

41. Bajpai MB, Asthana RK, Sharma NK, Chatterjee SK, Mukherjee SK: Hypoglycemic effect of Swerchirin from the hexane fraction of *Swertia chirayita*. *Planta Med* 1991, **57**, 102-104.

42. Saxena AM, Bajpai MB, Mukherjee SK: Swerchirin induced blood sugar lowering of streptozotocin treated hyperglycemic rats. *Indian J Exp Biol* 1991, **29**, 674-675.

43. Saxena AM, Bajpai MB, Murthy PS, Mukherjee SK: Mechanism of blood sugar lowering by a Swerchirin-containing hexane fraction (SWI) of *Swertia chirayita*. *Indian J Exp Biol* 1993, **31**, 178-181.

44. Vartanian GS, Parsadanian GK, Karagezian KG: Effect of trihydroxyoctadecadiene acids from Bryonia alba L. on the activity of glycogen metabolism enzymes in alloxan diabetes. *Biull Eksp Biol Med* 1984, 97, 295-297.

45. Contreras C, Roman R, Perez C, Alarcon F, Zavala M, Perez S: Hypoglycemic activity of a new carbohydrate isolated from the roots of *Psacalium peltatum*. *Chem Pharm Bull* (*Tokyo*), 2005, 53, 1408-1410.

46. Ake N, Nguyen KH, Edvards L, Dao VP, Nguyen DT, Hans JR, Rannar S, Claes-Goran OS: A novel insulin-releasing substance, Phanoside, from the plant *Gynostemma pentaphyllum*, *J Biol Chem* 2004, 279, 41361-41367.

47. Witherup KM, McLaughlin JL, Judd RL, et al: Identification of 3-hydroxy-3-methyl glutaric acid (HMG) as hypoglycaemic principle of spanish moss (*Tillandsia usneoïdes*). *J Nat Prod* 1995, 58, 1285-1290.

48. Krenisky JM, Luo J, Reed MJ, Carney JR: Isolation and antihyperglycaemic activity of bakuchiol from *Otholobium pubescens* (Fabaceae), a Peruvian medicinal plant used for the treatment of diabetes. *Biol Pharm Bull* 1999, 22, 1137-1140.

49. Iwu MM, Igboko OA, Okunji CO, Tempesta MS: Antidiabetic and aldose reductase activities of biflavones of *Garcinia kola*. *J Pharm Pharmacol* 1990, 42, 290-292.

50. Yoshikawa M, Harada E, Murakami T, *et al.*: Escins-Ia, Ib, IIa, IIb and IIIa bioactive triterpene oligoglycosides from the seeds of *Aesculus hippocastanum* L: Their inhibitory effects on ethanol absorption, and hypoglycaemic activity on glucose tolerance test. *Chem Pharm Bull* (*Tokyo*), 1994, 42, 1357-1359.

51. Nojima H, Kimura I, Chen FJ, *et al.*: Antihyperglycaemic effects of N-containing sugars from *Xanthocecis zambesiaca*, *Morus bombycis*, *Aglaenema treubii* and *Castanospermum autrale* in streptozotocin-diabetic mice. *J Nat Prod* 1998, 61, 397-400

52. Luo J, Chuang J, Cheung J, *et al.*: Masoprocol (nordihydroguaiaretic acid): A new antihyperglycaemic agent isolated from the creosote bush (*Larrea tridentata*). *Eur J Pharmacol* 1998, 346, 77-79.

53. Gonzalez M, Zarzuelo A, Gamez MJ, Utrilla MP, Jimenez J, Osuna I: Hypoglycaemic activity of olive leaf. *Planta Med*, 1992, 58, 513-515.

54. Kako M, Miura T, Nishiyama Y, *et al.*: Hypoglycaemic effect of the rhizomes of *Polygala senega* in normal and diabetic mice and its main component, the triterpenoid glycoside senegin-II, *Planta Med*, 1996, 62, 440-443.

55. Yoshikawa M, Murakami T, Ueno T, *et al.*: Bioactive saponins and glycosides. I. *Senegae radix*. (1): Esenegasaponins a and b and Z-senegasaponins a and b, their inhibitory effect on alcohol absorption and hypoglycaemic activity. *Chem Pharm Bull (Tokyo)*, 1995, 43, 2115-2122.

56. Yoshikawa M, Murakami T, Matsuda H, *et al.*: Bioactive saponins and glycosides. II. *Senegae radix*. (2): Chemical structures and hypoglycaemic activity, and ethanol absorption inhibitory effect of Esenegasaponin c, Z-senegasaponins c, and Z-senegins II, III and IV. *Chem Pharm Bull (Tokyo)*, 1996, 44, 1305-1313.

57. Kako M, Miura T, Nishiyama Y, Ichimaru M, Moriyasu M, Kato A: Hypoglycaemic activity of some triterpenoid glycosides. *J Nat Prod* 1997, 60, 604-605.

Chapter 15

Scientific Evaluation of Traditional Medicine: Ethnopharmacology, Reverse Pharmacology, System Biology to Metabolomics

***Palpu Pushpangadan*[1], *R. Govindarajan*[2], *S.K. Srivastava*[2], *Ch.V. Rao*[2], *K. Narayanan Nair*[2], *A.K.S. Rawat*[2], *Shanta Mehrotra*[2], *A.K. Sharma*[3], *S. Rajasekharan*[4], *V. George*[4] and *P.G. Latha*[4]**

[1]*Amity Institute for Herbal and Biotech Products Development, VRA-173, Mannamoola, Peroorkada P.O., Trivandrum – 695 005, Kerala*

[2]*National Botanical Research Institute, Lucknow, U.P.*

[3]*Forest Research Institute, Dehradun, Uttaranchal*

[4]*Tropical Botanic Garden and Research Institute, Trivandrum – 695 562, Kerala*

The efforts to heal ailments and the desire to attain vitality and longevity prompted mankind from the very beginning to explore his natural surroundings. By trial, error, empirical reasoning or even experimentation the early man selected a number of therapeutic agents, mainly from plants and at times from animals and minerals for treating various ailments or to feel good. Innovative and creative members of succeeding generations have both incrementally improved the existing remedies and/or added new remedies. All ancient cultures of the world have thus evolved their own medical lore and practices which became the ethnomedical traditions or traditional medical wisdom of those cultures. In many eastern cultures such as those in India and China these experiences were systematically recorded and organized into regular system of medicine that later became the Materia Medica of these countries[1]. Traditional systems of medicine in India function via two streams, *viz.* the codified written traditions known as classical systems of medicine, such as Ayurveda, Siddha, Unani and Amchi, practiced mainly by the urban or elite group of society, and the oral tradition, also known as the 'Local health traditions' (LHT), which are, perhaps, very rich and diverse and practiced by traditional rural physicians (vaidyas), folk healers or tribal physicians.

Traditional Medicine and its Decline

The term Traditional Medicine (TM) is a heterogenous one that refers to the broad range of natural healthcare practices which existed before the emergence of modern scientific methods of healthcare in the 19th century.

However, all those systems of medicine that evolved before 19th century which continued to be practiced even after the emergence of modern medicine could be termed as TM[2]. World Health Organization (WHO) defined TM as the sum total of knowledge, skill and practices based on the theories, beliefs and experiences of different indigenous cultures, whether explicable or not, used in the maintenance of health and in the prevention, diagnosis, improvement or treatment of physical and mental illness or maintain wellbeing[3]. The term 'complementary medicine', 'alternative medicine' and 'non-conventional medicine' etc. are used interchangeably with traditional medicine. WHO has identified and enlisted more than 100 types of TM practices, which are currently in use throughout the world.

Until the beginning of the 19th century, all medical practices were what we now call traditional. The renaissance period brought great scientific upheavals that began to introduce Cartesian scientific materialism into all human activities and notably into the theory and practice of health care. Its method was to break up complex phenomena into their component parts and to deal with each one in isolation. This approach resulted in the search for a single cause for the diseases and correspondingly the modern pharmacological investigations were aimed at finding a single active principle that could be isolated from the medicinal plants. The introduction of this kind of abstract medicine in the from of basic chemicals and pharmaceuticals during the 18th and the 19th centuries has demonstrated methods for bringing quick relief in sufferings and had won instant admiration and popularity. This system known as allopathy or modern medicine made rapid advances during the 19th and 20th centuries as a result of the advances made in physical, biological, chemical and pharmacological sciences. New discoveries of sulfa drugs, synthetics, antibiotics, cortisones and other therapeutic agents emerged in quick succession and swept all other systems of medicine off their feet. Allopathic medicine is however expensive and available only to the affluent. The World Health Organization has estimated that 80 per cent of the world population relies on traditional medicine for primary health care. The Chiang Mai declaration of the health professionals and conservation specialists reaffirmed the WHO declaration of "Health for all by the year 2000" through the primary health care approach and emphasized the vital importance of Traditional Medicine in achieving this goal.

Revival of TM

20th century demonstrated the tremendous success of modern medical sciences, particularly in diagnosis, treatment and surgical measures of a number of diseases that were regarded as incurable in the past. Direct intervention through technological and molecular means has now become possible. Humankind is now harvesting the full benefit of the progress of modern medical science and technology. But we are also equally conscious about the inadequacy of modern medicine in dealing with many metabolic and degenerative disorders and other such ailments associated with old age. Also modern medicines have very strong side effects, high costs, and are not accessible to majority of human population. The oriental systems of TM have satisfactory management and even cure for many such ailments. Thus towards the end of 20th century there began a revival of interest in TM.

According to a survey conducted by WHO, the use of plant remedies is on the increase even in the developed countries especially among younger generation. In the industrialized countries, the consumers are seeking visible alternatives to modern medicine with its associated dangers of side effects and over medication. The leading US newspaper New York times dated 28.2.'03 reported that side effects of drugs kill more Americans annually than the World War II and Vietnam War combined. Investigations have revealed that in the US 51 per cent of FDA approved drugs have serious adverse effects not detected prior to their approval and that over 1.5 million people are sufficiently injured by prescription drugs annually that they require hospitalization[4]. Once in hospitals, the problem may be compounded. The incidence of serious and fatal adverse drug reaction (ADRs) in US hospitals is now ranked as between the 4th and the 6th leading causes of death in United States next to heart diseases, cancer, pulmonary diseases and accidents. The promotive and preventive aspects prevalent in oriental medicine, especially in the Indian (Ayurveda, Siddha, Unani and Amchi), and Chinese Systems of medicine are finding increasing popularity and acceptance in the developed countries. During the last decade, WHO's Health Assembly has passed a number of resolutions in response to such a resurgence of interest in the study and use of traditional medicine.

The mechanisation and undue objectification of human life and health care systems of the present era have culminated to an extreme excess between physician and patient by the interpolation of a third entirely mechanical thing, the machine, replacing the creative synthesizing role of the traditional physicians. This has resulted in the dehumanization of the medical system. In contrast to this scenario of the modern medicine, the traditional medicine attempts to embody a holistic approach *i.e.* viewing an individual in his totality within society and the ecological environment. It emphasizes the view point that ill health or disease is brought about by an imbalance or disequilibrium of man's physiological, psychological, behaviourial, ecological and spiritual environment and not just by an external pathogenic agent, be it a micro-organism or otherwise. No doubt, the modern medicine has accomplished great strides in developing many new life saving drugs. Modern health care system stressed more on the curative and to a lesser extent to the preventive aspects of diseases and very little has been done on the health promotive aspects. Problems of health have been replaced by problems of drugs and diseases. Instead of medicine for man, we have men for medicine. Modern medicine may help man to provide apparent physical health but is devoid of mental, social and spiritual health. Modern medicine is more concerned with the cure of disease but remains indifferent to health preservation. It is in this context that the relevance of the holistic approach of the traditional health care practice becomes important. There have been an ever increasing production and consumption of phytomedicines based on various traditional systems of medicine both in the developing and developed countries. A steady global market for many such herbal products is emerging.

Genesis of the Subject Ethnopharmacology

Ethnopharmacology as a scientific term was first introduced at an international symposium held at San Francisco in 1967 (Efron *et al.*, 1967)[5]. This was used while discussing the theme 'Traditional Psychoactive drugs' in this Symposium. But later Rivier and Bruhn (1979)[6] made an attempt to define Ethnopharmacology as "a multidisciplinary area of research concerned with observation, description and experimental investigation of indigenous drugs and their biological activities. It was later redefined by Bruhn and Holmstedt (1981)[7] as "The interdisciplinary scientific exploration of biologically active agents traditionally employed or observed by man". In its entirety, pharmacology embraces the knowledge of the history, source, chemical and physical properties, compounding, biochemical and physiological effects, mechanism of action, absorption, distribution, biotransformation, excretion and therapeutic and other uses of drugs. A drug is broadly defined as any substance (chemical agent) that affects life processes. Therefore, briefly, the main component of ethnopharmacology may be defined as pharmacology of drugs used in ethnomedicine[8]. The authors however felt that none of the above said definition captures the true spirit of this interdisciplinary subject. The authors, therefore, preferred to state the following. Ethno–(Gr., culture or people) pharmacology (Gr., drug) is about the intersection of medical ethnography and the biology of therapeutic action, *i.e.*, a transdisciplinary exploration that spans the biological and social sciences. This suggests that ethnopharmacologists are professionally cross-trained–for example, in pharmacology and anthropology–or that ethnopharmacological research is the product of collaborations among individuals whose formal training includes two or more traditional disciplines. In fact, very little of what is published as ethnopharmacology meets these criteria.

Nyman (1995)[9] has suggested that the objectives of Ethnopharmacology should focus on (1) the basic research aiming at giving rational explanation to how a traditional medicine works, and (2) the applied research aiming at developing a traditional medicine into a modern medicine (Pharmacotherapy) or to develop its original usage by modern methods (Phytotherapy).

The scientific evaluation and standardization of traditional remedies using exclusively the parameters of the modern medicine is both conceptually wrong and unethical. Evaluation of traditional remedies particularly those of the classical traditions has to be based on the theoretical and conceptual foundation of these classical systems of medicine, but may utilize the advancements made in modern scientific knowledge, tools and technology. In fact it is important to combine the best of elements of concept and practice from traditional medicines and modern medicines with the objective to improve the health care system of humankind. Such an integrated approach to study and develop holistic health care system is termed as the Ethnopharmacological approach. The concept of Ethnopharmacology research in India evolved in 1980s independently of this international initiative.

Ethnopharmacology research in India was initiated at Regional Research Laboratory (RRL), Jammu in 1985 by the then Director Dr. C.K. Atal along with his student Dr. P. Pushpangadan, the then chief coordinator of All India Co-ordinated

Project on Ethnopharmacology (AICRPE) and the senior author of this communication. Dr. Atal, however left RRL in mid 80s. But Dr.Pushpangadan and his students, colleagues and a few other enthusiasts, notably Dr. A.K. Sharma, Dr. S. Rajasekharan, Dr. V.George, Dr. P.G.Latha, Dr. K. Narayanan Nair, Dr. B.G. Nagavi, Shri. P.R. Krishna Kumar etc. continued their effort to develop ethnopharmacology research. They observed that subjecting the traditional herbal remedies including the remedies of the classical systems like Ayurveda, Siddha and Unani to the parameters of modern medicine is not only foolish, but suicidal. Both these systems are conceptually quite different. The concept of disease, its etiology, manifestation and approach to treatment etc. are all viewed on a holistic basis contrary to the reductionistic approach of modern medicine. Only an integrated approach that combines the best of theory, concepts and methods of the classical systems of medicine such as Ayurveda, Siddha and Unani with the modern scientific knowledge (Phytochemistry and Pharmacology), tools and technology can bring in the desired results.

The concept and methods of Ethnopharmacology research thus developed by the authors contain experts from diverse disciplines like Ayurveda, Siddha, scholars of Sanskrit and Tamil languages (who can correctly interpret the classical texts of Ayurveda and also its theoretical basis like 'Sankhya' and 'Vaiseshika' philosophy), ethnobotany/ethnomedicine, chemistry, pharmacognosy, pharmacology, biochemistry, molecular biology and pharmacy etc. The main objective of this approach was to develop appropriate techniques to evaluate the traditional remedies in line with the classical concepts of Ayurvedic pharmacy and pharmacology such as the 'Rasa', 'Guna', 'Veerya', 'Vipaka' and 'Prabhava', in other words 'Samagrah Guna' of the 'Draya Guna' concept of Ayurveda. The senior author was successful in convincing Prof. M.G.K. Menon way back in 1985 who then agreed to be the Chief Patron of the newly formed National Society of Ethnopharmacology. This society was formally registered in 1986 with the senior author as its first founder president. The first ethnopharmacology laboratory started functioning at Regional Research Laboratory, Jammu under the All India Coordinated Research Project on Ethnobiology (AICRPE) funded by the Ministry of Environment and Forest, Govt. of India. However, the first full fledged Ethnopharmacology Division was started in 1992 at Tropical Botanic Garden and Research Institute (TBGRI) where the author joined in 1990 as its Director. At TBGRI the team could successfully demonstrate the integrated approach and could develop novel scientifically verified standardized herbal drugs. Some herbal drugs developed at TBGRI after filing patents were released for commercial production. The Ethnopharmacology Society in association with TBGRI and with the financial assistance of DANIDA organized the first National Conference on Ethnopharmacology in Trivandrum, Kerala from 24th to 26th May 1993. Selected papers in this conference were compiled and published as 'Glimpses of Indian Ethnopharmacology' in 1995. The second national conference of Ethnopharmacology was organized at J.S.S College of Pharmacy, Mysore in 1997 and the third at Pankaj Kasthuri Ayurveda College, Trivandrum in 2004 and the 4th at Amala Cancer Research Institute, Thrissur in 2006. In 1999 Feb. the senior author moved from TBGRI, Trivandrum to National Botanical Research Institute (NBRI) Lucknow, a pioneer plant research institute under the umbrella of Council of Scientific and Industrial

Research (CSIR). International Society of Ethnopharmacology in association with National Society of Ethnopharmacology and National Botanical Research Institute (NBRI) have organized the Vth International Congress on Ethnopharmacology in November, 1999 at NBRI, Lucknow. At NBRI, the senior author has established a state of the art model of Ethnopharmacology laboratory and Herbal Product Development division where the latest analytical techniques such as HPTLC, High-Through put analysis, activity guided isolation techniques and similar other innovative new techniques in validating, formulating and standardizing the herbal products etc. were introduced.

Evidence Based Medicine (EBM) or Scientific Medicine

Evidence based medicine is the goal of modern medicine. The scientific world is looking for rational evidence of the therapeutic claims of drugs. Generally a reductionist approach is employed to prove the safety and therapeutic efficacy. This means studying the activity on known targets using receptor binding assays. However, we know that this approach has also got its limitation since no single active compound can adequately explain the clinical activity. A reason could be that synergism and pro drug cannot be detected by such reductionist approach and only an *in vivo* system biology approach alone could detect such activity.

The term 'evidence-based medicine' first appeared in the medical literature in a paper by Guyatt *et al.*, in 1992[10]. Generally there are three distinct areas of EBM. The first is to treat individual patients with acute and chronic pathologies by treatments supported in the most scientifically valid medical literature. According to the Centre for Evidence-Based Medicine, "Evidence-based medicine is the conscientious, explicit and judicious use of current best evidence in making decisions about the care of patients"[11,12]. The term "evidence based medicine" has gained substantial currency over the past few years and it has been described as a "paradigm shift" that will eventually "change medical practice of future"[13,14]. Thus, medical practitioners would select treatment options for specific cases based on the best research for each patient they treat. The second area is the systematic review of medical literature to evaluate the best studies on specific topics. This process can be very human-centred, as in a journal club, or highly technical using computer programmes for information techniques such as data mining. Increased use of information technology turns large volumes of information into practical guides. Finally evidence-based medicine can be understood as a 'medical movement' whose advocates work to popularize the method and usefulness of the practice in the public.

Multi-component botanical formulations can be standardized with newer technique such as DNA fingerprinting, High Performance Thin Layer Chromatography (HPTLC), liquid chromatography-mass spectroscopy etc.[15]. However, clinical studies of herbal medicine are more important for validating drug safety. Also suitable study in animal models will help in understanding the mechanisms of action or pharmacodynamics of the drug. However, for bringing more objectivity and also to confirm traditional claims, systematic clinical trials are necessary.

Evidence-based medicine categorize different types of clinical evidence and ranks them according to the strength of their freedom from the various biases that beset medical research. For example, the strongest evidence for therapeutic interventions is provided by systematic review of randomized, double blind, placebo controlled trials involving a homogenous patient population and medical condition. In contrast, patient testimonials, case reports and even expert opinion have little value as proof because of the placebo effect, the biases inherent in observation and reporting of cases, difficulties in ascertaining who is an expert, and more. Practicing evidence based medicine requires not only clinical expertise but also expertise in retrieving, interpreting and applying the results of scientific studies and in communicating the risks and benefits of different course of action to patients.

There is another school who believes that those traditional drugs having long history of clinical evidence do not require another clinical study/trial, but what is required is to provide a clinical toxicity study to ensure it is safe and a pharmacological evidence for the therapeutics (pharmacodynamics elucidating the therapeutic action).

Reverse Pharmacology

Reverse Pharmacology[16] is the term used in the scientific elucidation of the pharmacological action of the clinically proven/time tested traditional remedies. Ethnopharmacology is also considered to be a time saving cost effective method of new drug discovery. The classical drug discovery has become a very complex, capital-intensive and time taking process in spite of the technological support like High Throughput Screening (HTS) and combinatorial chemical synthesis etc. The pharmaceutical companies who invested in such drug discovery processes could not reap rewards in new lead discovery as expected.

Traditional medicine like Ayurveda, Siddha and Unani are in use for over hundreds of years and therefore clinical existence comes as a presumption. However, for bringing more objectivity and also to confirm traditional claims, systematic clinical trials are necessary. In Ayurvedic Medicine research, clinical experience, observations or available data becomes the starting point. In conventional drug research, it comes at the end. Thus the drug discovery based on Ayurveda follows a 'reverse pharmacology' path. Herbal drugs should also need to conform to the global standards such as dissolution time, microbial, pesticidal and heavy metal contaminations etc.

Reverse pharmacology comprises of three stages–experimental, exploratory and experimental[17]. Possessed with a pluralistic healthcare, India offers a goldmine for robust documentation of clinical observations of bio-dynamic effects of standardized traditional drugs. The exploratory studies would cover dose-activity in ambulant patients and in selected *in-vitro* and *in-vivo* models to evaluate the key target. These exploratory leads are evaluated critically for resource allocation and state-of-the-art experimental studies. The experimental stage involving relevant basic and clinical science would be employed to study the plant or a molecule at different levels of biological organization. This would define the safety, efficacy, preventive or therapeutic dimensions of the new or natural drug.

National Botanical Research Institute (NBRI), Lucknow in association with Deenadayal Research Institute (DRI) Chithrakoot organized a National workshop on "Ayurveda Research Scenario-challenges and opportunities and prospects for Excellence" from 24th to 26th May 2003 at Chithrakoot. The deliberations of this workshop led to various recommendations known as Chithrakoot declaration. Dr. R.A. Mashelkar, the then DG, CSIR, while presenting the declaration mentioned the concept of Golden triangle in which the traditional drugs, modern science/modern medicine are interlinked synergistically for new drug discovery and development[18]. Later, CSIR jointly with the Dept. of Ayurveda, Yoga and Naturopathy, Unani, Siddha and Homeopathy (AYUSH) and Indian Council of Medical Research (ICMR) launched a research programme under the 'Golden Triangle' concept. In this initiative the Department of AYUSH gives technical guidance regarding formulations to be used. CSIR carries out the preclinical studies on the formulations (suggested by AYUSH) and ICMR conducts the clinical trials. The objectives of the programme are[19]

1. To develop safe and effective standardized Ayurvedic products for the identified disease conditions.
2. To develop new Ayurvedic and plant based products effective in disease conditions of national/global importance.
3. To develop mechanism to make products affordable in the domestic market.
4. To use appropriate technologies for development of single and polyherbal products to make it globally acceptable.
5. To develop potential patentable products.

The fourteen areas of priority envisaged under this partnership are Rasayana, Joint disorders, Memory disorders, Menopausal syndrome, Bronchial allergy, Fertility and infertility, Cardiac disorders (cardioprotective and anti-atherosclerosis), Sleep disorders, Irritable Bowel Syndrome, Vision disorders, Urolithiasis and Benign Prostate Hypertrophy (BPH), Malaria/Filaria/Leishmaniasis, Diabetes and Bhasma toxicity. With regard to regulation of the plant based drugs ICMR has brought out ethical guidelines which would soon be legislated through a bill for Promotion and Regulation of Biomedical Research[19].

The reverse approach in pharmacology has been quite successfully applied in the past. For example, *Rauvolfia serpentina* was convincingly demonstrated to be an anti-hypertensive in 1931. But a drug, reserpine, emerged only after 20 years. This happened because the path of reverse pharmacology was random and quite discontinuous. Currently, Council of Scientific and Industrial Research (CSIR), India, through the New Millennium Indian Technology Leadership Initiative (NMITLI) has adopted the path of reverse pharmacology. The NMITLI team in the last four years has networked for R&D in a multi-institutional, multi-disciplinary endeavour to develop natural drugs for treating diabetes, arthritis and hepatitis. The results have been remarkable as to the hits and leads obtained.

Reverse pharmacology was only sporadically applied to new drug development. It is the need of the time to document unknown, unintended and desirable, novel, prophylactic and therapeutic effects in observational therapeutics. Several new classes of drugs have accidentally emerged by this path.

New Millennium Indian Technology Leadership Initiative (NMITLI) Herbal Project

Reverse pharmacology approach was adopted as a major initiative for developing standardized novel herbal formulation based on Ayurvedic wisdom and modern scientific knowledge. Under the NMITLI programme CSIR has launched a multiinstitutional programme in developing a globally acceptable herbal drug by a fast tract innovation driven method. Effective herbal drugs for treating Diabetes mellitus, Hepatitis and Arthritis have been included in this venture. Institutions that are part of CSIR Arthritis network include: ISHS, University of Pune: Central coordinating institution; CRD, Pune: clinical coordination; NBRI, Lucknow: Pharmacognosy; RRL, Jammu: Chemical profiling and advanced pharmacology; ARI, Pune: Animal pharmacology; IRSHA, Pune: In vitro Studies. For clinical studies institutes involved are: AIIMS, New Delhi; NIMS, Hyderabad; KEM and SPARC, Mumbai whereas the Industry partners include Dabur, Zandu, AVP, AVS and Nicholas Piramal[20]. The success of this initiative can be gauged by taking an example from work done under NIMITLI on Arthritis, wherein several exploratory controlled clinical drug studies on standardized Ayurveda derived herbal formulations to identify potentially promising candidates for further development and validation in rigorously designed Phases 2 and 3 clinical drug trials have been carried out. The senior author was associated with all the three NMITLI herbal drug programmes as one of its Co-ordinators.

Application of DNA Micro-arrays

The DNA array (micro array, gene array) is the latest molecular methodology applied to study the herbal medicines. The term DNA (gene) array refers to a solid surface to which is attached numerous small pieces of DNA representing short sequences of specific genes. The array may be macro-arrays which are usually fabricated membrane of nylon, or other relatively inert material, impregnated with scores or hundreds of pieces of DNA in the form of discrete spots. In contrast the micro array is usually a siliconized glass slide to which thousands of pieces of DNA fragments or oligonucleotides are precisely spotted by a robot[21] (Hudson and Altamirano 2006). Hudson and Altamirano demonstrated it in their pioneering study on DNA micro arrays that is relatively simple manipulation of cultured cells (mamalian or yeast) such as addition of fresh serum and medium could result in profound changes in the transcription profile, both qualitatively and quantitatively. This is obviously relevant to the use of herbal medicine, since the herbal drugs are mostly polyherbal mixtures comprising numerous potentially bio-active molecules, to all of which individual cells of superficial tissues might be exposed and hence modulated. Hudson and Altamirano have reviewed about 18 studies published in the period of 2001-2003 in which some form of herbal medicine has been evaluated in cell cultures or in animals, by means of DNA arrays[21]. There have been important studies on gene expression analysis, in response to herbal preparations, which involved examination of selected genes as well as gene arrays containing thousands of genes. Many of the array studies utilized Affymetrix or other commercial form of arrays or the custom prepared micro arrays on glass slides with wide variety of genes represented[21]. The science of proteomics is rapidly approaching the same level of analytical capability as genomics and soon we will be able to correlate transcription changes with protein changes for a given herbal preparation.

Ayugenomics

According to Ayurvedic concept every individual is constitutionally unique and therefore it is important to diagnose the constitutional nature ('Prakruti') of each and every individual and the prescription has to be made as per the unique constitutional nature of the patient/individual. This individualized concept and practice was changed to a common form only in the recent past of about a century or so with the transformation of Ayurveda into a commercial medical system. But interestingly, modern medicine is also beginning to evolve into an individualized/customized system with the emergence of our understanding of the human genome. For years physician have noted these differences, but had no way to predict them. The human genome analysis is now demonstrating the scientific basis of such variations (Patwardhan et al, 2004)[22,23]. Pharmacogenetics is the study of the hereditary basis for differences in response of a population to a drug. The same dose of a drug will result in elevated plasma concentrations for some patients, but not in others. Some patients will respond well to drugs, while others may not. The drug might show adverse effects in some but not in others. Population and enzyme polymorphisms are known. Large differences among racial groups also occur in GST, an enzyme involved in detoxification of environmental toxins. These differences affect susceptibility of individuals to various forms of cancers[23]. Several such critical evaluations of these aspects had led to the following observations. Instances of individual traits in disease manifestation and response to treatment have been now revealed after the human genome investigation. The importance of such individual variations in health and disease is in fact an important basic principle of Ayurveda which the ancient Ayurvedic masters like Charaka explained about 4000 years ago. Charaka observed that "every individual is different form the other and hence should be considered as a different entity as many variations are there in the universe and all are seen in human beings". Ayugenomics describes the basis of designer medicine[23]. An in-depth study and analysis of this Ayurvedic wisdom with modern genome study could yield much valuable information that may help in treating human disorders. There are over 5800 clinical signs and symptoms in Ayurveda and method for treating them in a customized manner based on the constitutional nature of the individual[24].

System Biology and Metabolomics

Conventional medicines provide data on specific action of drugs. But with the better understanding on cell biology it is now clear that biological system is just not an assembly of tissues, cells, genes or its products, the proteins. But what is important is the traffic and cross talk between them, *i.e.*, the biological function of the whole system *i.e.*, system biology. System biology is defined as "studying biology as an integrated system of genetic, protein, metabolic, cellular and pathway events that are influx and interdependent[25]. It was the advancement made in genomics that led to the development of system biology. It involves massive profiling experiments at different biological levels such as DNA, mRNA (transcriptomics), protein (proteomics) and metabolites (metabolomics)[26]. This kind of approach, in fact, accounts for the holistic approach of most of the oriental systems of medicine more particularly Ayurveda and Siddha. The latest advancements in molecular biology and genomics particularly after completion of Human Genome Project and development of novel diagnostic tools and technology etc. opened up a new world of possibilities providing a better insight into the mode of biological action of drugs by comparing the changes in the transcriptome, proteome and metabolome patterns when compared to those observed with known drugs[24]. Such an approach is now known as system biology and metabolomic approaches paving towards personalised medicines by measuring the activity in a living organism (which can be anything from cell culture, animals to patients) for extracts with different combinations of compounds that correlate with the activity. Good examples of this approach are the methods developed for urine analysis that allow the diagnosis of a variety of diseases[24] as well as measuring possible liver or kidney toxicity. Analysis of large numbers of urine samples of healthy persons and patients made by NMR has resulted in the identification of certain biomarkers for diseases[23]. This is known as metabolomics approach. Using system biology approach for the organism and combining this with metabolomics data for different extracts of medicinal plant or fraction thereof, it should be feasible to make correlations between the occurrence of certain compounds in the extract and their activity. This means that activity due to synergism and pro-drugs might be proved, and even the responsible compounds can be identified[24].

Metabolomics of plants is rapidly developing. It will be a key technology in systembiology approach, for studies of the activity of medicinal plants[24]. The ultimate goal of metabolomics is to qualitatively and quantitatively analyse all metabolomics in an organism. Various other methods for identifying the metabolic intermediates and their changes/variation on account of drug action etc. were experimented by other workers. Fiehn, 2002 and Fiehn *et al.*, 2001[27,28] have given some definitions for the analysis of metabolomes.

1. Metabolic profiling: aims at measuring a selected group of metabolites in an organism;
2. Metabolomics: aims at measuring all metabolites in an organism qualitatively and quantitatively; in studies of pathogenesis analyzing materials such as urine and serum, this is referred to as metabonomics;
3. Metabolic fingerprinting: aims at measuring a fingerprint of the metabolites in an organism, without identification of all compounds.

The major differences thus being in the choice of trying to qualitatively and quantitatively identify (all) compounds in an organism, or to use a differential display type of approach to identify differences and subsequently identity which compounds are responsible for these differences. In cases of looking at a single compound or a well defined group of compounds, one speaks of a targeted approach[26,27].

Such study may enable one to recognize the pro-drugs or synergism and may also lead to identification of new modes of action including new targets. The system biology and metabolomics may emerge as challenging areas of research for better understanding on herbal drug action and in drug development.

Future of Ethnopharmacology

A primary difficulty in defining and projecting a future for ethnopharmacology is to identify the objectives of a largely virtual field whose self-identified membership represents, in addition to commercial entities, a diverse suite of academic and applied disciplines. Departments or degree-granting programmes designated specifically as ethnopharmacology does not exist, it is primarily represented by published investigators trained in pharmacology, anthropology, ethnobotany, or pharmacognosy. Contributions are made as well by historians of science, clinicians, ethnographers, agronomists, biochemists, researchers in veterinary medicine and others. This multi–(but not trans-) disciplinarity has challenged efforts to harmonize objectives and integrate methodologies (Elisabetsky, 1986 [29]; Prinz, 1990 [30]; Etkin, 1996 [31], 2001[32]; Etkin and Ross, 1991 [33], 1997 [34]). For the future, one would hope that the multivocality of the various disciplines that contribute to ethnopharmacology will create a dynamic tension that encourages dialogue and collaboration.

1. Advances in laboratory and clinical sciences will continue, allowing ethnopharmacologists to characterize to a greater level of specificity: the constituents and activities of medicinal plants (and other substances); how variations in the collection and storage of plants, and the preparation and administration of medicines, affects pharmacologic profiles; interactions among constituents of single–and multiple-species medicinal preparations, and between traditional plant medicines and both pharmaceutical drugs and complementary and alternative medicines.
2. More comprehensive analysis will address the effects of ingesting phytochemicals in the maintenance/ improvement of body functions and/ or disease prevention. Such analysis may lead to observations that substantiate the dietary proscriptions and prescriptions that characterize some indigenous medical systems. It has been argued that the rapid acceptance and commercialization of nutraceuticals reflects a return to earlier health paradigms in which little distinction was made between food and medicine.
3. Dosage schedules for indigenous medicines will require clarification. Some traditional formulations (like some pharmaceuticals) are prescribed for substantial duration with no significant improvement expected for weeks or months. In view of the relatively low level of active constituents per dose of plant material, and the mode of preparation for home medicines, one might argue that traditional therapies involve the regular ingestion of low doses of active substance(s) over a significant period of time. In pharmacodynamic terms, it is likely that this pattern of disease intervention may be profoundly different from an acute (single administration) or sub-chronic (a few administrations) challenge to any given molecular target.

Nevertheless, traditional posology has rarely been taken into account in evaluating medicinal plant extracts or substances in new drug screening/ development programmes. Lack of information on the details of traditional use is in part related to practical matters: a research design that measures the effects of repeated interaction with tissues and/or molecular targets requires large quantities of testing materials. In vitro methodologies are, unfortunately, inadequate for these purposes. Nevertheless, the consequences of constant and repeated challenges to molecular targets will need to be taken into consideration at least in interpreting results, especially if the objective is an analysis integrated with results from in vivo models and traditional claims.

4. Application of the rigorous ethnographic field methodologies refined over the last several decades will continue to improve our comprehension of the cultural construction and social transaction of healing in diverse cultures. An integrated, theory–and issue-driven ethnopharmacology will move from multidisciplinary (parallel streams lacking integration), to interdisciplinary (some methodological and theoretical exchange across disciplines), to transdisciplinary methodologies that integrate the perspectives, objectives, and tools of diverse disciplines.
5. Drug discovery from natural products will remain an important goal for some ethnopharmacologists, with the understanding that pharmaceutical advances in this area have the potential to improve health in all world cultures.
6. Increasingly in the future ethnopharmacologists will have to respect and interact with national and local governments, as well as with the growing number and diversity of entities that have evolved over the last 10-15 years as indigenous groups have formalized their sociopolitical circumstances through local, national, and global representations. These interactions should be participatory collaborations that involve local peoples in all phases of research.
7. The existing, and future iterations of the U.N. Convention on Biological Diversity and other ethical issues will guide ethnopharmacology research design and application. The extension to indigenous peoples of intellectual property rights will continue to be complex, contentious, and politically nuanced. It will involve people and entities whose perceptions of, and access to, authority and resources is not equal. Issues of benefit sharing become increasingly abstract and, despite the growing magnitude of the literature on benefit sharing, the breadth of debate has contracted to center primarily on commercial bilateral contractual agreements, despite that most of the resources whose benefits could be shared are not amenable to those legal covenants. Further, many constituencies are excluded from such bilateral contractual benefit sharing, *e.g.*, countries and communities who could impart the same knowledge or resources.
8. In view of the obstacles described above, and to broaden our knowledge base, the trend will continue to base more ethnopharmacology research in

traditional pharmacopoeia of the West, as well as in botanicals marketed as complementary and alternative medicines and supplements. At the same time, attracted by the commercial success in the West, countries of the developing world will try to develop Western-like plant medicines based on local medicinal flora. One advantage of this trend is that such efforts stimulate the development of evidence-based new botanical medicines, with the requisite local development of all the necessary disciplines. A disadvantage is to standardize traditional medicines for the sake of marketing, obscuring the diversity of ways that botanicals are used by traditional peoples.

9. At the same time, ethnopharmacologists will strive harder in the future to connect to issues of social, as well as phytochemical and clinical, salience by assuring that the results of rigorous bioassays and medical ethnography be translated, integrated, and applied to the indigenous contexts in which people use those plants. Ethnopharmacology can contribute to the exploration of phytotherapeutical resources for use in the local contexts and countries of origin. Even where biomedicine is a significant primary care modality, local botanicals can be integrated into holistic health care settings that encourage sustainable resource management through medicinal plant gardens and home-based or cottage-industry preparation of botanical medicines.
10. Perhaps, the most demanding work for the future will be to build theoretical capacity in ethnopharmacology. To date, only a handful of researchers have contributed to this development, exploring such issues as:
    (a) How local ecological environmental knowledge both under girds and emerges from co-evolutionary people–plant–landscape relations.
    (b) How the apprehension and management of resources is culturally constructed and socially transacted in ways that influence knowledge asymmetries and health disparities.
    (c) How the multicontextual use of plants (in medicine, food, cosmetics, etc.) impacts health, as well as the conservation of cultural and biological diversify.

Conclusion

We are thus witnessing a new paradigm in medical research with the emergence of ethnopharmacology. The complexity of ingredients and the aspect of synergistic bioactivities of TM would be well explained/demonstrated by system biology approach that enables linking of the complex metabolic profile of herb with biological effects–herbal metabolic fingerprints with bioactive assays and multivariate statistical analysis would provide a method to involve the whole spectrum for the medical and the pharmaceutical approach. This was essentially the concept and philosophy of the oriental systems of medicine like Ayurveda, Siddha, Unani and the Chinese Traditional Medicine. System biology approach thus demonstrates a shift in focus from the reductionistic approach and strategy of modern medical research to the holistic approach and strategy of TM, more particularly Ayurveda. The drug therapy that used to be mostly symptomatic, will now aim at targets that are closer to the causes of diseases. Therapeutic progress, which used to be indirect, conjectural and coincidental is about to become more directed, definitive and intentional. At the same time as researchers are discovering new knowledge, they are developing new opportunities to advance medicine in an effort to move this field rapidly forward and to seek new ways in which these advances can provide better health and quality of life to patients. Science of Chronobiology teaches us to follow natures rhyme. Ayurveda emphasizes on this biohumoral variations during meals, across seasons and throughout one's life span. Application of this biohumoral rhyme in clinical practice is common.

References

1. Pushpangadan P, Govindarajan R: Need for scientific validation and standardization of TM to meet the Healthcare of the Third World in 21st century. In: Herbal medicine phytopharmaceuticals and other natural products. Trends and advances. Jointly published by Centre for S&T of the Non-aligned and other Developing Countries (NAM S&T Centre) and Institute of Chemistry, Colombo, Sri Lanka, 2006.
2. Pushpangadan P: Important Indian medicinal plants of global interest, International Conclave on Traditional Medicine. Produced and published by AYUSH and NISCAIR, CSIR, New Delhi. 2006, pp 67-73
3. WHO, 2003 http://www.who.int/mediacentre/factssheets/fs134/en
4. Lozarou J, *et al*: Incidence of adverse drug reactions in hospitalized patients. A meta-analysis of prospective studies. JAMA, 1998, 279, 1200-1205.
5. Efron DH, Holmstedt B, Kline NS (eds.): Ethnopharmacological Search for Psychoactive Drugs. Publ 1645, US Department of Health, Education and Welfare. Government Printing Office, Washington D.C. 1967
6. Rivier J, Bruhn JG: Editorial. *J Ethnopharmacol* 1979, 1, 1.
7. Bruhn JG, Holmstedt B: Ethnopharmacology, objectives, principles and perspectives. *In*: Beal JL, Reinhard E (eds) Natural products as medicinal agents. Hippokrates Verlag, pp 405-430, 1981.
8. Subramoniam A, Pushpangadan P: Ethnopharmacological validation of Traditional medicine/remedies. *In*: Pushpangadan P, Nyman U, George V (eds.), Glimpses of Indian Ethnopharmacology, TBGRI Publication, Trivandrum, 1995, pp 351-358
9. Nyman Ulf: Ethnopharmacological validation of Traditional medicine/remedies. *In*:. Pushpangadan P, Nyman U, George V (eds.), Glimpses of Indian Ethnopharmacology TBGRI Publication, Trivandrum, 1995, pp 343-350.
10. Guyatt G, Cairns J, Churchill D, *et al*.: 'Evidence-Based Medicine Working Group' "Evidence-based medicine, a new approach to teaching the practice of medicine". *JAMA*, 1992, 268, 2420-2425.

11. Glossary of terms in Evidence-Based Medicine (http://www.cebm.net/glossary.asp). Centre for Evidence-Based Medicine Retrieved on 2006-06-29

12. Guyatt GH, Sackett DL, *et al.*: Users guides to the Medical literature IX. A method of grading healthcare recommendations–*JAMA*, 1995, 274, 1800-1804.

13. Guyatt GH, Haynes B, Jaeschke R, Cook D, Greenhalgh T, Meade M, Green L, Naylor, CD, Wilson M, McAlister F, Richardson WS: Introduction:The philosophy of Evidence-Based Mdicine. *In*: Guyatt G, Rennie D (eds). User's Guides to the Medical Literature: A Manual for Evidence-Based Clinical Practice. Chicago, AMA Press, 2002, pp. 3-12.

14. Eisenberg, JM: Evidence-Based Medicine. Expert Voices. 2001.

15. Vaidya Pawan Kumar Godatwar: Evidence Based Medicine in the context of Ayurveda *J Ayurveda* 2007, 1, 4-7.

16. Vaidya A: Reverse Pharmacology approach 2002, CSIR NMITLI Herbal drugs development programme, 2002.

17. Vaidya A, *et al.*: Ayurvedic Pharmacoepidemiology–a new discipline *J Assoc Phys India* 2003, 51, 528

18. Mashelkar RA: Chitrakoot Declaration, National Botanic Research Institute and Deenadayal Research Institute Convention on Ayurveda. 2003

19. Kumar NK, Muthuswamy V, Ganguly NK: Initiative of Indian Council of Medical Research in Scientific validation of Traditional Medicine. International Conclave on Traditional Medicine 16.12.2000. New Delhi, Publ. Dept. of AYUSH and NISCAIR/CSIR, New Delhi. 2006.

20. Qazi GN: Drug discovery and development of Ayurveda, International Conclave on Traditional Medicine publ. Dept. of AYUSH& NISCAIR/CSIR, New Delhi. 2006.

21. Hudson J, Altamirano M: The application of DNA microarrays (gene array) to the study of herbal medicines. *J Ethnopharmacol* 2006, 108, 2-15.

22. Patwardhan B: Ayugenomics-Integration for customized medicine. *Indian J Nat Prod* 2003, 19, 16-23

23. Patwardhan B, Ashok DB, Vaidya MC: Ayurveda and natural products drug discovery. *Current Science* 2004, 86 (6), 789-799.

24. Patwardhan B: Traditional Medicine: A Novel Approach for Available, Accessible and Affordable Health Care. In: Sharma RK, Arora R (Eds.) Herbal Drugs A Twenty First Century Perspective, Jaypee Brothers, Medical Publishers (P) LTD. New Delhi. Pp. 8-27,2006

25. Verpoorte R, Choi YH, Kim HK: Ethnopharmacology and system biology. A perfect holistic match. *J Ethnopharmacol*, 2005, 100, 53-56.

26. Van der Greef *et al.*: The role of metabolomics in system biology. *In*: Metabolic profiling, Harrigan GG, Good acre R (Eds), Khuwer Academic Publications, Boston, USA, pp 171-188, 2003.

27. Fiehn O: Metabolomics–the link between genotypes and phenotypes. *Plant Molecular Biology* 2002, 48, 155-171.

28. Fiehn O, Kopka J, Dormann P, Altmann T, Trethewey RN, Willmitzer L: Metabolite profiling for plant functional genomics. *Nature Biotechnology*, 2000, 18, 1157-1161.

29. Elisabetsky, E: New directions in ethnopharmacology, *J Ethnobiol* 1986, 6, 121-128.

30. Prinz A: Misunderstanding between ethnologists, pharmacologists, and physicians in the field of ethnopharmacology. *In*: Fleurentin J, Cabalion P, Mazars G, Santos DJ, Younos C (Eds.), Ethnopharmacologie: Sources, Methodes, Objectifs (ORSTOM Editions), Metz, France, pp. 95–99, 1990.

31. Etkin NL: Ethnopharmacology: the conjunction of medical ethnography and the biology of therapeutic action. *In*: Sargent CF, Johnson TM (Eds.), Medical Anthropology: Contemporary Theory and Method (revised ed.), Praeger Publishers, New York, pp. 151-164, 1996.

32. Etkin NL: Perspectives in ethnopharmacology: forging a closer link between bioscience and traditional empirical knowledge, *J Ethnopharmacol* 2001, 76, 177-182.

33. Etkin NL, Ross PJ: Should we set a place for diet in ethnopharmacology?, *J Ethnopharmacol* 1991, 32, 25-36.

Chapter 16

Biological Diversity in *Curcuma*: A Review

Sharad Srivastava*, A.K.S. Rawat and Shanta Mehrotra

Pharmacognosy and Ethnopharmacology Division,
National Botanical Research Institute, Lucknow – 226 001, India

ABSTRACT

Curcuma rhizomes, commonly used as a spice worldover, are well documented for its medicinal properties in Indian and Chinese systems of medicine. It has been widely used for the treatment of several diseases. Epidemiological observations are suggestive that consumption of some *Curcuma* species may reduce the risk of some form of cancers and render other protective biological effects in humans. These biological activities of *Curcuma* have been attributed to its constituent curcumin that has been widely studied for its anti-inflammatory, anti-angiogenic, antioxidant, wound healing and anti-cancer effects, etc. As a result of extensive epidemiological, clinical, and animal studies several molecular mechanisms are emerging that elucidate the multiple biological effects of curcumin.

Due to its diversified uses, a vast review of this genus has been done to put all its activities at one place which will not only help researchers for further evaluation but also provide substantial information for its further exploitation to develop novel herbal formulations.

Keywords: Curcuma, Curcumin, Wound healing, Anti-oxidant, Angiogenesis, Pharmacology, Ethnobotany.

Introduction

Curcuma rhizomes have been the subject of research in several laboratories in India and abroad and efforts have been made to find out the active principle(s) with

* E-mail: Sharad_ks2003@yahoo.com, Phone No. 91-9415082210, Fax: 91-522-2207219.

a view to optimize the activity and to explain the mechanism of action at molecular level. A large number of publications and several reviews have appeared. However, both turmeric and its components are still attracting attention and many new properties are being discovered. Curcumin is perhaps the most important constituent, which has undergone systematic research to unravel its useful properties and to develop it as a modern drug.

The economic potential of the genus *Curcuma* is much diverse, other than the world-renowned spices, it has some other lesser known and less exploited spicy species. *Curcuma amada* is a good condiment with its unique 'mango flavour'. The leaves of *C. zedoaria* are used to flavour fish and other dishes in Java.Various pharmacological properties of many species of *Curcuma* are reported. Natives of different countries use the starch-rich rhizomes and root tubers of *Curcuma* sp. as food; Jain (1) in his study reported that the rhizomes of *Curcuma neilgherrensis* and *C. pseudomontana* are edible.

The cosmetics value of *C. longa* and *C. aromatica* are well known in India since ages. Traditionally, Indian women use the paste of the rhizomes of these species to improve complexion and to remove skin scars. Modern cosmetic industry is using these plants in various products. Curcumin, the yellow dye extracted from the rhizomes of *Curcuma longa* and *C. zedoaria* is used as food dye and also as fabric dye.

All the commercially available *Curcuma* sp. are critically studied and evaluated by various workers for their spice value, chemical profile, medicinal properties and crop management as well. Some important reviews on such works are being briefed here. Govindarajan (2,3) published critical reviews on turmeric *C. longa.* The taxonomic status of *Curcuma heyneana* was discussed by Firman *et al.* (4) based on essential oil analysis. Bone (5) complimented turmeric as 'the spice of life' while Khanna (6) considered turmeric as 'nature's precious gift'. Liberti (7) published a monograph on turmeric and Srimal (8) published a detailed review on its medicinal properties. Maheshwari *et al.* (9) have also published a review on multiple biological activities of curcumin.

Taxonomy and Morphology

The genus *Curcuma* comprising about fifty species, distributed in tropical and subtropical regions of Asia, belongs to the tribe Hedychieae (10) and consists of a rather homogenous group of rhizomatous perennials. The name originated from the Arabic word 'kurcum' meaning yellow, which probably refers to the colour of the rhizome or the flower. The genus is easily recognized by its inflorescence, a spike with prominent spiral bracts laterally fuse and form pouches, each subtending a cincinnus of flowers, and a cluster of often coloured sterile terminal bracts forming what is called 'coma' (11).

Many taxonomists have attempted subgeneric classification of this genus. Roxburgh (12) divided it into two sections, depending on lateral or central spikes while Horaninov (13) distinguished 3 sections namely *Exantha* (spikes always lateral), *Mesantha* (spikes invariably terminal) and *Amphiantha* (spikes both terminal and lateral). Baker (14) accepted sects. *Exantha* and *Mesantha* while rejecting sect.

Amphiantha and introduced a new section *Hitcheniopsis*, which differed from the rest of the genus in its spurless anthers. Schumann (15) rejected the sectional classification based on spike position but recognised two subgenera [subgen, *Eucurcuma* and subgen. *Hitcheniopsis* (Baker) Schum based on the presence or absence of spur on anthers.

However, authors of most Floras have continued to rely upon questionable characters like position of spikes, presence or absence of root-tubers and the colour of the coma for the identification of species in the genus and consequently the genus is badly in need of a taxonomic revision (16). Roxburgh (17) had already pointed out that the positional difference of spikes is a matter of flowering season, the early spikes being lateral and later ones terminal. Subsequently, Santapau (18,19) has corroborated this in the case of *C. pseudomontana*, who has also demonstrated that the colour of the coma is variable within the species and hence unreliable for species delimitation. Mangaly and Sabu (20), corroborate the protracted study on wild and cultivated materials in South India.

In India, except for a few ubiquitous species, the genus is mainly concentrated in the South West and Northeast part of the country and has not been revised since Baker (14) who reported 29 species. Tomlinson's (21) work based on the anatomical evidence, has much relevance in the classification of the order Zingiberales. Sherlija *et al.* (22) reported the rhizome anatomy of four species of *Curcuma*.

Ethnobotany

C. xanthorrhiza is useful in the treatment of liver disorders and has a promising kind of broad spectrum hepatoprotective agent which is traditionally used in Indonesia (23). *Curcuma longa* was used predominantly for endoparasites, internal and external injuries and pregnancy related conditions in ethnic community of Trinidad and Tobago. *Curcuma longa* is also used in traditional and medical treatment as well as dietary intake in Nepal (24). It is also used in skin ailments and cosmetics in Assam (25).

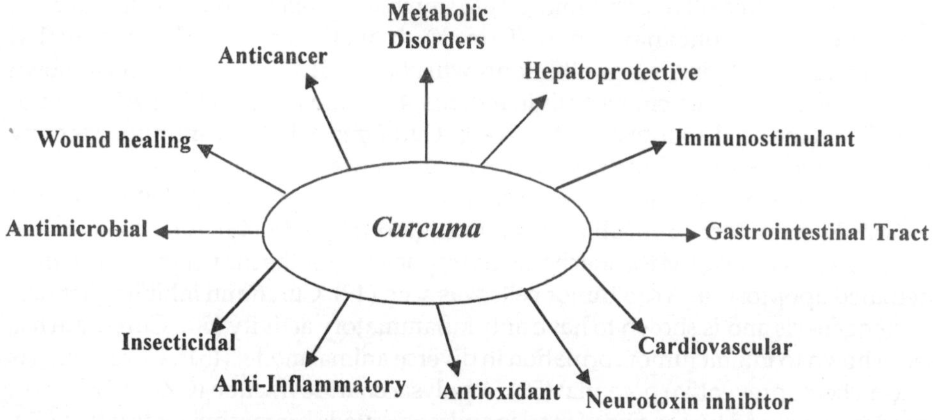

Figure 16.1: Diversified Potential of *Curcuma*

Biological Activities

Anticancer, Antitumor and Antiproliferative Activities

Genus *Curcuma* has much diverse pharmacological activities. Large number of reports are available showing either preventive or curative effect of curcumin, against cancer and tumorgensis. Anticancer activity has been demonstrated by several authors by measuring some marker enzymes (26, 27, 28, 29, 30, 31). Several authors (26, 27, 28, 32, 33, 34, 35) reported the anticancer and antitumour properties of *Curcuma longa*. Han (36) and Yu (37) evaluated Chinese anticancer drugs in which *Curcuma longa* is an ingredient. Itokawa *et al.* (38) reported the antitumour activity of *Curcuma xanthorrhiza*. Turmeric has shown to inhibit chemical carcinogeniesis (39). Extract of turmeric inhibited the aflatoxin production considerably (more than 90 per cent) at the concentration of 5-10 mg/ml (40). In *in vitro* study, curcumin, at 5 µM inhibited lipopolysaccharides (LPS) induced production of TNF-α (tumor necrosis factor-alpha) and IL-1 (interleukin-1) by a human monocytic macrophage cell line, monomac 6 (41). Turmeric in diet has been reported to prevent virus as well as chemical carcinogen-induced mammary tumors in mice and rats. Oral administration of curcumin (200 nmol/kg) inhibited the lung metastasis and increased the life span of mice with tumor induced by B16F10 melanoma cells (42). Cytotoxic, cytoprotective and chemopreventive effects of curcumin are well documented (29,31). Anto *et al.* (43) compared the cytotoxic and tumoricidal activities of eight synthetic curcuminoids in cultured L929 cells. All of them were cytotoxic and 50 per cent inhibition was achieved at around 1.0 µg/ml concentration, which was similar to that obtained with natural curcumin. Huang *et al.* (30) applied curcumin topically (1 to 3000 mmol) twice a week on CD-1 mice and demonstrated the inhibitory effect of all the doses against TPA-induced oxidation of DNA bases in epidermis but only 100 and 3000 mmol doses inhibited tumor promotion by TPA. They further demonstrated the inhibitory effect of curcumin (IC_{50} = 0.5-1.0 µM) on DNA and RNA synthesis in cultured HeLa cells. Curcumin in combination with genistein in the diet have the potential to reduce the proliferation of estrogen-positive cells (44). Curcumin is a potent antiproliferative agent for breast tumor cells. Dietary curcumin significantly inhibited the stem carcinogensis in mice (34). Curcumin (50 µM) inhibited proliferation of rat thymocytes stimulated with concanavalin A (Con A) as well as that of human Jurkat lymphoblastoid cells in the logarithmic growth phase (45). Curcumin has been shown to attenuate chemical carcinogenesis in rodents (46). Curcumin inhibited AK-5 tumor growth and induced apoptosis in AK-5 cells. Curcumin enhanced antitumor activity in combination with cisplatin (a widely used anticancer drug) against fibrosarcoma (47). *Curcuma domestica* and *C. xanthorrhiza* were found to possess inhibitory activity towards Epstein-Barr virus (EBV) activation induced by TPA (48). A redox signaling and caspase activation as the mechanisms responsible for the induction of curcumin mediated apoptosis in AK-5 tumor cells was seen (49). Curcumin inhibits chemical carcinogenesis and is shown to have anti-inflammatory activity (50). Curcumin has been shown to inhibit tumor formation in diverse animal models (51). Curcumin has cancer chemopreventive potential (52). A polysaccharide fraction (CZ-1-III) from *C. zedoaria*, decreased tumor size of mouse and prevented chromosomal mutation (53). Soybean lipoxygenase L1 catalysed the oxygenation of curcumin and that curcumin can act as a lipoxygenase substrate which inhibits cancer formation in mice (54). Curcumin has been shown to possess tumoricidal activity (55). Orally consumed curcumin significantly inhibited DMBA–and TPA-induced *tat* and *fos* gene expression in mouse skin (56). Curcumin enhanced PHIP-induced apoptosis and inhibited PHIP-induced tumorogenesis in the proximal small intestine of APC mice (57). Curcumin may suppress tumor promotion by blocking signal transduction pathways in the target cells.

Dietary curcumin may inhibit azoxymethanol induced colonic neoplasia in mice (58). Histopathological examination of the tumors showed that dietary curcumin inhibited the number of papillomas and sequamous cell carcinomas of the forestomach as well as the number of adenomas and adenocarcinomas of the duodenum and colon (29). Curcumin plays an important role in inhibition of Ehrlich ascites tumor in mice (59). Recently curcumin has been reported to be active against basophilic leukemia cells in presence of light (60). Curcumin inhibits colon cancer cell proliferation *in vitro* mainly by accumulating cells in the G2/M phase and the effect is independent of its ability to inhibit prostaglandin synthesis (61). Curcumin inhibited tumorigenesis during both initiation and promotion periods in several experimental animal models (30). Curcumin showed chemopreventive action when administered prior to, during and after carcinogen treatment of colon carcinogenesis (62). Curcumin induced apoptosis of several but not all cancer cells (63). Curcumin inhibits NMBA-induced esophageal carcinoma (64). Curcumin has shown anticarcinogenic activity in animals as indicated by its block of colon tumor initiation by azoxymethane and skin tumor promotion induced by phorbol ester TPA (65).

Antimicrobial and Antiviral Activities

The antimicrobial properties of *Curcuma* are well known and many researchers reported the antibiotic activities of *Curcuma*. Banerjee and Nigam (66, 67) reported the antibacterial and antifungal activity of various species of *Curcuma*. The *in vitro* antibacterial activity of alcoholic extract of turmeric, curcumin and its essential oil against Gram-positive bacteria has been reported. Shankar and Murthy (68) found antibacterial property of *C. longa*. Recently, curcumin was shown to be highly toxic to *Salmonella* but not to *E. coli* strain with capacity of DNA repair in presence of visible light (69). This indicated phototoxicity potential of curcumin (60) which might be useful in treatment of skin disorders like psoriasis, cancer, bacterial and viral infections. Photoactivation by visible light may be an advantage over psoralins, which get activated by UV-A only. Another interesting activity of curcumin is that of inhibiting the long terminal repeats of HIV-1 virus gene expression without significant effect on the cells (70). Turmeric has been tried clinically as eye drops in patients of conjunctivitis and the efficacy was comparable to soframycin. *C. xanthorrhiza* contains some principle(s) activating T and B cell-mediated immune functions (71). Curcumin is a modest inhibitor of the HIV-1 and HIV-2 proteases (72). Both the antibacterial and antifungal property in *Curcuma longa* was reported by Iyengar *et al.* (73). Mazumdar *et al.* (74) have reported the inhibitory activity of curcumin against HIV-1 integrase which is essential for integration of a double stranded DNA copy of the viral RNA into a host genome and for HIV replication. Thus, curcumin could be active as an anti-HIV drug. Thomas *et al.* (75) studied the antibacterial activity of 17 spp. of Zingiberaceae belonging to the genera *Alpinia, Curcuma, Kaempferia* and *Zingiber*. Antifungal property of *C. longa* was reported by Niaz *et al.* (76), Apisariyakul *et al.* (77) and Roth *et al.* (78). Curcumin (10 to 100 nM) inhibited *Tat* transactivation of HIV-1-LTR Lac Z by 70 to 80 per cent in He La cells (79). Curcumin was analysed for the immunodeficiency activity in Balb/c mice (80). Curcumin may inhibit Th1 cytokine profile in CD4+ T cells by suppressing 11-12 production in macrophages and prints to a possible therapeutic use to curcumin in the Th-1-mediated immune diseases (81). Curcumin have been proposed as HIV-1 integrase inhibitor (82). The antibacterial activity of xanthorrhizol, isolated from the methanol extract of *C. xanthorrhiza* roots was evaluated against oral microorganisms in comparison with chlorhexidine (83). Curcumins also showed a moderate activity against *Plasmodium falciparum* and *Leishmania major* (84).

Insecticidal Properties

Molluscicidal property of *C. longa* was reported by Maini and Morallo-Rejesus (85); Roth *et al.* (78). The insecticidal property of different species of *Curcuma* was reported by Pandji *et al.* (86). Cyclocurcumin from turmeric has been successfully used as nematocidal agent. Jurgens *et al.* (87) reported novel nematocidal agents from *C. comosa. C. aromatica* oil was evaluated against mosquitoes in mustard and coconut base oil (88).

Anti-inflammatory Activity

Curcumin showed anti-inflammatory effect in acute, subacute and chronic models of inflammation in mice and rat models. The oral ED_{50} in mice, against carrageenin-induced acute oedema was 100.2 mg/kg compared to 78 mg/kg of cortisone. In subacute cotton pellet and granuloma pouch tests in rats, it inhibited granuloma formation by 14 to 30 per cent at the dose range from 80 to 160 mg/kg, p.o. for 7 to 14 days. In adjuvant-induced arthritis in rats, curcumin had weaker (about 1/3) effect than phenylbutazone. It did not produce significant gastric irritation and had no effect on the cardiovascular or central nervous systems (89, 90, 91, 92, 93). Sodium curcuminate and volatile oil of *Curcuma* have also been investigated for anti-inflammatory activity (94, 95). The anti-inflammatory property of *Curcuma longa* was studied by several authors (31, 43, 96, 97, 98, 99, 100). Similar property was also reported in *C. xanthorrhiza* by Claeson *et al.* (101, 102). In acute carrageenin-induced oedema test in rats, the ED_{50} of sodium curcuminate was found to be 0.36 mg/kg i.p., compared to 47.8 per cent inhibition of the oedema by 10 mg/kg i.p. of hydrocortisone. Analogues of curcumin have also been prepared in an effort to increase the activity but none of the synthesized compounds was significantly better than the parent molecule (103). Clinically curcumin did not produce any side effect up to 1600mg/kg/day for 4 weeks in phase-I trials in male volunteers. Phase-II clinical trials have been conducted in patients with rheumatoid arthritis and osteoarthritis. Although curcumin was found weaker than phenylbutazone, no side effects were reported. Response was obtained also in osteoarthritis, but the number of patients was too small. Satoskar *et al.* (104) published the results of a double blind trial with curcumin in cases of acute inflammation comparing it with oxyphenylbutazone and placebo in which curcumin produced significant effect. Germacrone from methanol soluble extract of *C. xanthorrhiza* has been shown to possess anti-inflammatory activity (105). Curcumin has been shown to possess anti-inflammatory activity on the proliferation of blood mononuclear cells and vascular smooth muscle cells (58). Curcumin inhibited platelet aggregation induced by arachidonate, adrenalin and collagen, thus showing anti-inflammatory activity (106). A bioguided fractionation of anti-inflammatory plant extract as well as fractions of the roots of *C. xanthorrhiza,* which contain the known inducible nitric oxide synthase (INOS) inhibitor curcumin were assayed (107). Dehydrocurdione, a sesquiterpene isolated from *C. zedoaria* have anti-inflammatory potency related to its antioxidant effect (108). Curcumin could be used as a safe and effective drug in the treatment of idiopathic inflammatory orbital pseudotumors (109).

Cardiovascular Activity

Curcumin inhibited rat liver microsomal delta 5 and delta 6 desaturases (110). *C. xanthorrhiza* contains active principle(s) other than curcuminoids which can modify the metabolism of lipid and lipoproteins (111). Alpha-curcumene is one of the active principles exerting triglyceride-lowering activity in *C. xanthorrhiza* (71). Blood cholestrol was lowered significantly by dietary curcumin in streptozotocin-induced diabetic rats (112). The hypolipidimic effect of an ethyl acetate extract of the rhizome of *C. comosa* Roxb. was investigated in mice (113). Active compounds in *Curcuma* extracts may be protective in preventing lipoperoxidation of subcellular membranes in a dose dependent manner thus preventing the atherosclerosis (114). Intragastric administration of ethyl acetate extract of *C. comosa* rhizome (0-500 mg/kg per day) to hypercholestremic animals for 7 days decreased both plasma triglyceride and cholestrol levels in a dose-dependent manner (115). An ethanol–aqueous extract obtained from the rhizomes of *C. longa* is used in the management of cardiovascular diseases in which atherosclerosis is important (116). A daily oral administration of the hydroalcoholic extract decreases significantly the LDL and apolipoprotein B and increased the HDL and apo A of healthy subjects (117).

Effect on Gastrointestinal Tract

Several reports suggest that curcumin as well as turmeric increase bile flow (118). Essential oils of turmeric have also been found to increase the bile flow and found that sodium curcuminate decreased the amount of solids in the bile in low doses but increased the excretion of bile salts, bilirubin and cholesterol in high doses. The aqueous extract reduced the acid output, methanolic extract mainly decreased the pepsin output. In another study, gastric mucin content was found to be increased. The gastric and duodenal antiulcer properties of curcumin as well as of turmeric, in high doses, are also documented. However, some investigators have found it to be ulcerogenic. The gastric secretion was found to be reduced after 3 h in conscious rabbits by aqueous and methanolic extracts of turmeric. The antiulcer property was reported by Kositchaiwat *et al.* (119) in *Curcuma longa.* Mulky *et al.* (120) and Nagabhusan *et al.* (121) reported the antimutagenicity of *C. longa*. An oral dose of 500 mg/kg of ethanol extract of turmeric produced significant antiulcer effect in a variety of models in rat (122). The preventive action of curcumin on the formation of cholestrol gallstones in mice and hamsters has been reported. The regression of established cholesterol gallstones in mice by curcumin has also been observed.

Tocamphyl–a synthetic choleretic preparation from root extract of *C. longa* was investigated on pancreatic exocrine secretion and bile flow and on the release of some gastrointestinal hormones by administering it intraduodenally using anesthetized rats (123). Curcumin was able to modulate *in vitro* both expression and function of hepatic pgp (124). Concurrent treatment of turmeric extract gave a significant protection against CCl_4 induced liver damage in rats (125). Extracts of *Curcuma* have beneficial effects in biliary dyskinesia (126). The therapeutic efficiency of microsphere entrapped *C. aromatica* oil infused *via* hepatic artery was observed against transplanted rat hepatoma (127). Curcumin prevented cyclosporin-indused reduction of biliary bilirubin and cholestrol extraction and its influence on biliary excretion of cyclosporin (CS) and its metabolites in the bile fistula model in rats (128).

Hepatoprotective Activity

Curcumin and turmeric have been shown to protect liver against a variety of toxicants *in vitro* as well as *in vivo*. They include carbon tetrachloride, aflatoxin B-1, paracetamol (129) iron, and cyclophosphamide (130, 40, 27) in mouse, rat and duckling. Soni *et al.* (40) reported more than 80 per cent inhibition of mutagenesis induced by aflatoxin B-1 in *Salmonella thyphimurium* tester strains TA98 and TA100 by turmeric and curcumin at a concentration of 2 µg/plate. Turmeric in the diet (5 and 10 per cent) has been found to stimulate enzymes (arylhydrocarbon hydroxylase, UDP glucuronyl transferase, glutathiones–transferase) which metabolize xenobiotics (131). The effect of turmeric (4.0 g/kg/day) and curcumin (0.4 g/kg/day) on the hepatic levels of glutathion-S-transferase, acid soluble sulfhydryl (-SH), cytochrome b_5 and cytochrome P-450 enzymes after 14 or 21 days of administration in lactating dams and translactationally exposed F-1 pups was studied. All the enzymes examined were significantly elevated in lactating dams as well as in pups. Curcumin has been reported to strongly inhibit cytochrome 450-1A in liver, an isoenzyme involved in the bioactivation of several toxins including benzo [α] pyrene (132, 133, 134, 135). Schlepper and Winteroff (136) reported hepatoprotective activity of *C. longa*, and Lin *et al.* (137) that of *C. xanthorriza*. Hepatoprotective sesquiterpenes isolated from aqueous acetone extract of *C. zedoaria* rhizome were found to show potent protective effect on D-galactosamine (D-GalN)/Lipopoly saccharides (LPS) induced acute liver injury in mice.

Metabolic Disorders

Evidence for the hypocholesterolemic and hypolipidemic activities of curcumin has been provided when it was fed with diet to rats for 7 weeks at the concentration of 0.15 per cent (138). Ethanolic extract of *C. longa* has been shown to have hypoglycemic activity in normal as well as alloxan-induced diabetes in rats. In streptozotocin-induced diabetic rats fed with 0.5 per cent curcumin in diet for 8 weeks, a significant improvement in the metabolic status along with reduction in blood cholesterol, triglycerides and phopholipids were noted (112). Similar reduction in renal cholesterol and phospholipids was also observed. The authors observed a marked increase in hepatic cholesterol-7α-hydroxylase activity suggesting a higher rate of cholesterol catabolism under the effect of curcumin.

Immunostimulant Activity

Japanese workers have reported the isolation of polysaccharides, named ukonan A-D, from the hot water extract of *C. longa* rhizomes, which has been shown to stimulate reticulo-endothelial system in a carbon clearance test. They have also isolated a lipopolysaccharide from the roots of *Curcuma*, which is similar to bacterial lipopolysaccharides and is a immunostimulant. Experimentally (turmeric 4 mg/kg/day = curcumin 0.4 mg/kg/day) and clinically (equivalent to 20 mg/kg/day of curcumin), turmeric extract has been found to decrease serum lipid peroxides which play an important role in pathogenesis of normal senescence and age related diseases like atherosclerosis (139).

The inhibitory activity on the proliferation of vascular smooth muscle, (140), increased fibrinolytic activity (141), reduction in lipid peroxidation (110, 135) and antiplatelet (106, 138) activities may be the other important contributory factors.

In clinical trial conducted in China, turmeric (50 g/day) was found to be as effective as clofibrate, (141). Curcumin has also been reported to prevent the formation of cholesterol gallstones in mice and hamsters, when fed (0.5 per cent) along with lithogenic diets and also to dissolve the preformed cholesterol gallstones. Turmeric has been reported to increase the mitogenic response of splenic lymphocytes in rat and to alter the population of lymphocytes in mice (111). Dietary curcumin (40 mg/kg) in rats for 5 weeks enhanced IgG levels but did not affect delayed type of hypersensitivity and natural killer cell activity.

Effect on Respiratory System

Based on Ayurveda *Curcuma longa* is used against bronchial asthma, (142). The protective effect of curcumin (200 mg/kg for 7 days) on rat lung against the toxicity induced by cyclophosphamide has been observed. Antiallergic activity of *Curcuma* extract has also been reported (143).

Wound Healing Activity

Tissue repair and wound healing are complex processes that involve inflammation, granulation and tissue remodeling. Injury initiates a complex series of events that involves interactions of multiple cell types, various cytokines, growth factors, their mediators and the extra-cellular matrix proteins (ECM). Local application of turmeric is a household remedy in India for several conditions such as skin diseases, insect bites and chicken pox (144). Based on the ancient use of turmeric in wound healing, our earlier studies evaluated the effect of curcumin on enhancement of wound healing. We used full thickness punch wound model to study its effect on wound healing. Curcumin treated wound biopsies showed a large number of infiltrating cells such as macrophage, neutrophils and fibroblasts as compared to untreated wound. The presence of myofibroblast in curcumin treated wound demonstrated faster wound contraction (145). Migration of various cells represents potential sources of growth factors required for the regulation of biological processes during wound healing. Transforming growth factor (TGF-β1) is important in wound healing as it stimulates the expression of fibronectin (FN) and collagen by fibroblasts and increases the rate of formation of granulation tissue *in vivo* (146, 147). Curcumin treatment resulted in enhanced fibronectin (FN) and collagen expression (145). Furthermore, the treatment led to an increased formation of granulation tissue including greater cellular content, neo-vascularization and a faster re-epithelialization of wound in both diabetic as well as hydrocortisone impaired wounds (148) by regulating the expression of TGF-β1, its receptors and nitric oxide synthase during wound healing (149). Other studies involving systemic administration of curcumin have shown its beneficial effects by the enhancement of muscle regeneration after trauma *in vivo* by modulating NF-κB activity (150). Recent studies have suggested that curcumin inhibited the damage caused by hydrogen peroxide in human keratinocytes and fibroblasts (151) suggesting the antioxidant role in enhanced wound repair. Similarly, curcumin incorporated collagen matrix treatment showed increased wound reduction, enhanced cell proliferation and efficient free radical scavenging as compared with control and collagen treated rats (152). Curcumin pretreatment enhanced the synthesis of collagen, hexosamine, DNA, nitrite and histologic assessment of wound biopsy specimens showed improved collagen deposition and an increase in fibroblast and vascular densities suggesting that curcumin may be able to improve radiation-induced delay in wound repair (153). It has also been studied for antiulcer activity in acute ulcer model in rat by preventing glutathione depletion, lipid peroxidation and protein oxidation. Denudation of epithelial cells during damage of gastric lumen is reversed by curcumin through re-epithelialization. Furthermore, both oral and intraperitoneal administration of curcumin blocked gastric ulceration in a dose dependent manner. It accelerated the healing process and protected gastric ulcer through attenuation of MMP-9 activity and amelioration of MMP-2 activity (154). These studies clearly suggested that curcumin treatment resulted in faster closure of wounds, better regulation of granulation tissue formation and induction of growth factors. It suggests that it acts at different levels to enhance wound repair. Further studies are warranted to evaluate turmeric/curcumin as a potential therapeutic agent in clinical setting of wound healing.

The wound healing property of turmeric was investigated long back and its local application was found to be effective. A pilot study has been undertaken to prove the efficacy of turmeric for healing chronic ulcers and scabies (155). Curcuminoids also protected normal human keratinocytes from hypoxanthine/xanthine oxidase injury (156). An *in vivo* effect of curcumin was evaluated on wound healing in rats and guinea pigs (145). Antioxidative and hypolipidaemic action of curcumin is responsible for its protective role against ethanol induced brain injury (157). Curcumin also enhanced the wound repair in diabetic impaired healing (148).

Antioxidant Activity

Oxidative stress plays a major role in the pathogenesis of various diseases including myocardial ischemia, cerebral ischemia-reperfusion injury, hemorrhage and shock, neuronal cell injury, hypoxia and cancer. Curcumin, exhibits strong antioxidant activity, comparable to vitamins C and E (158). Curcumin with its proven anti-inflammatory and antioxidant properties has been shown to have several therapeutic advantages. It was shown to be a potent scavenger of a variety of reactive oxygen species including superoxide anion radicals, hydroxyl radicals (159) and nitrogen dioxide radicals. It was also shown to inhibit lipid peroxidation in different animal models (160). Curcumin protected oxidative cell injury of kidney cells (LLC-PK1) by inhibiting lipid degradation, lipid peroxidation and cytolysis (161) and also decreased ischemia-induced biochemical changes in heart in a feline model (162). Vascular endothelial cells treated with curcumin prevented oxidant mediated injury by increased heme oxygenase production (163). Curcumin was found to protect rat myocardium against isoprenaline (ISO) induced myocardial ischemic damage (164, 165, 166) and the protective effect was attributed to its antioxidant properties by inhibiting free radial generation (167). It caused a decrease in the degree of degradation of the existing collagen matrix and collagen synthesis, two weeks after the second dose of ISO. These effects were attributed to free radical scavenging properties and inhibition of lysosomal enzyme release by curcumin (166). Treatment with curcumin showed beneficial effects on renal injury by its ability to inhibit the expression of the apoptosis-related genes Fas and Fas-L (168).

A sum of approximately 26 compounds has been isolated from different *Curcuma* sp. having high antioxidant activity (169). Several authors have reported antioxidant property of *C. longa and C. xanthorrhiza* (158, 169, 33, 170, 171, 172). Turmerin from turmeric has been found to be an efficient antioxidant/DNA-protectant/antimutagen (173). In a cell free peroxidation system curcumin exerted strong antioxidative activity (42). Dietary turmeric lowers lipid peroxidation by enhancing the activities of antioxidant enzymes (159). The turmeric oxidant protein (TAP) has been isolated from the aqueous extract of turmeric (170). Three known curcuminods were evaluated for their antioxidative activity by using linolic acid on the substrate in an ethanol/water system (174). Free radical reactions have been studied with a variety of oxidants using Tx100 micells as a model membrane (175). *C. vera* a drug of traditional Chinese medicine was a natural source of antioxidative agent (176). Curcuminoid from C. *chunyujin* has shown antioxidant activity (177). Curcumin was shown to decrease the level of prostanoids in the tissue. Aqueous extract of C. *domestica* has potential antioxidative, antiinflammatory and antithrombotic effects (178). Curcuminoids isolated from C. *longa* protects the cells from beta A (1-42) through antioxidant pathway (179).

Toxicity Studies

Curcumin did not produce any toxicity either on single administration or on repeated oral administration over a period of 6 months in rat and monkey at doses up to 1800 and 800-mg/kg day, respectively. Investigators have also reported that when it was given orally in high doses (up to 5 g/kg) to rats, it did not cause toxic effects. Mathes and Ourisson (180) reported cytotoxic components from *C. longa* and *C. zedoaria*. Acute and chronic toxicity studies on the ethanolic extracts of the rhizomes of *C. longa* were carried out in mice. Curcumin has demonstrated phototoxicity to several species of bacteria under aerobic conditions (60). Chronic administration to rat over a period of 10 weeks at 750 mg/kg/day was found to be safe (159). Curcuminoids isolated from ethanolic extract of *C. zedoaria* were synthesized and demonstrated to be cytotoxic against human ovarian cancer OVCAR-3 cells (181).

Neurotoxin Inhibitory Activity

Cherdchu and Karlsson (182), Cherdchu *et al.* (183) and Rantanabanangkoon *et al.* (184) reported cobra neurotoxin inhibitory activity of *Curcuma* species. This neurotoxin inhibitor was found only in the water insoluble fraction of the rhizome extract. Potent antivenom against snakebite was isolated from *C. longa* commonly used in traditional Brazilian medicine (185).

Miscellaneous Effects

Srimal and Dhawan (93), Bone (5) and Srimal (8) reported a general study on various pharmacological activities of turmeric. Curcumin was found to inhibit the inflammation-induced nitrite formation in mouse peritoneal cells at concentrations of 2.5-10 µM (41). It also gave protection, at low doses, against the chromosomal damage caused by gamma radation. Prevention of cataractogenesis of rat eye lens treated *ex vivo* with curcumin (75 mg/kg, p.o. for 14 days) has been reported. The mechanism suggested was induction of glutathion-S-transferase isoenzyme rGST8-8 in lens epithelitum. In very high doses (> 14 g/kg), aqueous extract of turmeric has been found to have oestrogenic effect. Curcumin has been used as an important ingredient in 'Ksharsutra' which is an effective treatment for anal fistula.

Garg (186), Das (187) and Bhatnagar (188) reported contraceptive action of *Curcuma longa*. Deodhar *et al.* (189) reported antirheumatic property of *C. longa*. The clinical efficacy of a herboniveral formulation containing *C. longa* was undertaken in patients with osteoarthritis (190). Curcumin lowers the blood cholestrol levels and controls the diabetic nephropathy (112). Curcumin has been examined for its radioprotective property using the glyoxylase system, which is vital for various biological functions. Free radical scavenging and electron/hydrogen donations are probable attributes for the protective effect of curcumin (191). Curcumin administered orally to patients suffering from chronic antieri or ureitis (CAU) at a dose of 375 mg three times a day for 12 weeks, all the patients who received curcumin alone improved (192).

Phytochemistry

Turmeric is well known since long time for its bright yellow hue. It has been used as a colouring agent, as a dye in wool and jute industry, and as food additive. Curcumin (diferuloylmethane), which gives yellow colour to turmeric rhizomes, is one of the active ingredients responsible for the biological activity. The first report on the yellow dye in turmeric was by Daube in 1870 (3). Later Srinivasan (193) and Janaki and Bose (194) reported studies on pigments of turmeric. The yield of Curcumin in one sample was reported to be 2 per cent but it ranges between 2.5-5.0 per cent on dry weight basis. Some studies on the pigment 'curcumin' are by Sastry (195), Lahiri (196), Balakrishanan *et al.* (197), Tonnesen and Karisen (198), Rouseff (199), Faruq and Haque (200), and Zachariah and Babu (201). Apart from curcumin, some other curcuminoids, proteins and carbohydrates are also present. A study on the curcumionids in turmeric was reported by Verghese (202) and two new curcuminoid pigments were reported from turmeric by Nakayama *et al.* (203). The synthesis of curcumin is known and its structure was determined. Different methods of curcumin

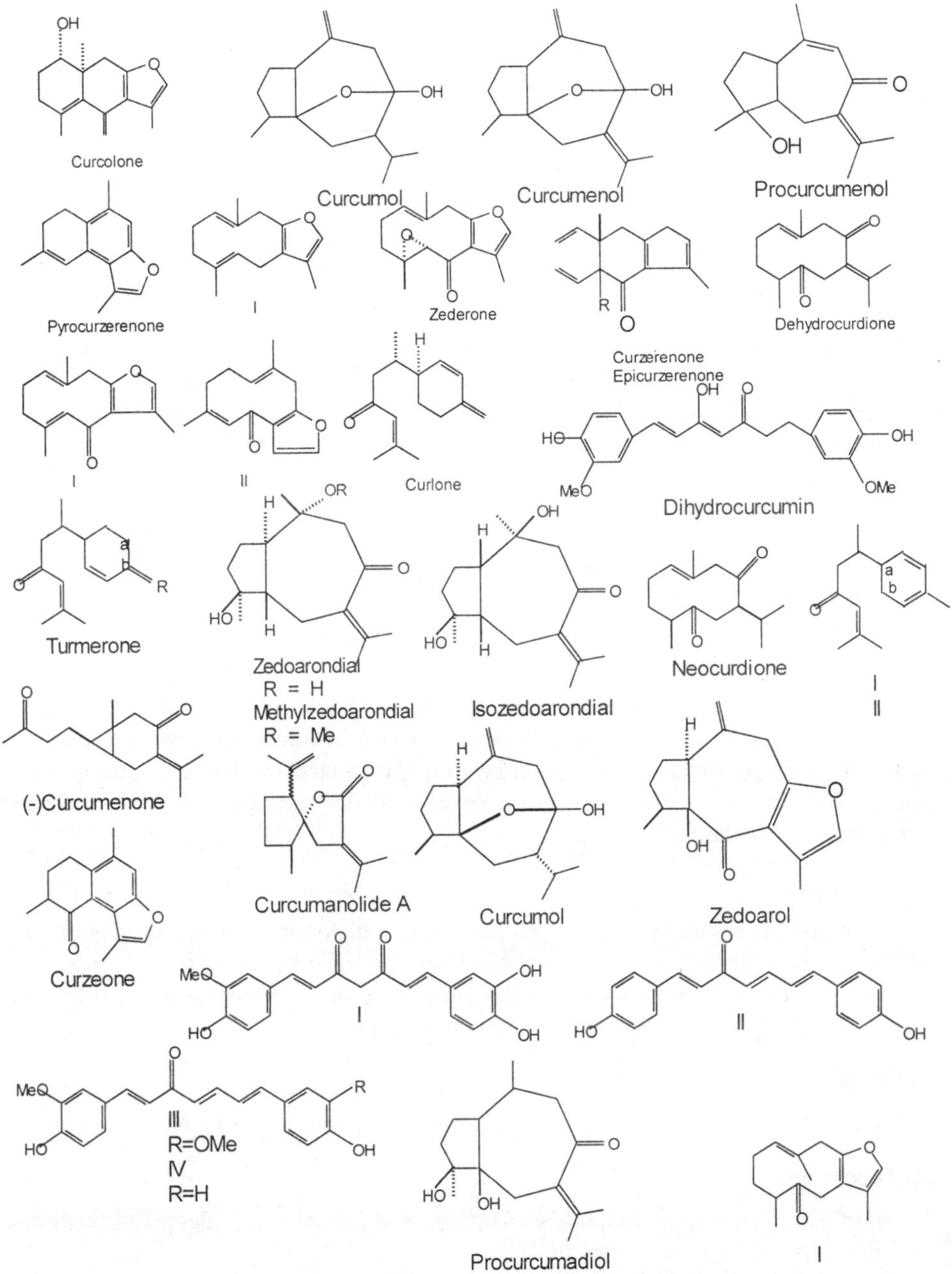

Figure 16.2: Chemical Constituents Isolated from *Curcuma* Species

evaluation were discussed by Jacob and Verghese (204), Chi and Kim (205), Gaitonde and Sapre (206), Dwivedi *et al.* (207) and Longyun *et al.* (208). Sanagi (209) reported various methods of curcumin extraction. The constituents of turmeric *Curcuma longa* were reported by many workers (210, 211, 130, 212, 213, 214, 203, 215, 216) (Figure 16.2). Zwaving and Bos (217) reported the essential oils analysis of *C. longa* and 4 other species of *Curcuma.* Uehara *et al.* (218) and Suksamran *et al.* (219) reported phytochemical studies on *C. xanthorrhiza;* Ohkura *et al.* (220) on *C. wenyujin*, Firman *et al.* (4) on *C. hayneana. C. kwangsiensis*, Ky *et al.* (221) on *C. trichosantha*, Ma *et al.* (222) on *C. zedoaria*, Dung *et al.* (223) on *C. pierreana*, Dung *et al.* (224) on *C. haemandii*, Kojima *et al.* (225) and Bordoloi (226) on *C. aromatica*, Wong *et al.* (227) on *C. mangga* and Sirat *et al.* (228) and Jirovetz *et al.* (229) on *C. aeruginosa* and Behura (230) on *C. longa, C. caesia* and *C. amada.*

The rhizomes of *C.aromatica* contain α-pinene, β-pinene, camphene, 1,8-cineole, isofuranogermacrene, borneol, isoborneol, camphor, germacrone and tetramethylpyrazine. Isolation of antiarrhytmic compounds, dipotassium magnesium dioxalate, from the bulbs has been done. Three new sesquiterpenes–isozedoarondiol, methylzedoarondiol and neocurdione were isolated along with some other compounds and the absolute structure of zedoarondial was determined by X-ray analysis. Detection of germacrone, xanthorrhizol, curcuphenol and hydroxyisogermafurenolide in essential oil by GC was reported. (-) curdione, the antipode of the antitumor principal of *C. aromatica* was synthesised. Eleven minor sesquiterpenes were isolated from the rhizome. Analysis of essential oils of five *Curcuma* species was carried out (217).

A wide range of sesquiterpenoids have been synthesised and structures have been established. A new guaiane, zedoarondiol, was isolated from fresh rhizomes of *C. zedoaria* and its structure was elucidated from spectral evidence. A quantitative and qualitative analysis of the essential oil was performed by GC-MS and a 12 step synthesis of curdione was done.

Conclusion

The present review reveals a vast diversity of different *Curcuma* species and its utilities in therapeutics. This will be useful source of information to the researchers in developing more and more scientifically validated herbal formulations from *Curcuma* species particularly by curcumin and its derivatives.

Acknowledgement

Authors are thankful to the Director, NBRI for providing all the facilities.

References

1. Jain SK: *Dictionary of Indian Folk Medicine and Ethnobotany*. Deep Publications, Paschim Vihar, New Delhi. 1991.

2. Govindarajan VS: Ginger–Chemistry, Technology and Quality Evaluation, part I and II CRC *Critical Reviews in Food Science and Nutrition*. 1982, 17, 1-258.

3. Govingarajan VS: Turmeric–Chemistry, Technology and Quality. CRC *Critical Reviews in Food Science and Nutrition*. 1980, 14, 119-301.

4. Firman K, Kinoshita T, Itai A and Sankawa U: Terpenoids from *Curcuma heyneana*. *Phytochem*. 1988, 27, 3887-3891.

5. Bone K: Turmeric–The spice of life. *British J Phytotherapy*. 1991, 2, 51-60.

6. Khanna NM: Turmeric–Nature's precious gift. *Curr Sci.*, 1999, 76, 1351-1355.

7. Liberti, L., Turmeric–a monograph. *Nat Prod*. 1993, V, 1-2.

8. Srimal RC: Turmeric, a brief review on medicinal properties. *Fitoterapia*. 1997, 68, 483-493.

9. Maheshwari RK, Singh AK, Gaddipati J and Srimal RC: Multiple biological activities of curcumin, a short review. *Life Sciences*. 2006, 78, 2081–2087.

10. Smith RM: *Synoptic keys to the genera of Zingeberaceae pro parte*. Dept. Publ. Ser. 2. Roy. Bot. Gard. Edinbergh, 1981.

11. Mangaly JK and Sabu M: A taxonomic revision of the South Indian species of *Curcuma* Linn. (Zingiberaceae). *Rheedea*. 1993, 3, 139-171.

12. Roxbergh W: *Flora Indica*. Serampore, 1820.

13. Horaninov: *Prodromus Monographiae Scitaminiearum* Petropoli (St. Petersburg), 1862.

14. Baker JG: Scitamineae in J.D. Hooker's, *Flora British India*, London, 6, 198-264, 1890-1892.

15. Schumann K: Zingeberaceae, in, Englar A, Das Pflanzenreich IV-46 (Heft 20), Berlin, 1904, 1-458.

16. Larsen K and Smith RM: A new species of *Curcuma* from Thailand. *Notes Roy Bot Gard Edinburgh*. 1978, 30, 269-272.

17. Roxbergh W: Descriptions of several of the monandrous plants of India. *Asiatic Res.* 1810, 11, 318-362.

18. Santapau H: *Curcuma pseudomontana* Grah. *J Bombay Nat Hist Soc*. 1945, 45, 618-623.

19. Santapau H: On a common species of *Curcuma* of Bombay and Salsette Islands. *J Bombay Nat Hist Soc*. 1952, 51,135-139.

20. Mangley JK and Sabu M: *Curcuma pseudomontana* Garh. (Zingeberaceae), A revised description *J Econ Tax Bot*. 1987, 10, 159-162.

21. Tomilinson PB: Phylogeny of Scitamineae–morphological and anatomical consideration. *Evolution*. 1962, 16,192-213.

22. Sherlija KK, Ramashree AB, Unnikrishnan K and Ravindran PN: Comparative rhizome anatomy of four species of *Curcuma*. *J Spices and Aroma Crops*. 1998, 7,103-109.

23. Lin SC, Lin CC, Lin YH, Supriyatana S and Teng CW: Protective and therapeutic effects of *Curcuma xanthorrhiza* on hepatotoxin–induced liver damage. *American J Chin Med*. 1995, 23, 243-254.

24. Eigner D and Scholz D: *Ferula asa-foetida* and *Curcuma longa* in traditional medical treatment and diet in Nepal. *J Ethnopharmacol.* 1999, 67, 1-6.

25. Saikia AP, Pykala VK, Sharma P, Goswami P and Bora U: Ethnobotany of medicinal plants used by Assamese people for various skin ailments and cosmetics. *J Ethnopharmacol.* 2006, 106, 149-157.

26. Kuttan R, Sudheeran PC and Joseph CD: Tumeric and Curcumin as topical agents in cancer therapy. *Tumori.* 1987, 73, 29-31.

27. Soudamini KK and Kuttan R: Cytotoxic and tumor reducing properties of Curcumin. *Indian J Pharmacol.* 1988, 20, 95-101.

28. Soudamini KK and Kuttan R: Inhibition of chemical carcinogenesis by Curcumin. *J Ethnopharmacol.* 1989, 27, 227-233.

29. Huang MT, Lou YR, Ma W, Newmark HL, Reuhl KR and Conney AH: Inhibitory effects of dietary curcumin on forestomach, duodenal and colon carcinogenesis in mice. *Cancer Res.* 1994, 54, 5841-5847.

30. Huang MT, Newmark HL and Frenkel K: Inhibitory effects of curcumin on tumorigenesis in mice. *J Cell Biochem Suppl.* 1997, 27, 26-34.

31. Rao TS, Basu N, Seth SD, Siddiqui HH: *Ind J Physiol Pharmacol.* 1984, 28, 211.

32. Azuine MA and Bhide SV: Adjuvant chemoprevention of experimental cancer, Catechin and dietary tumeric in forestomach and oral cancer models. *J Ethnopharmacol.* 1994, 44, 211-217.

33. Anto RJ, George J, Babu K, Rajasekharan KN and Kuttan R: Antimutagenic and anticarcinogenic activity of natural and synthetic curcuminoids. *Mutation Res.*1996, 370, 127-131.

34. Limtrakul P, Lipigorngoson S, Namwong O, Apisariyakul A and Dunn FW: Inhibitory effect of dietary curcumin on skin carcinogenesis in mice. *Cancer lett.* 1997, 116, 197-203.

35. Nishio H, Yanaka K, Konoshima T, Takayasu J, Satomi Y, Nishino A and Iwashima A: Curcumin, a major colouring agent of food additive *'turmeric'* interacts with Ca calmodulin complex, and inhibit tumour promoter induced phenomena. *Oncology.* 1992, 11, 65-69.

36. Han R: Recent progress in the study of anticancer drugs originating from plants and traditional medicine in China. *Chinese Med. J.* 1995, 108, 729-731.

37. Yu R: Taking the path of combining traditional Chinese medicine with Western medicine in cancer research and control. *Chinese Med. J.* 1995, 108,732-733.

38. Itokawa H: Antitumour agents isolated from higher plants. Abst. III. International Congress on Ethnopharmacology and its Contemporary Utilization, Beijing, China, 6-10 September 1994. A-14.

39. Azuine MA, Kayal JJ and Bhide SV: Protective role of aqueous turmeric extract against mutagenicity of dried-acting carcinogens as well as benzo [alpha]

pyrene-induced genotoxicity and carcinogenicity. *J Cancer Res Clin Oncol.* 1992, 118, 447-52.

40. Soni KB, Rajan A and Kuttan R: Reversal of aflatoxin induced liver damage by turmeric and curcumin. *Cancer Lett.* 1992, 66, 115-121.
41. Chan MM: Inhibition of tumour4 necrosis factor by curcumin, a phytochemical. *Biochemical Pharmacology.* 1995, 49, 1551-1556.
42. Ammon HP, Safayhi H, Mack T and Sabieraj J: Mechanism of antiflammatory actions of curcumin and boswellic acids. *J Ethnopharmacol.* 1993, 38, 113-119.
43. Anto RJ, Kuttan G, Babu KVD, Rajasekharan KN and Kuttan R: Anti-inflammatory activity of natural and synthetic curcuminoids. *Amala Res Bull.* 1996, 16, 73-77.
44. Verma SP, Salamone E and Goldin B, Curcumin and genistein, plant products, show synergistic inhibitory effects on the growth of human breast cancer MCF-7 cells induced by estrogenic pesticides. *Biochem Biophys Res Commun.* 1997, 233,692-696.
45. Sikora E, Bielak-Zmijewska A, Piwocka K, Skierski J and Radziszewska E: Inhibition of proliferation and apoptosis of human and rat T lymphocytes by curcumin, a curry pigment. *Biochem Pharmacol.* 1997, 54, 899-907.
46. Piper JT, Singhal SS, Salameh MS, Torman RT, Awasthi, YC and Awasthi S: Mechanisms of anticarcinogenic properties of curcumin, the effect of curcumin on glutathione linked detoxification enzymes in rat liver. *The International Journal of Biochemistry and Cell Biology.* 1998, 30, 445-456.
47. Navis I, Sriganth P and Premalatha B: Dietary curcumin with cisplatin administration modulates marker indices in experimental fibrosarcoma. *Pharmacol Res.* 1999, 39, 175-179.
48. Vimala S, Norhanom AW and Yadav M: Anti-tumour promoter activity in Malaysian ginger rhizobia used in traditional medicine. *Br J Cancer.* 1999, 80,110-116.
49. Bhaumik S, Anjum R, Rangaraj N, Pardhasaradhi BV and Khar A: Curcumin mediated apoptosis in AK-5 tumor cells involve the production of reactive oxygen intermediates. *FEBS Lett.* 1999, 456, 311-314.
50. Singhal SS, Awasthi S, Pandeya U, Piper JT, Saini MK, Cheng JZ and Awasthi YC: The effect of curcumin on glutathione-linked enzymes in K562 human leukemia cells. *Toxicol Lett.* 1999, 109, 87-95.
51. Chun KS, Sohn Y, Kim HS, Kim OH, Park KK, Lee JM, Moon A, Lee SS and Surh YJ: Anti-tumor promoting potential of naturally occurring diarylheptanoids structurally related to curcumin. *Mutat Res.* 1999, 428, 49-57.
52. Surh Y: Molecular mechanism of chemopreventive effects of selected dietary and medicinal phenolic substances. *Mutat Res.* 1999, 428, 305-327.
53. Kim KI, Kim JW, Hong BS, Shin DH, Cho HY, Kim HK, Yang HC: Antitumor genotoxicity and anticlastogenic activities of polysaccharide from *Curcuma zedoaria*. *Mol Cells.* 2000, 10, 392-398.

54. Skrzypczak-Jankum E, McCabe NP, Selman SH and Jankum J: Curcumin inhibits lipoxygenase by binding to its central cavity, theoretical and X-ray evidence. *Int J Mol Med*. 2000, 6, 521-526.

55. Bhaumik S, Jyothi MD and Khar A: Differential modulation of nitric oxide production by curcumin in host macrophages and NK cells. *FEBS Lett*. 2000, 483, 78-82.

56. Limtrakul P, Anuchapreeda S, Lipigorngoson S and Dunn FW: Inhibition of carcinogen induced c-Ha-ras and c-fos proto-oncogenes expression by dietary curcumin. *BMC Cancer*. 2001, 1, 1.

57. Collett GP, Robson CN, Mathers JC and Campbell FC: Curcumin modifies Apc (min) apoptosis resistance and inhibits 2-amino 1-methyl-6-phenylimidazol [4,5-b] pyridine (PhIP) induced tumour formation in Apc(min) mice, *Carcinogenesis*. 2001, 22, 821-825.

58. Huang MT, Deschner EE, Newmark HL, Wang ZY, Ferraro TA, Conney AH: Effect of dietary curcumin and ascorbyl palmitate on azoxymethanol-induced colonic epithelial cell proliferation and focal areas of dysplasia. *Cancer Letters*. 1992, 64, 117-121.

59. Ruby AJ, Kuttan G, Babu KD, Rajasekharan KN and Kuttan R: Anti-tumour and antioxidant activity of natural curcuminoids. *Cancer Lett*. 1995, 94(1), 79-83.

60. Dahl TA, Bilski P, Reszka KJ and Chingnell CF: Photocytotoxicity of curcumin. *Photochem Photobiol*. 1994, 59, 290-294.

61. Hanif R, Qiao L, Shiff SJ and Rigas B: Curcumin, a natural plant phenolic food additive, inhibits cell proliferation and induce cell cycle changes in colon adenocarcinoma cell lines by a prostaglandin-independent pathway. *J Lab Clin Med*. 1997, 130, 576-584.

62. Kawamori T, Lubet R, Steele VE, Kelloff GJ, Kaskey RB, Rao CV and Reddy BS: Chemopreventive efffect of curcumin, a naturally occuring anti-inflammatory agent, during the promotion/progression stages of colon cancer. *Cancer Res*. 1999, 59, 597-601.

63. Anto RJ, Maliekal TT and Karunagaran D: L-929 cells harboring ectopically expressed RelA resist curcumin-induced apoptosis. *J Biol Chem*. 2000, 275, 15601-15604.

64. Ushida J, Sugie S, Kawabata K, Pharm QV, Tanaka T, Fujii K, Takeuchi H and Ito Y: Chemopreventive effect of curcumin on N-nitrosomethylbenzylamine-induced esophageal carcinogenesis in rats. *Jpn J Cancer Res*. 2000, 91, 893-898.

65. Lin JK, Pan MH and Lin-Shiau SY: Recent studies on the biofunctions and biotransformations of curcumin. *Biofactors*. 2000, 13, 153-158.

66. Banerjee A and Nigam SS: Anti bacterial efficacy of the essential oils derived from the various species of the genus–*Curcuma* Linn. *J Res Ind Med Yoga Homoeo*. 1977, 12, 89-96.

67. Banerjee A and Nigam SS: Antifungal efficacy of the essential oils derived from the species of the genus–*Curcuma* Linn. *J Res Ind Med Yoga Homoeo*. 1978, 13, 63-70.

68. Shankar TNB and Murthy VS: Effect of turmeric (*Curcuma longa*) fractions on the growth of some intestinal and pathogenic bacteria *in vitro. Indian J Exp Biol.* 1979, 17, 1363-1366.

69. Tonnesen HH, Vries H, Karlson J and Henegouwen GB: Studies on curcumin and curcuminoids, Investigation of the photobiological activity of curcumin using bacterial indicator systems. *J Pharma Sci*. 1987, 76, 371-373.

70. Li GJ, Zhang, LJ, Dezube BJ, Crumpacker CJ, Pardee AB: *Proc Nat Acad Sci.* USA, 1993, 90, 1839.

71. Yasni S, Imaizumi K, Sin K, Sugano M, Nonaka G and Sidik: Identification of an active principle in essential oils and hexane-soluble fractions of *Curcuma xanthorrhiza* Roxb. showing triglyceride-lowering action in rats. *Food and Chemical Toxicology*. 1994, 32, 273-278.

72. Sui Z, Salto R, Li J, Craik C, Ortiz de Montellano PR: Inhibition of the HIV-2 proteases by curcumin and curcumin boron complexes. *Bioorganic and Medicinal Chemistry*. 1993, 1, 415-422.

73. Iyengar MA, Rao MPR, Bairy I and Kamath MS: Antimicrobial activity of the essential oil of *Curcuma longa* leaves. *Indian Drugs*. 1995, 32, 249-250.

74. Mazumder A, Raghavan K, Weinstein J, Kohn KW and Pommier Y: Inhibition of human immunodeficiency virus type-1 integrase by curcumin. *Biochem Pharmacol.* 1995, 49, 1165-1170.

75. Thomas E, Shanmugam J and Rafi MM: Antibacterial activity of plants belonging to Zingiberaceae family. *Biomedicine*. 1996, 16, 15-20.

76. Niaz I, Kazmi AR and Jilani G: Effect of turmeric derivatives on radial colony growth of different fungi. *Sarhad J Agri*, 1994, 10, 571-573.

77. Apisariyakul A, Vanittananakom N and Buddhasukh D: Antifungal activity of turmeric oil extracted from *Curcuma longa* (Zingiberaceae). *J Ethnopharmacol*. 1995, 49, 163-169.

78. Roth BN, Chandra A and Nair MG: Novel Bio-activities of *Curcuma longa* constitutents. *J Nat Prod*. 1998, 61, 542-545.

79. Barthelemy S, Vergnes L, Moynier M, Guyot D, Labidalle S and Bahraoui E: Curcumin and curcumin derivatives inhibit Tat-mediated transactivation of type 1 human immunodeficiency virus long terminal repeat. *Research in Virology*. 1998, 149, (1), 43-52.

80. Antony S, Kuttan R and Kuttan G: Immunomodulatory activity of curcumin. *Immunol Invest*. 1999, 28, 291-303.

81. Kang BY, Song YJ, Kim KM, Choe YK, Hwang SY and Kim TS: Curcumin inhibits Th1 cytokine profile in CD4+T cells by suppressing interleukin-12 production in macrophages. *Br J Pharmacol*. 1999, 128, 380-384.

82. De-Clercq E: Current lead natural products for the chemotherapy of human immunodeficiency virus (HIV) infection. *Med Res Rev.* 2000, 20, 323-349.

83. Hwang JK, Shim JS and Pyun YR: Antibacterial activity of xanthorrhizol from *Curcuma xanthorrhiza* against oral pathogens. *Fitoterapia.* 2000, 71, 321-323.

84. Rasmussen HB, Christensen SB, Kvist LP, Karazmi A: A simple and efficient separation of the curcumins, the antiprotozoal constituents of *Curcuma longa. Planta Med.* 2000, 66, 396-398.

85. Maini PN and Morallo-Rejesus BM: Toxicity of some volatile oils against golden snail (*Pomacea* spp.). *Philipp J Sci.* 1992, 121, 391-397.

86. Pandji C, Grimm C, Wray V, Witte L and Proksch P: Insecticidal constituents from four species of Zingiberaceae. *Phytochem.* 1993, 34, 415-419.

87. Jurgens TM, Frazier EG, Schaeffer JM, Jones TE, Zink DL, Borris RP, Nanakora W, Beck HT and Balick MJ: Novel nematocidal agents from *Curcuma comosa. J Nat Prod.* 1994, 57, 230-235.

88. Das NG, Nath DR, Baruah I, Talukdar PK and Das SC: Field evaluation of herbal mosquito repellents. *J Commun Dis.* 1999, 31, 241-245.

89. Srimal RC, Khanna NM, Dhawan BN: *Ind J Pharmacol.* 1971, 3, 10.

90. Srimal RC and Dhawan BN: *J Pharm Pharmacol.* 1973, 25, 447.

91. Srimal RC and Dhawan BN: *'Development of Unani Drugs from Herbal sources and the role of elements in their mechanism of action'.* RB Arora (Ed.). Hamdard National Foundation Monograph, Hamdard National Foundation, New Delhi. 1985, pp 131-142.

92. Srimal RC: *Science Today.* 1986, 20, 26.

93. Srimal RC and Dhawan BN: Pharmacological and clinical studies on *Curcuma longa. Hamdard Med.* 1987, 30, 131-142.

94. Ghatak N, Basu N, *Ind J Exper Biol.* 1972, 10, 235.

95. Rao TS, Basu N and Siddiqui HH: Anti-inflammatory activity of Curcumin analogues. *Indian J Med Res.* 1982, 75, 574-578.

96. Wagh KR and Shingatgeri MK: Plants and Medicine, Anti-inflammatory effect of *Curcuma longa* Linn. in rats. *Capsule.* 1981, 20, 39-40.

97. Khung N, Rastogi G and Grover K: Anti-inflammatory and analgesic activities of *Curcuma longa. Indian J Pharmacol.* 1986, 18, 59-60.

98. Matsuda H, Ninomiya K, Morikawa T and Yoshikawa M: Inhibitory effect and action mechanism of sesquiterpenes from Zedoariae Rhizoma on D-galactosamine/lipopolysaccharide-induced liver injury. *Bioorg Med Chem Lett.* 1998, 8, 339-344.

99. Iyengar MA, Rao MPR and Gurumadhava Rao S: Anti-inflammatory activity of volatile oil of *Curcuma longa* leaves. *Indian Drugs.* 1994, 31, 528-531.

100. Razago Z and Gabor M: Effects of Curcumin and nordihydroguairetic acid on mouse ear oedema induced by croton oil or dithranol. *Pharmazie*. 1995, 50, 156-157.

101. Claeson P, Panthog A, Tuchinda P, Reutrakul V, Kanjanapothi D, Taylor WC and Santisuk T: Three non-phenolic diarylheptanoids with anti-inflammatory activity from *Curcuma xanthorrhiza. Planta Med.* 1993, 59, 451-454.

102. Claeson P, Pongprayoon U, Sematong T, Tuchinda P, Reutrakul V, Soontornsaratuna P and Taylor WC: Non-phenolic linear diarylheptanoids from *Curcuma xanthorriza*, A novel type of topical anti-inflammatory agents, structure–activity relationship. *Planta Med.* 1996, 62, 236-240.

103. Mukhopadhyaya A, Basu N, Ghatak N, Gujral PK: *Agents Actions*. 1982, 12, 508.

104. Satoskar RR, Shah SJ and Shenoy SG: *Intl J Clin Pharmacol Ther Toxicol*. 1986, 24, 651.

105. Ozaki Y: Antiflammatory effect of *Curcuma xanthorrhiza* Roxb, and its active principles. *Chem Pharm Bull.* 1990, 38, 1045-1048.

106. Srivastava R, Puri V, Srimal RC and Dhawn BN: *Arzneim Forch*. 1986, 36, 715.

107. Dirsch VM, Stuppner H and Vollmar AM: The Griess assay, suitable for a bio-guided fractionation of anti-inflammatory plant extracts. *Planta Med.* 1998, 64, 423-426.

108. Yoshioka T, Fujii E, Endo M, Wada K, Tokunaga Y, Shiba N, Hohsho H, Shibuya H and Muraki T: Antiinflammatory potency of dehydrocurdione, a zedoary-derived sesquiterpene. *Inflamm Res.* 1998, 47, 476-481.

109. Lal B, Kapoor AK, Agarwal PK, Asthana OP and Srimal RC: Role of curcumin in idiopathic inflammatory orbital pseudotumours. *Phytother Res.* 2000, 14, 443-447.

110. Shimizu S, Jareonkitmongkol S, Kawashima H, Akimoto K and Yamada H: Inhibitory effect of curcumin on fatty acid desaturation in Mortierella alpina IS-4 and rat microsomes. *Lipids*. 1992, 27, 509-512.

111. Yasni S, Imaizumi K, Nakamura M, Aimoto J and Sugano M: Effect of *Curcuma xanthorrhiza* Roxb. and curcuminoids on the level of serum and liver lipids, serum apolipoprotein A-1 and lipogenic enzymes in rats. *Food and Chemical Toxicology*. 1993, 31, 213-218.

112. Babu PS and Srinivasan K: Hypolipidemic action of curcumin, the active principle of turmeric (*Curcuma longa*) in streptozotocin induced diabetic rats. *Mol Cell Biochem.* 1997, 166, 169-175.

113. Piyachaturawat P, Teeratagolpisal N, Toskulkao C and Suksamaran A: Hypolipidemic effect of *Curcuma comosa* in mice. *Artery*. 1997, 22, 233-241.

114. Quiles JL, Aguilera C, Mesa MD, Ramirez-Tortosa MC, Baro L and Gil A: An ethanolic-aqueous extract of *Curcuma longa* decreased the susceptibility of liver microsomes and mitochondria to lipid peroxidation in atherosclerotic rabbits. *Biofactors*. 1998, 8, 51-57.

115. Piyachaturawat P, Charoenpiboonsin J, Toskulkao C and Suksamrana A: Reduction of plasma cholesterol by *Curcuma comosa* in hypercholesterolaemic hamsters. *J Ethnopharmacol.* 1999, 66, 199-204.

116. Ramirrez-Tortosa MC, Mesa MD, Aguilera MC, Quiles JL, Baro L, Ramirez-Tortosa CL, Martinez-Victoria E and Gil A: Oral administration of a turmeric extract inhibits LDL oxidation and has hypocholesterolemic effects in rabbits with experimental atherosclerosis. *Atherosclerosis.* 1999, 147, 371-378.

117. Ramirez-Bosca A, Soler A, Carrion MA, Diaz-Alperi J, Bernd A, Quintanilla C, Quintanilla AE and Miquel J: An hydroalcoholic extract of curcuma longa lowers the apo B/apo A ratio. Implications for atherogenesis prevention. *Mech Ageing Dev.* 2000, 119, 41-47.

118. Ozaki Y and Soedigdo S: *Soyakugaku Zassi.* 1988, 42, 333.

119. Kositchaiwt C, Kositchaiwat S and Havanondha J: *Curcuma longa* Linn. in the treatment of gastric ulcer comparison to liquid antacid, a controlled clinical trial. *J Med Assoc Thailand,* 1993, 76, 601-605.

120. Mulky N, Amonaar AJ and Bhide SV: Antimutagenicity of curcumins and related compound, the structural requirement for the antimutagenicity of curcumins. *Indian Drugs.* 1987, 25, 91-95.

121. Nagabhushan M, Amonkar AJ and Bhide SV: *In vitro* antimutagenicity of Curcumin against environment mutagens. *Food Chem Toxicol* 1987, 25, 545-547.

122. Rafatullah S, Tariq M, Al-Yahya MA, Mossa JS and Ageel AM: Evaluation of turmeric (*Curcuma longa*) for gastric and duodenal antiulcer activity in rats. *J Ethnopharmacol.* 1990, 29, 25-34.

123. Imamura M, Yamauchi H and Chey WY: Effect of intraduodenal infusion of pancreatic exocrine secretion and gastrointestinal hormone release in rats. *Int J Pancreatol.* 1994, 15, 187-193.

124. Romiti N, Tongiani R, Cervelli F and Chieli E: Effects of curcumin on P-glycoprotein in primary cultures of rat hepatocytes. *Life Sci.* 1998, 62, 2349-2358.

125. Deshpande UR, Gadre SG, Raste AS, Pillai D, Bhide SV and Samuel AM: Protective effect of turmeric (*Curcuma longa* L.) extract on carbon tetrachloride-induced liver damage in rats. *Indian J Exp Biol.* 1998, 36, 573-577.

126. Niederau C and Gopfert E: The effect of chelidonium and turmeric root extract on upper abdominal pain due to functional disorders of the biliary system. *Med Klin (Munich),* 1999, 94, 425-430.

127. Wu W, Deng R and Ou Y: Therapeutic efficacy of microsphere-entrapped *Curcuma aromatica* oil infused via hepatic artery against transplanted hepatoma in rats. *Zhonghua Gan Zang Bing Za Zhi.* 2000, 8, 24-26.

128. Deters M, Siegers C, Hansel W, Schneider KP and Hennighausen G: Influence of curcumin on cyclosporin-induced reduction of biliary bilirubin and cholesterol excretion and on biliary excretion of cyclosporin and its metabolites. *Planta Med.* 2000, 66, 429-434.

129. Donatus IA and Vermeulen NP: Cytoxic and cytoprotective activities of curcumin. Effects on paracetamol-induced cytotoxicity, lipid peroxidation and glutathione depletion in rat hepatocytes. *Biochem Pharmacol.* 1990. 39, 1869-1875.

130. Kiso, Y, Suzuki Y, Oshima Y and Hikino H: Stereostructure of curlone, a sesquiterpenoid of *Curcuma longa* rhizomes. *Phytochem.* 1983, 22, 596-597.

131. Goud VK, Polasa K, Krishnaswamy K: *Plants Food for Human Nutri.* 1993, 44, 87.

132. Oetari S, Sudibyo M, Commandeur JNM, Samhoedi R, Vermeuleri NPE: *Biochem Pharmacol.* 1996, 51, 39.

133. Kiso Y, Suzuki Y, Watanabe N, Oshima Y and Hikino H: Liver protective drugs. Part 8. Antihepatotoxic principles of *Curcuma longa* rhizomes. *Planta Med.* 1983, 49, 185-187.

134. Miquel J, Martinez M, Diez A, De-Juan E, Soler A, Ramirez A, Laborda J and Carrioa M: Effects of turmeric on blood and liver lipoperoxide levels of mice, lack of toxicity. *Age.* 1995, 18, 171-174.

135. Reddy AC, Lokesh BR: Studies on the inhibitory effects of curcumin and eugenol on the formation of reactive oxygen species and the oxidation of ferrous iron. *Molecular and Cellular Biochemistry.* 1994, 137, 1–8.

136. Schlepper O and Winterhoff H: *Curcuma domestica* Val., Choleretic activity in the isolated perfused rat liver (IPRL). Abstr. 6th International Congress on Ethnopharmacology, 3-7 September 2000, Switzerland. P4B/19.

137. Lin SC, Lin CC, Lin YH, Supriyatana S and Teng C W: Protective and therapeutic effects of *Curcuma xanthorrhiza* on hepatotoxin–induced liver damage. *American J Chin Med.* 1995, 23, 243-254.

138. Srivastava KC, Bordia A and Verma SK: Curcumin, a major component of food spice turmeric (*Curcuma longa*) inhibits aggregation and alters eicosanoid metabolism in human blood platelets. *Prostaglandins, Leukotrienes and Essential Fatty Acids.* 1995, 52, 223-227.

139. Miquel J, Martinez M, Diez A, De-Juan E, Soler A, Ramirez A, Laborda J and Carrioa M: Effects of turmeric on blood and liver lipoperoxide levels of mice, lack of toxicity. *Age.* 1995, 18, 171-174.

140. Huang HC, Jan TR and Yeh SF: Inhibitory effect of curcumin, an anti-inflammatory agent, on vascular smooth muscle cell proliferation. *European J Pharmacol.* 1992, 221, 381-384.

141. Chang H and Butt PP: *Pharmacology and Application of Chinese Materia Medica.* World Scientific Publishing Company, Singapore, 1987.

142. Jain JP, Naqvi SMA and Sharma KD: Clinical trial of volatile oil of *Curcuma longa* Linn. (Haridra) in cases of bronchial asthma (Tamaka swasa). *J Res Ayur Siddha.* 1990, 11, 20-30.

143. Yano S, Terai M, Shimizu KL, Fatagami Y, Horie S, Tsuchiya S, Ikegami F, Sekine T and Yamamoto Y: Antiallergic activity of extracts from *Curcuma longa.* Active components and mechanism of actions. *Phytomedicine.* 1996, 3, 58.

144. Nadkarni KM: *Curcuma longa. In:* Nadkarni KM (Ed.), *Indian Materia Medica.* Popular Prakashan Publishing Company, Bombay, 1976, pp. 414-416.

145. Sidhu GS, Singh AK, Thaloor D, Banaudha KK, Patnaik GK, Srimal RC, Maheshwari RK: Enhancement of wound healing by curcumin in animals. *Wound Repair and Regeneration.* 1998, 6, 167-177.

146. Varga J, Rosenbloom J, Jimenez SA: Transforming growth factor beta (TGF beta) causes a persistent increase in steady-state amounts of type I and type III collagen and fibronectin mRNAs in normal human dermal fibroblasts. *Biochemical Journal.* 1987, 247, 597-604.

147. Quaglino D, Nanney LB, Kennedy R, Davidson JM: Transforming growth factor-beta stimulates wound healing and modulates extracellular matrix gene expression in pig skin. I. Excisional wound model. *Laboratory Investigation.* 1990, 63, 307-319.

148. Sidhu GS, Mani H, Gaddipati JP, Singh AK, Seth P, Banaudha KK, Patnaik GK and Maheshwari RK: Curcumin enhances wound healing in streptozotocin induced diabetic rats and genetically diabetic mice. *Wound Repair Regen.* 1999, 7, 362-374.

149. Mani H, Sidhu GS, Kumari R, Gaddipati JP, Seth P and Maheshwari RK: Curcumin differentially egulates TGF-β1, its receptors and nitric oxide synthase during impaired wound healing. *BioFactors.* 2002, 16, 29-43.

150. Thaloor D, Miller KJ, Gephart J, Mitchell PO, Pavlath GK: Systemic administration of the NF-êB inhibitor curcumin stimulates muscle regeneration after traumatic injury. *American J Physiology Cell Physiology.* 1999, 277, C320-C329.

151. Phan TT, See P, Lee ST, Chan SY: Protective effects of curcumin against oxidative damage on skin cells in vitro, its implication for wound healing. *J Trauma.* 2001, 51, 927-931.

152. Gopinath D, Ahmed MR, Gomathi K, Chitra K, Sehgal PK, Jayakumar R: Dermal wound healing processes with curcumin incorporated collagen films. *Biomaterials.* 2004, 25, 1911-1917.

153. Jagetia GC, Rajanikant GK: Curcumin treatment enhances the repair and regeneration of wounds in mice exposed to hemibody gammairradiation. *Plastic and Reconstructive Surger.* 2005, 115, 515-528.

154. Swarnakar S, Ganguly K, Kundu P, Banerjee A, Maity P, Sharma AV: Curcumin regulates expression and activity of matrix metalloproteinases–9 and–2 during prevention and healing of indomethacin-induced gastric ulcer. *J Biol Chem.* 2005, 280, 9409-9415.

155. Charles V and Charles SX: The use and efficacy of *Azadirachta indica* ADR ('Neem') and *Curcuma longa* ('Turmeric') in scabies. A pilot study. *Trop Geogr Med.* 1992, 44, 178-181.

156. Bonte F, Noel-Hudson MS, Wepierre J and Meybeck A: Protective effect of curcuminoides on epidermal skin cells under free oxygen radical stress. *Planta Med.* 1997, 63, 265-266.

157. Rajakrishnan V, Viswanathan P, Rajasekharan KN and Menon VP: Neuroprotective role of curcumin from *Curcuma longa* on ethanol-induced brain damage. *Phytother Res.* 1999, 13, 571-574.

158. Toda S, Miyase T, Arichi H, Tanizawa H and Takino Y: Natural antioxidants III. Antioxidative components isolated from rhizome of *Curcuma longa* L. *Chem Pharm Bull,* 1985, 33, 1725-1728.

159. Reddy AC and Lokesh BR: Effect of dietary turmeric (*Curcuma longa*) on iron-induced lipid peroxidation in the rat liver. *Food Chem Toxicol.* 1994, 32, 279-283.

160. Sreejayan Rao MN: Curcuminoids as potent inhibitors of lipid peroxidation. *J Pharm Pharmacol.* 1994, 46, 1013-1016.

161. Cohly HH, Taylor A, Angel MF, Salahudeen AK: Effect of turmeric, turmerin and curcumin on H_2O_2-induced renal epithelial (LLCPK1) cell injury. *Free Radical Biology and Medicine,* 1998, 24, 49-54.

162. Dixit RS and Perti SL: Indigenous insecticides Part III–insecticidal properties of some medicinal and aromatic plants. *Bull Reg Lab Jammu.* 1963, 1, 169-172.

163. Motterlini R, Foresti R, Bassi R, Green CJ: Curcumin, an antioxidant and anti-inflammatory agent, induces heme oxygenase-1 and protects endothelial cells against oxidative stress. *Free Radical Biology and Medicine.* 2000, 28, 1303-1312.

164. Nirmala C, Puvanakrishnan R: Protective role of curcumin against isoproterenol induced myocardial infarction in rats. *Molecular and Cellular Biochemistry.* 1996b, 159, 85-93.

165. Nirmala C, Puvanakrishnan R: Effect of curcumin on certain lysosomal hydrolases in isoproterenol-induced myocardial infarction in rats. *Biochemical Pharmacology.* 1996, 51, 47-51.

166. Nirmala C, Anand S, Puvanakrishnan R: Curcumin treatment modulates collagen metabolism in isoproterenol induced myocardial necrosis in rats. *Molecular and Cellular Biochemistry.* 1999, 197, 31-37.

167. Manikandan P, Sumitra M, Aishwarya S, Manohar BM, Lokanadam B and Puvanakrishnan R: Curcumin modulates free radical quenching in myocardial ischaemia in rats. *Inter J Biochem Cell Biol.* 2004, 36, 1967-1980.

168. Jones EA, Shahed A, Shoskes DA: Modulation of apoptotic and inflammatory genes by bioflavonoids and angiotensin II inhibition in ureteral obstruction. *Urology.* 2000, 56, 346-351.

169. Matsuda T, Jitoe A, Isobe J, Nakatani N and Yonemori S: Antioxidative and anti-inflammatory curcumin related phenolics from rhizomes of *Curcuma domestica. Phytochem.* 1993, 32, 1557-1560.

169. Nakatani N: Phenolic antioxidants from herbs and spices. *Biofactors.* 2000, 13(1-4), 141-146.

170. Selvam R, Subramanian L, Gayathri R and Angayakanni N: The anto-oxidant activity of turmeric (*Curcuma longa*). *J Ethnopharmacol.* 1995, 47, 59-67.

171. Grinberg LN, Shalev O, Tonnesen HH and Rachmi-Lewitz EA: Studies on curcumin and curciminoids XXVI. Antioxident effects of curcumin on the red blood cell membrane. *Inter J Pharmaceutics*. 1996, 132, 251-257.

172. Matsuda T, Isobe J, Jitoe A and Nakatani N: Antioxidative curcuminoids from rhizomes of *Curcuma xanthorrhiza*. *Phytochem*. 1992, 31, 3645-3647.

173. Srinivas L, Shalini VK and Shylaja M: Turmerin, a water soluble antioxidant peptide from turmeric [*Curcuma longa*]. *Arch Biochem Biophys*. 1992, 292, 617-623.

174. Osawa T, Sugiyama Y, Inayoshi M and Kawakishi S: Antioxidative activity of tetrahydrocurcuminoids. *Biosci Biotechnol Biochem*. 1995, 59(9), 1609-1612.

175. Priyadarsini KL: Free radical reaction of curcumin in membrane models. *Free Radical Biol Med*. 1997, 23, 838-843.

176. Stano J, Granaci D, Neubert K and Kresanek J: Curcumin as a potential antioxidant. *Ceska Slov Farm*. 2000, 49, 168-170.

177. Huang J, Ogihara Y, Gonda R and Takeda T: Novel biphenyl ether lignans from the rhizomes of *Curcuma chuanyujin*. *Chem Pharm Bull*. 2000, 48, 1228-1229.

178. Rilantono LI, Yuwono HS and Nugrahadi T: Dietary antioxidative potential in arteries. *Clin Hemorheol Microcirc*. 2000, 23, 113-117.

179. Kim DSHL, Park SY and Kim JK: Curcuminoids from *Curcuma longa* L. (Zingiberaceae) that protect PC12 rat pheochromocytoma and normal human umbilical vein endothelial cells from betaA(1-42) insult. *Neuroscience Letters*. 2001, 303, 57-61.

180. Matthes HWD and Ourisson G, Cytotoxic components of *Zingiber zerumbet, Curcuma zedoaria* and *C. domestica*. *Phytochem*. 1980, 19, 2643-2650.

181. Syn WJ, Shen CC, Don MJ, Ou JC, Lee GH and Sun CM: Cytotoxicity of curcuminoids and some novel compounds from *Curcuma zedoaria*. *J Nat Prod*. 1998, 61, 1531-1534.

182. Cherdchu C and Karlsson E: Protolytic independent Cobra neurotoxin inhibiting activity of *Curcuma sp.* (Zingiberaceae). *Southeast Asian J Trop Med Public Health*, 1983, 14, 176-180.

183. Cherdchu C, Srisukawat K and Ratanabanangkoon K: Cobra neurotoxin inhibiting activity found in the extract of *Curcuma sp.* (Zingiberaceae). *J Med Assoc Thai*. 1978, 61, 544-554.

184. Ratanabanangkoon K, Cherdchu C and Chudapongse C: Studies on the cobra neurotoxin inhibiting activity in an extract of *Curcuma sp.* (Zingiberaceae) rhizome. *Southeast Asian J Trop Med Public Health*. 1993, 24, 178-185.

185. Ferreira LA, Henriques OB, Andreoni AA, Vital GR, Campos MM, Habermehl GG, de Moraes VL: Antivenom and biological effects of ar-turmerone isolated from *Curcuma longa* (Zingiberaceae). *Toxicon*. 1992, 30, 1211-1218.

186. Garg SK: Effect of *Curcuma longa* (Rhizomes) on fertility in experimental animals. *Planta Med*. 1974, 26, 225-227.

187. Das BVD: Methods for sterilization and contraception in ancient and mediaeval India. *Ayurvigyana*. 1982, 3, 10-14.

188. Bhatnagar U: Antifertility effect of *Curcuma lònga* extracts in female albino rats. *Indian J Physiol Allied Sci*. 1995, 49, 179-184.

189. Deodhar SD, Sethi R and Srimal RC: Preliminary study on antirheumatic activity of curcumin (difernloyl methane). *Indian J Med Res*. 1980, 77, 632-634.

190. Kulkarni RR, Patki PS, Jog VP, Gandage SG and Patwardhan B: Treatment of osteoarthritis with a herbomineral formulation, a double-blind, placebo-controlled, cross-over study. *J Ethnopharmacol*. 1991, 33, 91-95.

191. Chodhuary D, Chandra D and Kale RK: Modulation of radioresponse of glyoxalase system by curcumin. *J Ethnopharmacol*. 1999, 64, 1-7.

192. Lal B, Kapoor AK, Asthana OP, Agarwal PK, Prasad R, Kumar P and Srimal RC: Efficacy of curcumin in the management of chronic anterior uveitis. *Phytother Res*. 1999, 13, 318-322.

193. Srinivasan KR: The colouring matter in tumeric. *Curr Sci*. 1952, 21, 311.

194. Janaki N and Bose JL: Improved method for the isolation of Curcumin from Turmeric (*Curcuma longa* L.), *J Indian Chem Soc*. 1967, 11, 985-986.

195. Sastry BS: Curcumin content of turmeric. *Res and Ind*. 1970, 15, 258-260.

196. Lahiri K: Natural colouring agents, A Pharmaceutical overview. *East Pharm*. 1980, 23, 25-30.

197. Balakrishnan KV, Chandran CV, George KM, Pillai OGN, Mathulla T and Varghese J: Evaluation of *Curcuma*. *Perfum and Flavor*. 1983, 8, 46-49.

198. Tonnesen HH and Kaisen J: Studies on curcumin and curcuminoids V. Alkaline degradation of curcumin. *Food Tech Abstr*. 1985, 20, 3948.

199. Rouseff RL: High Performance liquid chromatographic separation and spectral characterization of the pigments in turmeric and annatto. *J Food Sci*. 1988, 53, 1823-1826.

200. Faruq MO and Haque MZ: Chemical investigations on Bangladeshi turmeric Part I. Preparation of synthetic dyes from curcumin. *Bangladesh J Sci Indust Res*. 1990, 25, 110-117.

201. Zachariah TJ and Babu NK: Effect of storage of fresh tumeric rhizomes on oleoresin and curcumin contents. *J Spices and Aroma Crops*. 1992, 1, 55-58.

202. Verghese J: Curcuminoids, the magic dye of *C. longa* L. rhizome. *Indian Spices*, 1999, 36, 19-26.

203. Nakayama R, Tamura Y, Yamanaka H, Kikuzaki H and Nakatani N: Two curcuminoid pigments from *Curcuma domestica*. *Phytochem*. 1993, 33, 501-502.

204. Jacob CV and Varghese J: ASTA method of curcumin evaluation, need for change in adoption of standard. *Indian Spices*. 1981, 18, pp 21.

205. Chi HJ and Kim HS: Curcumin content of cultivated turmeric in Korea. *Korean J Pharmacogn.* 1983, 14, 67-69.

206. Gaitonde RV and Sapre SP: Quantitative standardization of Curcumin derived from rhizomes of *Curcuma* species and *Costus speciosus. Indian J Nat Prod.* 1989, 5, 18-19.

207. Dwivedi AK, Raman M, Seth RK and Saria JPS: Combined thin layer chromatography–densitometry for the quantitation of curcumin in Pharmaceutical dosage forms and in serum. *Indian J Pharmaceutical Sci.* 1992, 54, 174-177.

208. Longyun L, Zhang Y, Quin S and Liao G: Ontogeny and curcumin accumulation of *Curcuma longa.* Abstr. III International Congress on Ethnopharmacology and its contemporary utilization, Beijing, China. 6-10 September, 1994. D-47.

209. Sanagi MM, Admed UK and Smith RM: Application of Supercritical fluid extraction and supercritical fluid chromatography to the analysis of *Curcuma longa* Linn. *In:* Proc. 7th Asian Symposium on Medicinal Plants, Spices and other Natural Products, Manila. 1992, pp. 2-7.

210. Kalique A and Amin MN: Examination of *Curcuma longa* L. I. constituents of the rhizome. *Nutr Abstr.* 1969, 39, 305.

211. Moon CK, Park NS and Koh SK: Studies on the lipid components of *Curcuma longa*. I. The composition of fatty acids and sterols. *Chem Abstr.* 1977, 87, 114582t.

212. Ogbeide ON, Eduaveguavoen OI and Paravez M: Identification of 2 hydroxy methyl anthraquinone in *Curcuma domestica. Pakistan J Sci.* 1985, 37, 15-17.

213. Hu J, Han X, Ji T, Yang Z, Wu X, Xie J and Guo Y: Formation of *Curcuma* lactone and determination of its molecular structure. *Kexue Tongbao.* 1987, 32, 816-820.

214. Ohshiro M, Kuroyangi M and Ueno A: Structures of sesquiterpenes from *Curcuma longa. Phytochem.* 1990, 29, 2201-2205.

215. Mc Carron M, Mills AJ, Whittaker D, Sunny TP and Varghese J: Comparison of the monoterpenes derived from green leaves and fresh rhizomes of *Curcuma longa* L. from India. *Flavour and Frag J.* 1995, 10, 355-357.

216. Sharma RK, Misra BP, Sarma TC, Bordoloi AK, Bordoloi AK, Pathak MG and Leclereq P A: Essential oils of *Curcuma longa* L. from Bhutan. *J Essent Oil Res.* 1997, 9, 589-592.

217. Zwaaving J H and Bos R: Analysis of the essential oils of five *Curcuma* species. *Flavour and Frag J.* 1992, 7, 19-22.

218. Uehara S, Yasuda I, Takeya K and Itokawa H: Terpenoids and curcuminoids of the rhizome of *Curcuma xanthorrhiza* Roxb. *Shoyakugaku Zasshi.* 1992, 112, 817-823.

219. Suksamrarn A, Eiamong S, Piyachaturawat P and Charoenpiboonsin J: Phenolic diaryl heptanoids from *Curcuma xanthorrhiza. Phytochem.* 1994, 36, 1505-1508.

220. Ohkura T, Gao J, Nishishita T, Harimaya K, Kawamata T and Inayama S: Identification of sesquiterpenoid constituents in the essential oil of *Curcuma wenyujin* by capillary gas chromatographic mass spectrometry. *Shoyakugaku Zasshi*. 1987, 41, 102-107.

221. Ky PT, Van de Ven LJM, Leclercq PA and Dung NX: Volatile constituents of the essential oil of *Curcuma trichosantha*. *J Essent Oil Res*. 1994, 6, 213-214.

222. Ma X, Yu X and Han J: Application of off-line supercritical fluid extraction–gas chromatography for the investigation of chemical constituents in *Curcuma zedoaria*. *Phytochemical Analysis*, 1995, 6, 292-296.

223. Dung NX, Tuyet NTB and Leclercq PA: Volatile constituents of the rhizome stem and leaf of *Curcuma pierreana* Gagnep. from Vietnam. *J Essent Oil Res*. 1995, 7, 261-264.

224. Dung NX, Truong PX, Ky PT and Leclercq PA: Volatile constituents of the leaf, stem, rhizome, root and flower oils of *Curcuma harmandii* Gagnep. from Vietnam. *J Essent Oil Res*. 1997, 9, 677-681.

225. Kojima H, Yanai T, and Toyota A: Essential oil constituents from Japanese and Indian *Curcuma aromatica* rhizome. *Planta Med*. 1998, 64, 380-381.

226. Bordoloi AK, Sperkova J and Ledercq PA: Essential oils of *Curcuma aromatica* Salisb. from Northeast India. *J Essent Oil Res*. 1999, 11, 537-540.

227. Wong KC, Chong TC and Chee SG: Essential oil of *Curcuma mangga* Vol. and Van Zijp rhizomes. *J Essent Oil Res*. 1999, 11,349-351.

228. Sirat, H. M., Jamail, S. and Hussain, J., Essential oil of *Curcuma aeruginosa* Roxb. from Malaysia. *J Essent Oil Res*. 1998, 10, 453-458.

229. Jirovetz L, Buchbauer G, Puschmann C, Shafi MP and Nambiar MKG: Essential oil analysis of *Curcuma aeruginosa* Roxb. leaves from South India. *J Essent Oil Res*. 2000, 12, 47-49.

230. Behura S: Gas chromatographic evaluation of *Curcuma* essential oils. *In*: Spices and aromatic plants–challenges and opportunities in the new century. Indian Society for Spices, Calicut. pp. 291-292, 2000.

Chapter 17

Therapeutic Potential of Medicinal Mushrooms Occurring in South India Amelioration of Oxidative Stress-Induced Hepato-Renal Damages: A Pre-Clinical Evaluation

T.A. Ajith[1] *and K.K. Janardhanan*[2*]

[1]*Department of Biochemistry, Amala Institute of Medical Sciences, Amala Nagar, Thrissur, Kerala – 680 555, India*

[2]*Department of Microbiology, Amala Cancer Research Centre, Amala Nagar, Thrissur, Kerala – 680 555, India*

**E-mail: kkjanardhanan@yahoo.com*

ABSTRACT

Oxidative stress resulting from the metabolisms of xenobiotics is one of the major etiological factors responsible for the organ damage and failure. Supplementation of antioxidants is a promising approach to ameliorate such organ damages. Antioxidants have a wide range of biochemical activities; these include inhibiting the generation of reactive oxygen species directly or indirectly, scavenging free radicals and altering the intracellular redox potential. Several natural antioxidants have been used to ameliorate many of the xenobiotics induced toxicities. Medicinal mushrooms represent a major untapped source of powerful antioxidants, a novel group of pharmaceutical agents that remain to be explored. Evaluations of the therapeutic application and clinical use of medicinal mushrooms occurring in South India has not received adequate attention. However, the investigations carried out at Amala Cancer Research Centre during the recent years can be considered as the major contribution in this area. Among the medicinal properties of mushrooms evaluated, *Phellinus rimosus* and *Ganoderma lucidum*, two-wood inhabiting macrofungi, offer promising leads for developing new pharmaceutical agents against oxidative stress mediated organ damages. Results of our studies on experimental animals revealed that ethyl acetate extract of *P. rimosus* and methanol extract of *G. lucidum* significantly and dose dependently protected hepato-renal toxicities either by preventing the CCl_4 / cisplatin-induced depletion of antioxidant status or by their direct antioxidant activities. The pre-clinical trials of these mushrooms have demonstrated their therapeutic potentials against toxins-induced hepatic or renal cell damages.

Keywords: *Antioxidant, Free radicals, G. lucidum, Medicinal mushrooms, P. rimosus, Xenobiotics.*

Introduction

Reactive oxygen species (ROS) are generated by ionizing radiations, by certain exogenous chemicals and from the redox cycle following the cellular metabolism. Irrespective of their origin, ROS may interact with cellular biomolecules, such as DNA, leading to modification and potentially serious consequences for the cell. Oxidative DNA damage is an inevitable consequence of cellular metabolism, with a propensity for increased levels following toxic insult. The appropriate pro-oxidant/ antioxidant balance can be shifted towards the pro-oxidant when the production of oxygen species is increased or when the levels of antioxidants are diminished in oxidative stress. Oxidative stress has been implicated in the pathogenesis of Alzheimer's disease, Huntington's disease and Parkinson's disease [1]. Numerous studies have established a relationship between levels of oxidative DNA damage and cancer [1,2].

Exposure to drugs and chemicals often induce toxicity to living organisms. Many organs are capable of metabolizing chemicals to toxic reactive intermediates and free radicals. Liver and kidneys are the major organs that are exposed to such toxic metabolites and free radicals. Antioxidants have a wide range of biochemical activities; these include inhibiting the generation of reactive oxygen species directly or indirectly, scavenging free radicals and altering the intracellular redox potential [3]. Several natural antioxidants have been used to ameliorate many of the xenobiotics induced toxicities.

Mushrooms represent a major and as yet largely untapped source of powerful new pharmaceutical products. Attempts have been made in many parts of the world to explore the use of mushrooms and their metabolites for the treatment of a variety of human sufferings [4]. Among the approximately known 10,000 species of mushrooms 300 possess significant pharmacological properties [5]. Many pharmaceutical substances with potent and unique valuable properties have been isolated recently from mushrooms.

Higher basidiomycetes mushrooms are unlimited source of anticancer and immunostimulatory polysaccharides [4]. Six hundred and fifty one species from 182 genera of higher basidiomycetes were reported to possess pharmacologically active polysaccharides in their fruiting bodes [5]. Medicinal mushrooms useful against cancer are known is China, Russia, Japan, Korea and United States. They have been traditionally used in China and Japan for the treatment of a variety of cancers. Extracts and powders of mushrooms in the form of capsule and sugar coated tablets are being marketed. Many pharmaceutical substances with potent and unique valuable properties isolated recently from mushrooms are being used worldwide. However, attempts to explore the medicinal value of mushrooms occurring in India are fragmentary. Investigations carried out in our laboratory showed that extracts of the fruiting bodies of a number of mushrooms possessed significant antioxidant activities and were able to protect the oxidative stress induced organ damages. Among the mushrooms evaluated, the effect of ethyl acetate extract of the fruiting bodies of *Phellinus rimosus* and methanol extract of *Ganoderma lucidum* to ameliorate the chemical induced hepato-renal damage in experimental animals was highly significant.

Phellinus species are polypore macrofungi, mostly tropical and 18 species are known from Kerala, India. One of the species, *P. linteus* is reported to possess in vitro antioxidant, anti-angiogenic and xanthine oxidase inhibiting activities [6]. *Phellinus rimosus* (Berk) Pilat is found growing on jackfruit tree trunks in Kerala. Our earlier investigations showed that ethyl acetate and methanol extracts of *P. rimosus* possessed profound antioxidant, anti-inflammatory, antitumor and antibacterial activities [7,8,9,10].

Ganoderma lucidum (Fr) Karst is also a wood inhabiting macrofungus, commonly known as Reishi or Ling Zhi. In Chinese folklore, fruit bodies of *Ganoderma* have been regarded as panaceae for all type of diseases. Our earlier investigations showed that extracts of the fruiting bodies of *G. lucidum* occurring in south India possessed profound antioxidant, anti-inflammatory and antitumor properties [11,12]. Recently we also reported the anticancer and radioprotective effects of this mushroom [13,14].

Hepatoprotective Activity of Mushroom Extracts

Hepatoprotective activity of ethyl acetate extract of *P. rimosus* and methanol extract of *G. lucidum* extract was evaluated using Carbon tetrachloride (CCl_4) induced hepatotoxicity in female Sprague Dawley rats (160 ± 20 g). Chronic exposure to CCl_4 (CCl_4 in paraffin oil 1:5, v/v; 1.5 ml/kg body wt., i.p; 3 times in a week for 5 weeks) significantly elevated the serum glutamate oxaloacetate transaminase (GOT) and glutamate pyruvate transaminase (GPT) activities compared to the normal group of animals. The altered ratio of SGPT to SGOT in animals administered with CCl_4 alone clearly confirmed the hepatotoxic status of the animals. Administration of the ethyl acetate extract of *P. rimosus* (25 and 50 mg/kg body wt.) and methanol extract of *G. lucidum* (500 and 1000 mg/kg body wt) orally one hour before each CCl_4 administration significantly lowered the serum GOT and GPT activities in a dose dependent manner. Similarly the serum alkaline phosphatase (ALP) activity was elevated significantly in the CCl_4 treated control group of animals. The inhibition of ALP activity or transaminases by the extracts at high doses was found to be more effective. The pretreatment of the extract prevented the elevation of SGPT, SGOT and serum ALP consequent to CCl_4 treatment, which indicated the hepatoprotective activity of the extracts (Table 17.1).

The activities of hepatic antioxidant status such as superoxide dismutase (SOD), catalase (CAT) and glutathione peroxidase (GPx) were decreased significantly in the CCl_4 treated group of animals compared to the normal animals. The treatment with the extracts of *P. rimosus* and *G. lucidum* enhanced the reduced activity of these enzymes in the liver (Table 17.2). CCl_4 administration also enhanced lipid peroxidation. The level of lipid peroxidation was significantly lowered by the mushroom extracts (Figure 17.1)

Table 17.1: Effect of Ethyl Acetate Extract of *P. rimosus* (PR) and Methanol Extract of *G. lucidum* (GL) on Serum GOT, GPT and ALP Activities in Rats with Chronic CCl_4 Administration

Groups	*Treatment (mg/kg)*	*SGPT (IU/l)*	*SGOT (IU/l)*	*ALP (IU/l)*
Normal	Vehicle	116.5 ± 16.2	65.5 ± 5.4	179.9 ± 40.0
Control (CCl_4/Paraffin oil, 1:5)	—	959.8 ± 25.6*	231.1 ± 21.5*	437.3 ± 30.8*
PR + CCl_4	25	516.7 ± 79.2[a]	103.5 ± 7.1[a]	259.8 ± 16.5[a]
"	50	240.8 ± 16.9[a]	82.3 ± 4.7[a]	210.5 ± 7.8[a]
GL + CCl_4	500	410.2 ± 81.1[a]	130.0 ± 17.1[a]	310.1 ± 22.2[a]
"	1000	365.0 ± 35.0[a]	84.3 ± 7.7[a]	230.0 ± 9.8[a]

Values are mean ± S.D, n=6 animals

*$p<0.05$ (LSD) significantly different from normal.

[a]$p<0.01$ (Dunnett's *t*-test) significantly different from control group.

Table 17.2: Effect of Ethyl Acetate Extract of *P. rimosus* (PR) and Methanol Extract of *G. lucidum* (GL) on Hepatic SOD, CAT and GPx Activities in Rats with Chronic CCl_4 Administration

Groups	*Treatment (mg/kg)*	*SOD (U/mg protein)*	*CAT (U/mg protein)*	*GPx (U/mg protein)*
Normal	Vehicle	20.2 ± 2.9	64.5 ± 4.5	22.5 ± 2.2
Control (CCl_4/Paraffin oil, 1:5)	—	14.5 ± 2.1*	46.3 ± 4.8*	16.9 ± 0.8*
PR + CCl_4	25	17.2 ± 0.3[b]	53.9 ± 2.6[a]	18.8 ± 1.7[ns]
"	50	19.1 ± 0.8[a]	60.9 ± 3.7[a]	20.5 ± 0.4[a]
GL + CCl_4	500	18.4 ± 1.1[b]	50.5 ± 4.2[b]	17.5 ± 0.9[ns]
"	1000	20.2 ± 1.8[a]	60.1 ± 3.1[a]	21.4 ± 0.6[a]

Values are mean ± S.D, n=5 animals

*$p<0.05$ (LSD) significantly different from normal.

[a]$p<0.01$ [b]$p<0.05$ significant (Dunnett's *t*-test) and ns non-significantly different from control group.

Nephroprotective Activity of Mushroom Extracts

Nephrotoxicity was induced in male Swiss albino mice (30 ± 2 g) using cisplatin (16 mg/kg). Cisplatin administration dramatically enhanced serum urea and creatinine levels. Extracts of *P. rimosus* (25 and 50 mg/kg) and *G. lucidum* (250 and

500 mg/kg) were effective to prevent the renal damage as evident from the serum level of urea and creatinine (Table 17.3).

Table 17.3: Effect of Ethyl Acetate Extract of *P. rimosus* (PR) and Methanol Extract of *G. lucidum* (GL) on Renal Urea and Creatinine Levels in Mice Treated with Cisplatin

Groups	*Treatments (mg/kg)*	*Urea (mg/dl)*	*Creatinine (mg/dl)*
Normal	Vehicle	67.4 ± 8.7	0.43 ± 0.06
Control (cisplatin)	16	317.2 ± 22.4*	3.93 ± 0.58*
PR + cisplatin	25	102.6 ± 6.6[a]	0.99 ± 0.18[a]
"	50	77.1 ± 4.5[a]	0.53 ± 0.15[a]
GL + cisplatin	250	148.6 ± 5.6[a]	1.08 ± 0.08[a]
"	500	99.1 ± 11.1[a]	0.44 ± 0.06[a]

Values are mean ± S.D, (n=6 animals)

*p<0.01 (LSD) significantly different from normal.

[a]p<0.01(Dunnett's *t*-test) significantly different from control group.

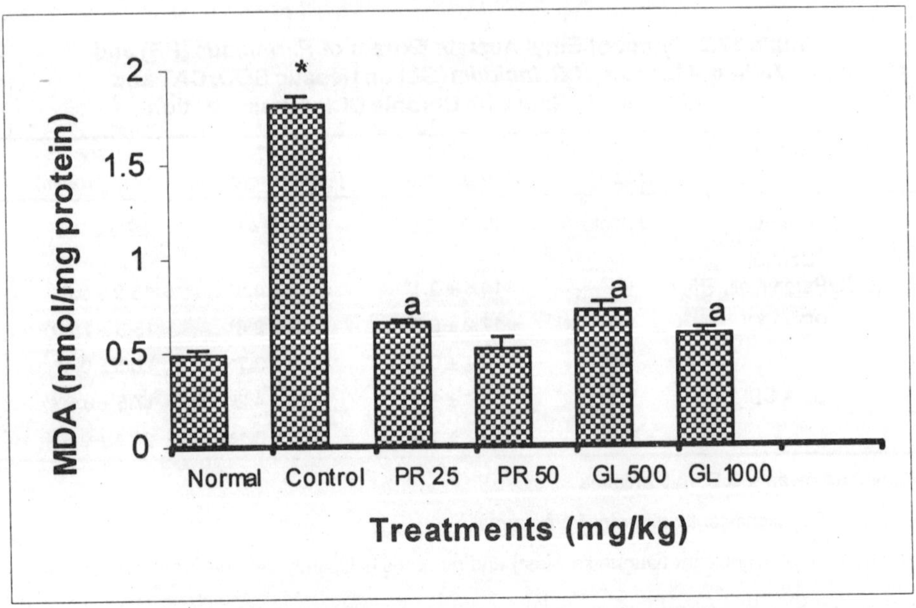

Figure 17.1: Effect of Ethyl Acetate Extract of *P. rimosus* (PR) and Methanol Extract of *G. lucidum* (GL) on Hepatic MDA Level in Rats After Chronic CCl_4 Administration. Values are mean ± S.D, n=5 animals, *p<0.01 (LSD) significantly different from normal, [a]p<0.01 (Dunnett's *t*-test) significantly different from control group.

The activities of renal antioxidant status such as superoxide dismutase (SOD), catalase (CAT) and glutathione peroxidase (GPx) were decreased significantly in the cisplatin treated group of animals compared to the normal animals. Treatment of extracts prior to the cisplatin challenge significantly enhanced the depleted renal antioxidant status (Table 17.4). Cisplatin treatment also increased the renal lipid peroxidation level and the administration of mushroom extracts effectively lowered the lipid peroxidation (Figure 17.2). The mushroom extracts also profoundly enhanced the renal GSH level (Figure 17.3).

Discussion

CCl_4 is metabolized by Cyt P-450 system to give the trichloromethyl radical ($CCl_3\cdot$). Trichloromethyl radical reacts with oxygen to form trichloroperoxy radical (CCl_3O_2), both these products induce the peroxidation of lipids [15]. The products of pėroxidation are known to inhibit protein synthesis and activity of certain enzymes. Liver contains high concentrations of both CAT and GPx. The chronic treatment of the CCl_4 decreased the activity of CAT and GPx. Further the activity of SOD and the level of GSH were also declined in the liver. The declined antioxidant status is responsible for the increased lipid peroxidation, which leads to loss of membrane

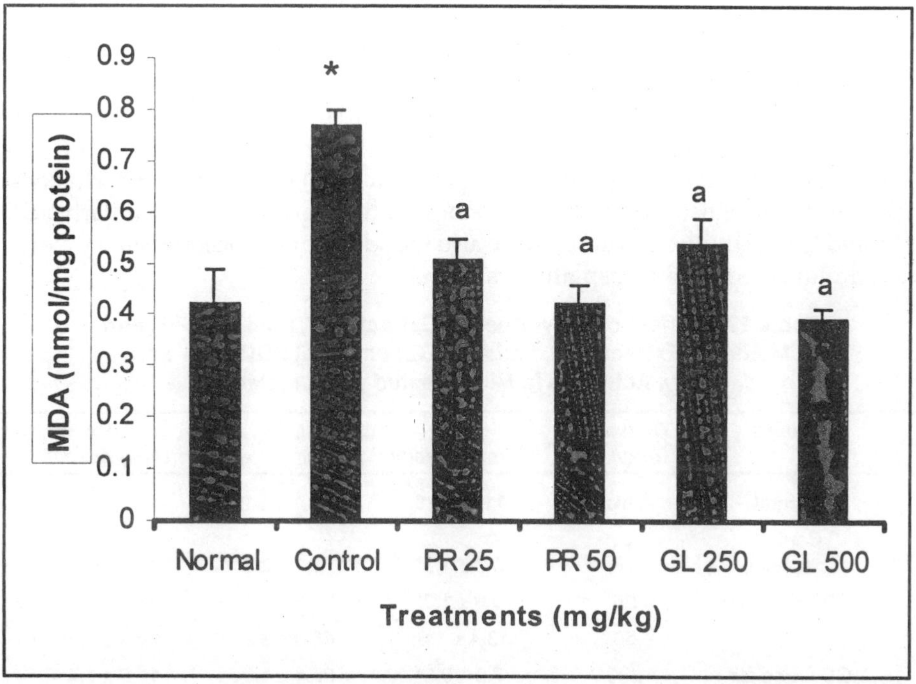

Figure 17.2: Effect of Ethyl Acetate Extract of *P. rimosus* (PR) and Methanol Extract of *G. lucidum* (GL) on Lipid Peroxidation level (MDA) in Mice Treated with Cisplatin. Values are mean ± S.D, n=6 animals, *p<0.01 (LSD) significantly different from normal. [a]p<0.01 (Dunnett's *t*-test) significantly different from control group.

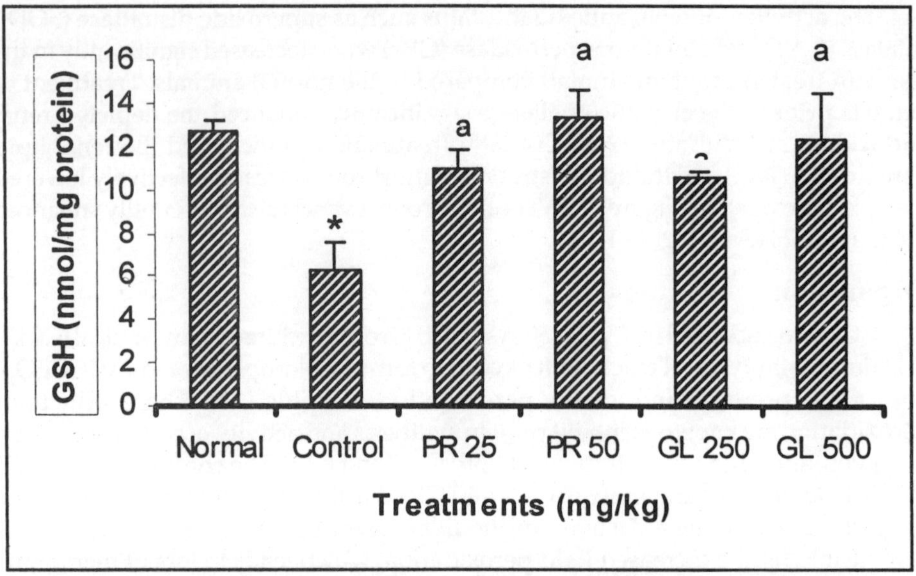

Figure 17.3: Effect of Ethyl Acetate Extract of *P. rimosus* (PR) and Methanol Extract of *G. lucidum* (GL) on Renal GSH Level in Mice with Cisplatin Administration. Values are mean ± S.D, n=6 animals, *p<0.01 (LSD) significantly different from normal. [a]p<0.01 Dunnett's *t*-test) significantly different from control group.

fluidity, integrity and finally cell functions of liver [16,17]. This may results in the leakage of enzymes and toxic metabolites from liver to circulation. Treatment of extract (50 mg/kg of *P. rimosus* and 1000 mg/kg of *G. lucidum*) prior to the CCl_4 challenge more effectively enhanced the activity of these antioxidant enzymes. Similarly SOD, CAT and GPx activities in kidney were also found to be enhanced when the extract was administered prior to cisplatin challenge.

Table 17.4: Effect of Ethyl Acetate Extract of *P. rimosus* (PR) and Methanol Extract of *G. lucidum* (GL) on Renal SOD, CAT and GPx Activities in Mice Treated with Cisplatin

Groups	*Treatment (mg/kg)*	*SOD (U/mg protein)*	*CAT (U/mg protein)*	*GPx (U/mg protein)*
Normal	Vehicle	11.8 ± 1.0	48.1 ± 5.9	26.3 ± 3.2
Control (cisplatin)	16	6.7 ± 1.2*	14.7 ± 2.3*	5.6 ± 1.8*
PR + cisplatin	25	9.9 ± 1.2[a]	32.8 ± 3.5[a]	13.1 ± 2.3[a]
"	50	13.4 ± 1.5[a]	46.3 ± 3.3[a]	22.4 ± 2.3[a]
GL + cisplatin	250	8.8 ± 0.9[a]	30.4 ± 1.9[a]	11.5 ± 1.4[a]
"	500	13.3 ± 0.6[a]	42.0 ± 2.1[a]	22.5 ± 2.0[a]

Values are mean ± S.D, (n=6 animals)

*p<0.01 (LSD) significantly different from normal.

[a]p<0.01(Dunnett's *t*-test) significantly different from control group.

Impairment of renal function resulted in the elevation of urea and creatinine levels. The treatment of the extract prior to the CCl_4 or cisplatin injection increased the liver/renal SOD, CAT and GPx activities and effectively prevented the radical mediated loss of membrane integrity. The level of hepatic reduced glutathione (GSH) was elevated and the level of MDA was declined significantly in the extracts treated animals when compared to the control group of animals. Hence the treatment of mushroom extracts showed reduced serum transaminases/ALP activities in CCl_4 administered animals or urea and creatinine levels in cisplatin injected animals.

The role of GSH in the formation of conjugates with electrophilic drug metabolites most often formed by cytochrome P-450 linked monooxygenase is well established [18]. Studies with a number of models show that the hepato-renal toxicities of xenobiotics are often produced by GSH depletion [19,20]. The decreased concentration of GSH increases the sensitivity of organs to oxidative and chemical injury. The oxidation–reduction (redox) state of the pool of cellular thiols plays a central role in antioxidant defense and in the regulation of a large number of signal transduction pathways and metabolic functions [21]. Exogenous GSH could offer protection against CCl_4 or cispltain induced organ damage in animals [22]. The treatment of extracts before the CCl_4 or cisplatin injection prevented the decline of hepatic/renal GSH levels. Moreover, GSH protects these organs by forming the substrate for the activity of GPx and can also react directly with various aldehydes produced during the peroxidation of membrane lipids. Treatment of rat with extract plus CCl_4 enhances the activity of Se-GPx (selenium dependent GPx) compared to the CCl_4 alone treated animals. The enhanced GPx activity could partially protect the bio-membrane from oxidative attack.

Besides the antioxidant activity, glutathione has many physiological functions including detoxification of xenobiotics, modulation of redox-regulated signal transduction, storage and transport of cysteine, regulation of cell proliferation, synthesis of deoxyribonucleotide, regulation of immune response, and regulation of leukotriene and prostaglandin metabolism. GSH is able to increase the activation of cytotoxic T cells *in vivo*. The normal functioning of T lymphocytes is dependent upon cellular supplies of cysteine.

The concentration of MDA as a result of lipid peroxidation shows an increase in the CCl_4/cisplatin treated group. The decreased SOD activity can cause the initiation and propagation of lipid peroxidation in the cisplatin treated group. This decreased activity in cisplatin treated group may be either due to loss of copper and zinc, which are essential for the activity of enzyme or reactive oxygen species-induced inactivation of enzyme [23, 24]. The activity of CAT and GPx also decreased in the cisplatin treated group, which in turn increased the H_2O_2 and lipid peroxides. *P. rimosus* extract treatment is found to prevent the lipid peroxidation by enhancing the renal antioxidant enzymes.

Previous studies have demonstrated the significant *in vitro* radical scavenging activity of the ethyl acetate extract of *P. rimosus* and methanol extract of *G. lucidum* [9,12]. The presence of polyphenols and terpenes in these extracts might be responsible for this property [25]. Direct radical scavenging activity of the extract might also be involved in the hepatoprotective activity against acute or chronic CCl_4 exposure and nephroprotective activity against acute cisplatin administration.

Conclusion

Compelling evidence has shown that oxidative stress, resulting from an imbalance between pro-oxidant and antioxidant systems in favour of the former, largely contributes to immune system deregulation and complications observed in end-stage renal disease (ESRD) patients treated with haemodialysis, nerodegenerative diseases, diabetes mellitus, aging, inflammation and cancer. Natural antioxidants have been used to ameliorate many of the xenobiotics induced toxicities and are at the center of recent investigations. In the last decade medicinal mushrooms were intensively investigated for their medicinal effects in *in vivo* and *in vitro* models and several pharmacologically active substances were identified. Ethyl acetate extract of *P. rimosus* and methanol extract of *G. lucidum* significantly and dose dependently protected hepato-renal toxicities either by preventing the CCl_4/cisplatin-induced decline of antioxidant status or by their direct antioxidant activities. The pre-clinical trials reveal that of these mushrooms are promising sources of therapeutic agents against toxins-induced hepatic or renal cell damages.

References

1. Cooke MS, Evans MD, Dizdarglu M, Lunec J: Oxidative DNA damage: Mechanisms, mutation and disease. *The FASEB J*, 2003, 17, 1195-1214.
2. Cerutti PA, Trump BF: Inflammation and oxidative stress in carcinogenesis. *Cancer Cells*, 1991, 3, 1-7.
3. Hirose M, Imaida K, Tamano S, Ito N: Cancer chemoprevention by antioxidants. In: Ho CT, Oswa T, Huang MT, Resen RT (eds): Food Phytochemicals II: Teas, Spices and Herbs, American Chemical Society, Washington, 1994.
4. Jong SC, Birmingham JM: Edible mushrooms in Biotechnology. *Proceed Asian Mycol Symp*. Seoul, Korea. 1992, 18-35.
5. Miles S, Chang ST: Mushrooms biology concise basics and current developments. World Scientific, Singapore. 1997, 194-197.
6. Song YS, Kim SH, Sa JH, Jin C, Lim CJ, Park EH: Anti-angiogenic, antioxidant and xanthine oxidase inhibition activities of the mushroom *Phellinus lintus*. *J Ethnopharmacol*, 2003, 88, 113-116.
7. Ajith TA, Janardhanan KK: Antioxidant and anti-inflammatory activities of methanol extract of *Phellinus rimosus*. *Ind J Exp Biol*, 2001, 39,1166-1169.
8. Ajith TA, Janardhanan KK: Antioxidant and antihepatotoxic activities of *Phellinus rimosus* (Berk) Pilat. *J Ethnopharmacol*, 2002, 81, 387-391.
9. Ajith TA, Janardhanan KK: Cytotoxic and antitumor activities of a polypore macrofungus, *Phellinus rimosus*. *J Ethnopharmacol*, 2003, 84,157-162.
10. Sheena N, Ajith TA, Mathew T, Janardhanan KK: Antibacterial activity of three macrofungi, *Ganoderma lucidum*, *Navesporous floccosa* and *Phellinus rimosus* occurring in South India. *Pharmceutical Biol*, 2003, 41,564-567.

11. Jones S, Janardhanan KK: Antioxidant and antitumor activity of *Ganoderma lucidum* (Curt.: Fr.) P. Karst.-Reishi (Aphyllophoromycetideae) from South India. *Int J Med Mushr*, 2000, 2, 195-200.
12. Sheena N, Ajith TA, Janardhanan KK: Anti-inflammatory and anti-nociceptive activities of *Ganoderma lucidum* occurring in South India. *Pharmaceutical Biol*, 2003,41, 301-304.
13. Ajith TA, Janardhanan KK: Chemopreventive activity of a macrofungus *Phellinus rimosus* against N-nitrosodiethylamine induced hepatocellular carcinoma in rat. *J Ex. The. Oncol*, 2006, 5, 309-321.
14. Pillai TG, Salvi VP, Maurya DK, Nair CKK, Janardhanan KK: Prevention of radiation-induced damages by aqueous extract of *Ganoderma lucidum* occurring in Southern parts of India. *Curr Sci*, 2006, 91,341-344.
15. Ahr HJ, King LJ, Nastainczyk W, Ullrich V: The mechanism of reductive dehalogenation of halomethane by liver cytochrome P450. *Biochem Pharmacol*, 1982, 31, 383-387.
16. Halliwell B, Gutteridge JMC: In: Halliwell B, Gutteridge JMC (Eds.): Free radicals in Biology and Medicine Clarendon Press, Oxford, 1989.
17. Smith SM, Grishsm MB, Nancy EA, Granger DA, Kvietys PR: Gastric mucosal injury in the rat. Role of iron and xanthine oxidase. *Gastroenterol*, 1987, 92, 950-956.
18. Rana SVS, Allen T, Singh R: Inevitable glutathione, then and now. *Ind J Exp Biol*, 2002, 40, 706-716.
19. Mitchell JR, Jollow DJ, Potter WZ, Gillette JR, Brodie BB: Acetaminophen induced hepatic necrosis. Protective role of glutathione. *J Pharmacol Exp Ther*, 1973, 187, 211-215.
20. Jollow DJ, Mitchell JR, Zampaglione N, Gillete JR: Bromobenzene induced liver necrosis. Protective role of glutathione and evidence for 3,4-bromobenzene oxide as the hepatotoxic metabolite. *Pharmacol*, 1974, 11, 151-156.
21. Sies H: Glutathione and its role in cellular functions. *Free Radic Biol Med*, 1999, 29, 916-921
22. Rana S, Tyal MK: Influenze of zinc, vit-B12 and glutathione on the liver of rats exposed to carbon tetrachloride. *Industrial Health* (Japan), 1981, 19, 65-69.
23. Sharma RP: Interactions of cisplatin with cellular zinc and copper in liver and kidney tissues. *Pharmacol Res Commun*, 1985, 17, 197-206.
24. DeWoskin RS, Riviere JE: Cisplatin-induced loss of kidney copper and nephrotoxicity is ameliorated by single dose diethyldithiocarbamate, but not mesna. *Toxicol Appl Pharmacol*, 1992, 112, 182-189.
25. Shahidi F, Jaitra PK, Wanasundra: Phenolic components in herbs have been reported to be effective natural antioxidants. *Crit Rev Food Sci Nutr*: 1992, 32, 67-71.

Chapter 18

Traditional Medicine and the Intellectual Property Rights (IPR) Regime of 21st Century

Palpu Pushpangadan

Amity Institute for Herbal and Biotech Products Development, TC 10/910(1), VRA-173, Mannamoola, Peroorkada, Trivandrum – 695 005, Kerala, India

E-mail: palpuprakulam@yahoo.co.in

Food and medicine have always been indispensable companions of humans ever since evolution. Search for food that gives him energy, nutrition and health and agents that could alleviate pain and discomforts and also his longing for eternal health, longevity and vitality etc. prompted humans to develop diverse ways and means to achieve the same. The early humans explored their immediate surroundings and used his instinct and indulgence and learned many lessons that led to the developments of various food articles and art of healing. Most of the articles that man selected for healing are derived from the plant kingdom and such plants are called medicinal plants. Humans also tried and selected many animal products and minerals as healing agents. However, conscious selection of plants, animals and minerals for medicinal use probably began with the dawn of human civilization. Early humans by trials or error or even by experimentation did clinical trials for selecting therapeutically useful articles from these sources. The knowledge thus gained was passed on to the succeeding generations. Innovative members of the succeeding generations made incremental improvements or added new body of knowledge. Over millennia that followed the most effective agents were selected by such processes and that became part of the ethnomedical traditions. All human communities inhabited in different regions of the world have thus developed their own ethnomedical traditions. These efforts have gone in history by the name medicine.

The medical wisdom what is practiced and passed on to the succeeding generation is known as 'Traditional medicine" (TM) or Ethnic medicine (EM). All health care practices and treatment of disease practiced by traditional communities or local people in the world over is termed as TM. In fact all medicinal practices of the whole humankind before the advent of modern medicine in the 19th century were all

TM (Pushpangadan, 1996, 2002). In many eastern cultures such as those of India, China and the Arab world the TM was systematically recorded and incorporated into regular systems of medicine and that became the Materia Medica of TM of those countries.

World Health Organization (WHO) defined TM as "the sum total of the knowledge, skills and practices based on the theories, beliefs and experiences of indigenous cultures whether explicable or not used in the maintenance of health and in the prevention, diagnosis, improvement or treatment of physical and mental illness". The term 'complementary medicine', 'alternate medicine', and 'non-conventional medicine' etc. are used interchangeably with 'traditional medicine' in some countries.

In 1976 the World Health Assembly took note of the vital role that Traditional Medicine play in health service, particularly in the remote areas and drew attention to the manpower reserve that constituted the traditional practitioners (resolution WHA 29.72). In 1977 the WHO adopted a resolution to declare that the main social target of Governments in the coming decades should be the attainment by all people of the world, a level of health permitting them to lead socially and economically productive life known popularly as the goal of 'health for all' by 2000 AD. Resolution WHA 30.49 urged countries to utilize their traditional system of medicine. The Alma Ata conference of WHO in 1978 further declared that the primary health care is the key in attaining this goal and identified the vital role of the traditional medicine in achieving the same.

It has been estimated that 80 per cent of the people living in developing countries are almost fully dependent on traditional medical practices for meeting their primary health care needs, and higher plants are known to be the main source of drug therapy in traditional medicine. Since about 80 per cent of the total world's population resides in developing countries, about 64 per cent of the total population of the world utilizes plants as drugs *i.e.*, 3.2 billion people (Farnsworth, 1990).

TM in India

The Indian subcontinent is endowed with one of the richest expertise in TM. The TM in India functions through two social streams. One is the local folk stream (the local health traditions) which is prevalent at villages and tribal settlements in the country. The carriers of these traditions are house wives, thousands of traditional birth attendants, bone setters, practitioners in acupressure, eye treatment, snake bites treatment etc. and the traditional village level herbal physician, the 'vaidyas' or tribal physicians in the tribal areas. These local health traditions thus represent an autonomous community system of health delivery at the village level which runs parallel to the state supported system. Its potential goes largely unnoticed because of the dominant western medicine (Pushpangadan, 1995, 1996, 2002, 2005).

A second level of traditional health system is the scientific or classical system. This consists of codified and organized medical wisdom with sophisticated theoretical foundations and philosophical explanations and is expressed in thousands of regional manuscripts covering treatises on all branches of medicine and surgery.

Systems like Ayurveda, Sidha, Unani, Amchi and Tibetan are the expressions of this stream.

Ayurveda is perhaps the oldest (2500 BC) among the organized traditional medicine. It has gone through several stages of development in its long history. It spread with Vedic and Hindu culture as far east as Indonesia and to the west it influenced the ancient Greeks, who developed a similar form of medicine. The Buddhists added many new insights to it and they took it along with their religion to many different countries. In this way, Ayurveda became the basis of the healing traditions of Tibet, Sri Lanka, Burma, Japan and other Buddhist lands and influenced Chinese and Greek medicine. Ayurveda is thus a rich tradition, adaptable to many different times, cultures and climates.

Ayurvedic healing has two levels; one for the layman and self care, the other for the health care professional, the physician. The first involve self discipline wherein an individual leads a life style termed under 'swasthavrutha', who take food and nutrition according to his constitutional nature, age, climate and profession. This also include personal and civic hygiene, taking health promotive food and medicine form the Rasayana group (rejuvenating) of drugs. It also covers various time tested simple herbal remedies for treating common ailments. It is important to realize that many of our diseases can best be treated by us. Often a few simple therapies done as part of our daily regime can be effective. It is only when our life style is out of harmony that more severe diseases arise, and more specialized and complicated health care becomes necessary.

The second level provides some of this specialized Ayurvedic medical knowledge and outlines more technical and more sophisticated and complicated remedies handled by health care professionals.

According to Ayurveda there are three primary life forces or three biological humors in the body–'Vata', 'Pitta' and 'Kapha'. They correspond primarily to the elements of air, fire and water. Ayurvedic diagnosis and treatment of diseases are based on these biological humors. The proportion of the humors varies according to the individual. One humor will usually predominate and its nature will make its mark upon the organism in terms of its appearance and disposition. Most diseases arise from the inborn predominant humor and the Ayurvedic medicine prescribe methods for balancing or correcting such constitutional imbalances. This constitutional approach is the essence of Ayurveda. It gives Ayurveda immense power for disease prevention, health maintenance, longevity enhancement, and the treatment of disease. Interestingly the constitutional approach of Ayurveda is now supported by the modern genomic studies which has demonstrated that human individual has their own unique genetic constitution which led to the development of nutrigenomics and pharmacogenomics

Ayurvedic masters explained that the process of life is in constant state of flux and not in a static condition and that in this dynamic process a continual adjustment with the environment is necessary for the health and well being. Sushruta and Charaka, the authors of the classical Ayurvedic texts 'Sushruta Samhita' (BC 2500) and 'Charaka Samhita' (BC 1500) respectively, commented that if an organism fails to adjust and adapt either due to some innate deficiencies or due to overwhelming force of the environment the result is the diseased condition.

Charaka seems to have a combined role of philosopher and physician where as Sushruta tried to free medicine from priestly dimension and he created an atmosphere of independent thinking and investigation which later characterized the Greek Medicine. Sushruta can be acknowledged as one of the greatest medical scientists rather surgeons or physicians in the ancient India, who, for the first time changed the art of surgery into a practical science in the remote antiquity. Sushruta thus deserves to be known as the Father of Surgery.

During the second century BC Vagbhatta a Buddhist from Sind, wrote 'Ashatanga Samhita', that combined the essence of both the texts, of Charaka and Sushruta. One of his descendants Vagbhatta Junior (8th century) presented all the knowledge of Ayurveda as it existed during his time in a lucid manner in his 'Ashtangahritaya Samhita'. He dealt with surgery in detail as presented in the Sushruta Samhita. During the medieval period Ayurvedic literature remained mostly stagnant except for the work of Madhavacharya of 8th century. The successive onslaught of the early foreign invaders caused total devastation of the medical education institutions in India. Ayurveda suffered greatly on this account. The continued growth and development of the Ayurvedic medicine was thus adversely affected. It is still not fully recovered from this stagnation.

Siddha medicine practiced mainly in Tamil Nadu and part of Kerala is considered to be the oldest system of medicine in India dating back to 4000 BC. This system traces its origin to 'Sidhars', (saintly figures) who get revelations/enlightments in medicine through yoga practice and Sidha (spiritual achievement). All Sidha literature are in Tamil. It has also been referred to as the Agasthyar system, and its exponent is sage Agasthya. The system developed in the prevedic Dravidian culture (4000 BC) and after the introduction of Ayurveda the two systems seem to have developed parallel with similar principles and doctrines. Siddha specializes, to a larger extent on iatrochemistry and the usage of metals and minerals is much advocated in addition to that of medicinal plants.

The Unani system originated in Greece around 400 BC and its name can be traced from the Arabic name for Greece, 'Unan'. A number of Greek (*e.g.* Hippocrates, Aristotle, Herophilus) and Arabic (*e.g.* Ib-Bin Sina, Al-Mamum, Ibn Masawayh, Rhazas) philosophers have contributed to this system. Ayurvedic influence in the Greek as well as the Unani system can be noticed particularly in the humoral concept of health and diseases. Unani was introduced in India about 1000 years ago with the coming of Mughal invaders.

The Amchi system or the Tibetan system of medicine is prevalent in different Himalayan regions, from Lahul Spiti and Leh-Ladhak to Shillong and Sikkim and can trace its origin to the Ayurvedic system. Its therapy, however, makes use of more of animal and mineral products in addition to the herbs. Use of spring and mineral waters, moxibustion, mysticism and spiritual healings are also common in Amchi system.

While the classical traditions are documented in the form of texts or palm leaf manuscripts, most of the local health traditions of village physicians and the tribal medicine are oral in tradition. Of late, the traditional tribal communities in the world over are fast being engulfed in the rising tide of modernization and they are giving up their age old medicinal practices.

Decline of Traditional Medicine

The introduction of abstract medicine in the form of base chemicals and pharmaceuticals during the 18th and 19th centuries has demonstrated method for bringing quick relief from sufferings and this won instant admiration and popularity. This system known as allopathy made rapid advances during the 19th and 20th centuries as a result of the advances made in biological, chemical, and pharmacological sciences. New discoveries of sulpha drugs, synthetics, antibiotics, cortisones and other chemotherapeutic agents in quick succession swept all other systems of medicine by their feet. Universal adoption of modern medicine based on sound experimental data, toxicity studies and human clinical trials in turn obliterated the use of most of the traditional systems of medicine and the practice of traditional medicine eventually receded more or less to the country side.

The plant kingdom has long served as the main resource base for the traditional medicines. This began to change in the 1930s with the advent of synthetic chemistry and was cemented in the 1950s with the introduction of laboratory-bred 'wonder drugs' such as the antibacterials, sulfonamides or sulfa drugs. Predictably, the American pharmaceutical industry quickly lost interest in natural products as sources of potential new medicines. When Schultes, the renowned American Ethnobotanist, returned to Harvard in 1939 after completing ethnobotanical research among the Indians of Southern Mexico, he was unable to find an American drug firm or even a single American chemist willing to work with him. They dismissed him by saying they didn't want to waste their time looking at these folk medicines. Finally, he has to send his materials to a sympathetic young Swedish chemist for analysis. This chemist, Albert Holfmann, later became famous as the inventor of LSD. Less widely known, however, is that he isolated the hallucinogenic alkaloid psilocybin from mushrooms of Schulte's Mexican collections. From this natural model he synthesized the cardiac betablocker visken, which has improved the quality of life for millions of people with heart problems.

Synthetic drugs like the sulfonamides and diazepam (a sedative) have led some chemists to the illusion that synthetic chemistry is the sole future of new drug discovery. Chemists having synthesized a few compounds began to consider themselves to be better chemists than nature. In fact, nature had conceived of diazepam long before the modern-day chemists. Several years ago scientists found that tiny amounts of these drugs occur naturally in wheat and potatoes. Similarly, Dr. Norman Farnsworth of the University of Illinois, a leading figure in natural product chemistry, enjoys pointing out how proud chemists were thirty years ago when they synthesized an antidote for accidental poisoning by organophosphorus insecticides. Later it was found that the substance occurred naturally in electric eels (Pushpangadan, 1996).

Revival of Traditional Medicine

Today we find a renewed interest in traditional medicine. During the past decade, there has been an ever increasing demand especially from the developed countries for more and more plant drugs containing medicinally useful alkaloids, polyphenolics, steroids, glycosides and terpenoid derivatives. The revival of interest in natural drugs, especially derived from plants, started in the the 1980s, mainly because of the widespread belief that 'green' medicine is healthier than synthetic products. This has led to the rapid spurt of demand for health products like herbal teas, ginseng etc. and also there has been an increasing preference towards the utilization of natural flavours, dyes, preservatives etc. rather than the less expensive synthetics. A classical example for this trend is clear from the vanilla industry where there is a large demand for the much more expensive natural vanillin isolated from the Vanilla plant. According to a survey conducted by WHO, the uses of medicinal plant remedies are on the increase even in the developed countries especially among younger people. In the industrialized countries, the consumers are seeking visible alternatives to modern medicine with its danger of over medication or harmful side effects of synthetic drugs. The promotive and preventive medicines widely prevalent in oriental systems, especially the Indian (Ayurveda, Siddha and Unani) and the Chinese systems of medicine, are finding increasing popularity and acceptance in the developing and developed countries.

Quality of TM, particularly the commercially produced TM and its safety etc. have become a matter of great concern. Diverse TM practices have been developed in different cultural backgrounds and were highly individualized. Converting them in to a commercial system has resulted in its quality deterioration. Quality evaluation and national policy and laws for regulation of TM was almost absent. It was against this background WHO TM strategy 2002-2005 was developed, with four primary objectives, framing policy, enhancing safety, efficacy and quality ensuring access and promising national use. Resolution on TM was adopted at the fifty sixth World Health Assembly held in May 2003. The resolution requested WHO to support Member States by providing internationally acceptable guidelines and technical standards and also evidence based information to assist Member States in formulating policy regulations for safety, efficacy and quality of TM (WHO, 2005).

Intellectual Property Rights and TM

Intellectual Property (IP) means the creative products emanating from the exercise of human mind/brain and IPRs are the legal rights governing these rights granted to individual(s) or corporate bodies to have monopolistic ownership or control. Such IP exercise of human brain/mind such as thoughts, inventions, processes, ideas having innovative and inventive steps capable of industrial applications. The holder of IPR gets an exclusive right over the use. The IPR is intangible, has the characters of a property, can be transferred or sold or licensed like a property and can be protected against any wrongful infringement. IPR is essentially a concept and practice developed by the industrialized western countries in 19th century to allow monopolistic ownership or control over intangible products. Such concepts and practices were almost alien to third world countries. The traditional communities in the world over generated knowledge and practices and shared freely with all without any monetary benefits. Traditional communities treated bioresources and associated knowledge system developed by the innovative members of the community as common property to be shared and cared for the benefit of all and never intended for trading or commercializing it. But the colonial powers who reached the third world began to access the local resources and the associated TK and with the intervention of S&T converted it into marketable commodity and made it as their private property with IPR and did not share the profit from the people from whom they obtained the resources and associated TK. It was in this background that the epoch making Earth Summit was convened at Rio-de-Janeiro in June 1992 by the UN wherein over 151 countries signed the Convention on Biological Diversity (CBD).

CBD entered into force in December 1993 and to date it has been ratified by over 188 countries. It has created a new international regulatory frame work in accession of genetic resources and for promoting fair and equitable sharing of benefits accrued from the use of biodiversity and associated TK. It has been suggested that, if corporate bodies can secure IPR protection of their innovative products they developed from the lead they obtained from TK, then the providers of such knowledge that is the traditional communities are also entitled to IPR protection of their TK. This was first discussed in the first International Congress on Ethnobiology (ISE) held in 1988 at Belem, Brazil which came out with the Belem declaration. Belem declaration outlined explicitly the responsibilities of scientists, sociologists, anthropologists and environmentalists in addressing the rights of traditional communities. Later, the second ISE congress held in 1990 at Kuming, China, established a global action plan calling for specific and urgent action to stop destruction of biological and cultural diversity as mandated in the Declaration of Belem. This was followed by the establishment of the Global Coalition for Bio-cultural Diversity to unite indigenous people's scientific organizations, and development of groups to implement a forceful strategy for use of traditional knowledge. The coalition group formed a working group on IPR, now called as Working Group of Traditional Intellectual Resource Rights (WGTRR). It has attempted to build a concept on IPR protection and compensation, while recognizing the traditional resources-both tangible and intangible. The term 'property' was dropped because property of traditional people frequently has intangible spiritual manifestation, and, although workth of protection is in alienable or can be long human being. Therefore, the term 'Traditional Resource Right' (TRR) was adopted to reflect the necessary rethinking. The concept of TRR can accommodate a wide range of relevant international agreement as a basis for 'sui generis' system of protection for indigenous people and their resources that is, a system that is unique and does not belong to an existing category of IRR (Posey 1996).

Developing an enabling and equitable legal framework for regulated access to biological resources and associated knowledge system has been a major concern for many countries particularly the megadiversity countries of the south. This concern has loomed large ever since the ratification and adoption of Convention on Biodiversity (CBD) on 29th Dec 1993. The World Trade Organization (WTO) which came into being in June 1995 administered TRIPs which argued for effective protection of all innovations involving inventive step and having industrial application. TRIPs have also included a provision under Article 273 (b) to exclude patentability "plants and animals rather than microorganisms and essentially biological processes for the production of plants or animals other than non-biological processes". The same provision also guarantees the protection of plant varieties either by patents or an effective *sui generis* system or by a combination thereof.

The existing inequities in international legal framework particularly of the CBD and WTO-TRIPs, and also the disproportionate distribution of Biodiversity and associated TK, and biotechnologies across the world have been the major impediments to implementing a dynamic and transparent mechanism for regulating and monitoring Access and Benefit Sharing (ABS) for IPR protection of TK. ABS is an important which needs to be addressed along with protection of TK as with genetic resources. To deal with the issues relating to ABS, an ad hoc open ended working group was established by the conference of parties of CBD and this Working Group in its meeting held in Bonn 2001 developed a guideline on access and benefit sharing meant to assist parties and stakeholders with the implementation of the access and benefit sharing provisions of the convention. At the 3rd meeting of the Working Group held in Feb 2005 and subsequently in Feb 2006 made negotiations for an international regime on access to genetic resources and associated TK. It also addressed other approaches including considerations of an international certificate of origin/source/legal provenance; and measures including consideration of their feasibility, practically and cost to support compliance with prior informed consent (PIC), of the contracting party providing such resources and mutually agreed terms on which access was granted to contracting parties with use of genetic resources and associated TK. The regime is expected to be negotiated before the end of 2010. ABS has become a rather contentious subject of wide ranging discussions and details at various international forums under the aegis of CBD, WTO-TRIPs, WIPO, UN-FAO, UNEP etc.

The Indian legislations which deals with TK protection are (1) Protection of Plant Varieties and Farmers Right Act (PPVFR Act), 2001 (2) Biological Diversity Act (BD Act) 2002 and the Patent (Amendment) Act 2005. The PPVFR Act was enacted to make India TRIPs complaint with respect to grant IP protection of plant varieties and also TK as per CBD. The BD Act seeks to establish national sovereignty over the bio-resources and associated TK and provides regulation for its sustainable use and access of its components and associated TK and ensuring fair and equitable sharing of benefits arising out of its use. The Patent Act 2005 contains provisions for revocation of patent claims or prevent grant of wrong patents world wide based on India's biological diversity and TK, wherein (1) the complete specifications does not disclose or wrongly mention the source or geographical origin of biological material used for the invention (2) the invention so far as claimed in any claim of the complete specification is anticipated having regard to the knowledge, oral or otherwise available within any local or indigenous community in the country.

There has been misappropriation of TK more particularly associated with TM during past many years. Patents were granted on products developed from leads obtained from TK/TM without the involvement or consent of the holders of such TK/TM. The grant of wrong patents linked to TM which is either based on what is already a part of the TK of the developing world, or a minor valuation thereof has been causing great concern to the developing world (Gupta, 2006). The development of Traditional Knowledge Digital Library (TKDL) in India is indeed an outcome of the legal battle that Council of Scientific and Industrial Research (CSIR) waged from India for a re-examination of US Patent No. 5401504, which was granted for the wound healing properties of Turmeric filed by two US based Indians. In a land mark decision, United State Patent and Trademark Office (USPTO) revoked this patent after ascertaining the fact that there was no novelty, the innovation being used in India for centuries and there are documentary evidence for the same. This was the first time that a patent based on TK of a developing country was challenged successfully and USPTO revoked the patent. The case of revocation of the patent granted to W.R.Grace company and US Department of Agriculture on Neem by European patent office were again on the same ground on its use having been known in India. To prevent the wrongful patenting of the codified TM of the country, TKDL project was launched in June 2001 collaboratively between the Department of Ayurveda, Yoga and Naturopathy, Unani, Siddha and Homeopathy (AYUSH) and CSIR in order to prevent misappropriation of disclosed TK contained in the codified TM texts.

Defensive protection of disclosed TK through TKDL is only the first step within a comprehensive TK protection policy of India (Gupta, 2006). Defensive measures must be supplemented by positive measures, such as benefit sharing, in order to safeguard the interest of TK holders. Besides the codified documented TM, India has a very rich and diverse oral tradition on TM, the protection of which is a very difficult task. The oral traditions of TM, the medicinal wisdom of Traditional communities developed and updated/improved over thousands of years is currently threatened of extinction on account of the fast changing life styles of the traditional communities. In India an effort has been made to document such a knowledge system of the tribal communities of the country by launching on All India Coordinated Programme on Ethnobiology (AICPPE) in 1982 by Govt. of India.

It was Dr. M.S. Swaminathan way back in 1976 who recognized the intrinsic potential TK, particularly those of the tribal communities of India or danger of its possible loss due to fast change in the life style that is taking place in these communities. He then mooted the idea of documenting a protecting knowledge. AICRPE was finally launched by Govt. of India in which the author functioned as the chief coordinator. It was operated at 27 centres in the country and about 600 scientists drawn from botany, zoology, sociology, anthropology, Ayurveda, Chemistry, pharmacology worked over 16 years (1982-1998) and generated a rich bank of information. It has documented the use of over 10,000 wild plants by the tribes of India out of which over 8000 plant species are sued for medicine besides many other products of animal and mineral origin. This data is now being digitized, but not put in public domain for want of its IPR protection.

Prior Informed Consent System and Benefit–Sharing Procedures: The NIF Model

The National Innovation Foundation (NIF), an autonomous society established under the Department of Science and Technology, Government of India in 2000, works for recognizing, respecting and rewarding innovations and outstanding traditional knowledge at the grass roots. NIF and the HONEY BEE Network under SRISTI (Society for Research and Initiatives for Sustainable Technologies and Institutions), an NGO based at Ahmedabad, have been scouting for documenting local innovations and linking their innovations for further valorization with Science and Technology experts, investors and entrepreneurs. NIF maintains a separate National Register for green Grassroots Technological Innovations and Traditional Knowledge. Until 2003, NIF has scouted about 37000 innovations and traditional knowledge examples from over 350 districts of India. Scouting and documentation; value addition and R&D through a network of S&T experts, institutions, people's organizations, and rural and urban innovators for developing business and micro-ventures at local levels based on valorization of grass root level innovations; intellectual property rights management; information and technology dissemination; and benefit sharing are the various steps involved in the NIF Programme on building of value chain of grass root innovations (Gupta 1999, 2001, 2003).

NIF has developed a model for facilitating the Prior Informed Consent (PIC) system for local innovators and traditional knowledge holders (see website www.nifindia.org, www.sristi.org/honeybee.html for NIF Update and Explanatory note for PIC addressed to the Innovators and the Traditional knowledge holders). The PIC models seek the innovators' or traditional knowledge holders' consent for partial or full disclosure of their innovation and disseminate them through print and web media, and provide NIF mediation for value addition, patenting or other kinds of IPR generation based on the local innovation or traditional knowledge, and for fixing criteria and the terms and conditions for sharing monetary or non-monetary benefits, if any, arising from the value addition, micro-venture development, patenting on a local innovation or traditional knowledge. The PIC process with regard to traditional knowledge holder and other grass root innovations is a quite complex one. This cannot be compared with the formal PIC process recommended for other ABS model involving Government agencies, R&D institutions and other organizations. The awareness, capacities and exposure level of the local innovators to the modern regimes of IPR scientific validation, management, trade policies, etc. is either minimum or low. Empowering these communities with knowledge and awareness on the values and potentials of the rich treasure-trove of knowledge they hold is an important exercise, which NIF has been successfully accomplishing through their scouting programmes, awareness campaigns, competitions and awards distribution conducted for successful innovators. NIF suggests the innovator or the knowledge holder to share their information on the following conditions:

1. With restrictions imposed
2. On commercial basis on terms for technology transfer, up front payments, royalties, license fees, etc.
3. On non-cost basis for personal application or household use only.
4. With further research and value addition in it
5. Any other conditions.

The PIC model of NIF has both advantages and disadvantages. The whole process of disclosure and dissemination of the local innovations, either partially or fully, needs to be examined, whether they affect adversely in eventual exclusion of potential innovations from possible valorization and IPR claims and also any possible misappropriation of such potentially useful innovations by others, and thereby depriving the local innovator of his/her intellectual property and customary rights.

The benefit sharing mechanism suggested by NIF's PIC models include four kinds of benefits *viz.* 1. *Monetary-Individual (MI)*–includes: monetary awards, license fees or royalty from commercial exploitation of technology or traditional knowledge, or any other monetary gain by entrepreneurial process. This will be firstly paid to the individuals, who may in turn share part of this with the community, innovation promotion fund and institutions helping the value chain; 2. *Monetary-Collective (MC)*–covers: trust funds, micro-venture funds, common property infrastructure, etc to be shared with the communities; 3. *Nonmonetary-Individual (NMI)* such as recognition, a citation in a public function, dissemination of one's creativity through media or in workshops or other public function, or using appellation on the product developed, business venture, etc.; 4. *Nonmonetary-Collective (NMC)*–includes: recognition to communities at appropriate levels for their collective wisdom, knowledge and social or cultural organizations, etc.

The NIF benefit-sharing procedures also suggest separate formula and modules for each kind of innovation on a case-to-case basis. Benefit sharing formula involving valorization with public or private R&D and the community or individual innovators needs to be evolved based on stakeholder consultations and on the degree of contributions by each stakeholder through an effective cost-benefit analysis. The existing complexities in the structure of the traditional knowledge domain itself, and also the very nature of the existing IPR system that accord protection only for the formal innovation based on the criteria of novelty, non-obviousness and utility, are some of the major impediments in evolving any uniform guidelines or model for access protection and benefit sharing involving traditional knowledge systems held in traditional communities or the grass root level innovators. However, NIF's efforts to networking with the grass root innovators so as to promote the local innovation and valorization of such knowledge, protection of the intellectual property rights, and equitable benefit sharing are gaining wider acceptance and credibility both nationally and internationally.

Community Registers and Peoples' Biodiversity Registers

The community gene bank and community agro biodiversity register programmes and Peoples Biodiversity Register (PBR) spearheaded by the MS Swaminathan Research Foundation (MSSRF), Chennai, the Foundation for Revitalization of Local Health Traditions (FRLHT), Bangalore, and the Centre for Ecological Sciences at Indian Institute of Science, Bangalore are examples of other useful mechanisms and methods to chronicle the biogenetic resources and associated knowledge systems of the traditional communities and local or rural people of the country. PBR is now accepted as a viable mechanism for documenting people's knowledge and biological resources under the Biodiversity Management Committees established under the

Indian Biological Diversity Act 2002. Development of comprehensive PBRs at local level is a highly rewarding exercise which would not only help to inventory and document the local biological and genetic resources along with the various actual uses and potential values of such resources, but also to conserve and sustainably use the biocultural diversity for gainful income generation and IPR generation through value addition and benefit-sharing processes (MSSRF, 1998; Ghate *et al.*, 2001; Kumar *et al.*, 2003; Sahai 2003a). PBR also ensures active involvement of the local and traditional communities in all decision-making processes related to biological diversity and traditional knowledge, including issues of access and benefit sharing. BMCs are entrusted with the preparation of PBRs and to assist the SBBs and NBA in matters on ABS related to local biogenetic resources and traditional knowledge.

The success story on compilation of community biodiversity registers and community gene bank programmes involving tribal communities of the Jeypore tracts of Orissa with the guidance and support from MSSRF is a good case study that demonstrates how the potential benefits of such community biodiversity programmes help enhance the livelihood options and security of the local and traditional people. This model of community agro-biodiversity programme has won the UN-Equator initiative Prize for poverty eradication and community empowerment at World Summit for Sustainable Development (WSSD) at Johannesburg in August 2002 (see *www.undp.org./equator initiative/ /equator prize_2002 html*).

Another community-based participatory conservation programme that has won international acclaim through the Equator Award of 2002 is the medicinal plant conservation and cultivation work achieved by Medicinal Plants Conservation Centre, (MPCC), Pune with the support of FRLHT (see *www.undp.org./equator initiative/ /equator prize_2002 html*).. The MPCC with an effective involvement of local communities has developed a decentralized system of nurseries, raising 50,000 plants of 50 different species and linking them with a network of herbal production centers. The propagation and cultivation of medicinal plants in nurseries have helped to reduce the pressures of collection from the wild and hence promoting the conservation of such valuable resources. The linkage with herbal production centers has helped to provide economic incentives to the communities involved in the MPCC programme. Such community network programmes on bio-resources conservation and management contribute significantly to the implementation of national policies and programmes on biodiversity, and intellectual property rights and access and benefit sharing involving genetic resources and traditional knowledge.

Indian Experiment in Benefit Sharing: "TBGRI Model" or "Kani Model" or "Pushpangadan Model" of Benefit Sharing

India has the distinction of being the first country in the world in experimenting a benefit-sharing model that implemented the Article 8(j) of CBD, in letter and spirit. It was the Tropical Botanic Garden and Research Institute (TBGRI) in Kerala (where the author was the then director from 1990-1999) that demonstrated that the indigenous knowledge system merits support, recognition and fair and adequate compensation. The model, which later on came to be known as "TBGRI Model" or "Kani Model" or "Pushpangadan Model", relates to the sharing of benefits with a forest dwelling Indian tribal community from whom a vital lead for developing a scientifically validated herbal drug (Jeevani) was obtained by a team of scientists led by the author who then functioned as the Principal Investigator and chief project coordinator of an All India Coordinated Research Project on Ethnobiology (AICRPE) sponsored by Govt. of India.

During the course of an ethnobotanical study on a forest dwelling tribe namely 'Kani' inhabiting in the southern Western Ghats located in the South Indian state Kerala, the author and his team came across with an unique tribal knowledge on the medicinal use of a lesser known wild plant namely *Trichopus zeylanicus* var. *travancoricus* having antifatigue property. The author and his research team then located at Regional Research Laboratory (RRL), Jammu carried out basic phytochemical and pharmacological properties and validated the tribal claim. He and his team later at TBGRI, Kerala developed a scientifically validated and standardized herbal formulation–which after necessary pharmacological, toxicological and clinical evaluation was released for commercial production in 1996. The author who was then the Director of TBGRI with the approval of competent authority agreed to share the benefits derived from this technology with the Kani tribe on a 1:1 basis. The Kani tribe received 50 per cent of license fee and continues to receive 50 per cent royalty.

The TBGRI Model has got wider acclaims, acceptance and popularity the world over, because it was the first of its kind that recognized the community rights and IPR of a traditional community by way of sharing equitably the benefits derived out of the use of a knowledge that has been developed, preserved and maintained by that community for many generations (Anand 1998, Anuradha, 1998, Bagla 1999, Gupta, 2002, Mashelkar, 2003). Further, it demonstrates the vast and as yet under–explored or untapped potentials of the Indian traditional knowledge systems, particularly the traditional health care practices of the local and indigenous people in India.

Kani tribe was then a totally unorganized forest dwelling semi-nomadic tribe. The prime concern in the beginning was therefore to evolve a viable mechanism enabling the tribe to receive such funds and utilizing the same for the welfare of the community. Several ways of sharing the benefits were discussed at many levels and it was finally decided to set up a trust fund of the tribe. The very idea of the trust fund had originated from very useful and protracted discussion that the author had with Prof. Anil K. Gupta, the founder and coordinator of SRISTI and Honey Bee Network. It took however, almost two years to transfer the benefits to the tribe. With the help of some local NGOs, the author and his colleagues along with some motivated government officials were able to educate and encourage the Kani tribe to form a registered trust, Kerala Kani Samudaya Kshema Trust (KKSKT) with only Kani adults as its members. The trust is fully owned and managed by the Kani tribe. Over 70 per cent of the Kani families of Kerala are now members of this Trust. In February 1999, the amount due to them (Rs. 6.5 lakhs) which was till then kept by TBGRI in a separate account was transferred to the Trust. As per the rules of the Trust the license fee and royalty received on account of the sale of the drug 'Jeevani' will be in a fixed deposit and only the interest accrued from this amount will be utilized for the benefits/ welfare of the members of the Kani tribe.

This model was thus developed and perfected over a period of about 12 years starting from 1987 to 1999 in full consultation with the Kani tribe. In fact, the whole process of this benefit sharing was started much before the CBD. It took almost 3 years for the Kani tribe to receive this benefit. The delay was mainly due to the inherent inability and absence of any organized mechanism for Kani tribe to receive such benefit. The secretary of Tribal and Scheduled Caste Department of Government of Kerala played a crucial role in the formation of the Kani Trust and also in effecting a smooth transfer of the amount due to the Kanis from TBGRI to the Kani Trust. The Kani Trust now continues to receive the royalty.

All along these years, starting from 1987, it was the mutual trust, respect, transparency and frequent interaction and communication between TBGRI and the Kani tribe that contributed to the success of this benefit-sharing model.

In addition to the license fee and royalty that Kani Trust is receiving, a large number of Kani families are now getting benefit from the cultivation of Arogyapacha and supply of the raw-material (*i.e.* the leaves of the plant) to the pharmaceutical company for the production of the drug. TBGRI has trained many tribal families for the cultivation of 'Arogyapacha' in and around their dwellings in the forest.

Impact on Kani on this Benefit Sharing

The sharing of benefits with the Kanis and formation of the Kani trust fund have started showing positive impacts in the sense that the tribal community is now becoming conscious about the values of and rights over their knowledge system and associated biological resources. These developments also have helped in bringing the Kani families to a single organizational framework, so that the benefits accrued from the trust fund could be utilized for the economic well being and social development in the Kani tribal hamlets. The Kani tribe is now a proud and dignified community. The trust has a concrete building of fully furnished 4 rooms (about 350 m^2) with fully furnished office room, conference hall, library cum reading room and a store room. The Kani community regularly meets at this building, discuss their problems and takes decisions for the welfare of the community. The Kani tribe, now is a confident and dignified community. They have initiated various welfare programmes for the benefit of their community. Looking back 10 years, it is unbelievable to see the kind of transformation of this otherwise timid, nomadic forest dwelling tribe who used to be scared of outsiders and foresters. They now stand up with dignity and claim their rights and privileges. The quality of their life has been tremendously improved. There are now many Kani boys and girls who have passed secondary school examinations and a few have even graduated. The trust recently acquired a 12 seated vehicle and a Kani young man now drives this vehicle from their hamlets to the nearest village markets and towns. The Trust was able to persuade the local authorities to construct a motorable road of over 10 Km inside the forest to the tribal village. Solar lamps are installed in their houses, they have a telephone connecting them to the outside world and some of their houses have television sets powered by solar energy.

The TBGRI Model is perhaps a unique experiment ever done, wherein the benefits accrued from the development of a product based on an ethno-botanical lead were shared with the holders of that traditional knowledge. Considering the significant outcome of this model in community empowerment, income generation and poverty eradication of a tribal community, Pushpangadan was awarded with the UN-Equator Initiative Prize (under individual category) at the World Summit on Sustainable Development held in Johannesburg in August 2002. Now with the CBD-Bonn and WIPO guidelines and our national legislation on Biodiversity in position, the TBGRI or Kani case study could be taken as an ideal model of equitable benefit sharing involving genetic resources and associated traditional knowledge.

21st century offers an excellent opportunity for megadiverse and TM rich countries like India to excel in offering a holistic healthcare programme for mankind. However, for achieving this leadership position in medicine, India need to build/strengthen her capacity in validating her TMs and explaining it in the contemporary scientific understanding and expertise and also in developing novel evidence based herbal remedies. It is well known that by doing so India could offer a very comprehensive and holistic programme for primary healthcare and also effectively deal with the lifestyle diseases, degenerative disorders for which there are no satisfactory cures in modern medical system. Ethnopharmacology, Reverse pharmacology and system biology are the scientific research areas required for reviving/revalidating and revitalizing the TMs of India. Such a creative research endeavour requires excellent expertise and teamwork of multi systems (like TMs modern science and modern medical science and associated technology) and multidisciplinary/transdisciplinary approach and state of art facility. A strict regulatory mechanism to oversea/control the quality, safety and standard of TM/HM are also important in reviving and revitalizing the TM/HM.

References

1. AICRPE (All India Coordinated Research Project on Ethnobiology), Final Technical Report, 1992-1998 (Ministry of Environment and Forests, Government of India, New Delhi)
2. Anand U: The wonder Drug (UBS Publishers Ltd., New Delhi.), 1998.
3. Anuradha RV: Sharing with the Kanis; a case study from Kerala, India Benefit-sharing case studies, Fourth Meeting of the Conference of Parties to the CBD, Bratislava, May, Secretariat of the Convention on Biological Diversity, Montreal. 1998.
4. Vaidya ADB, Kumar A, Rout A: Evidence based Ayurveda–Sorting Fact from Fantasy–In Ayurveda and its Scientific Aspects: Opportunities for Globalization. Published jointly by Department of Ayurveda, Yoga and Naturopathy, Unani, Siddha and Homoeopathy and CSIR, New Delhi, 2006.
5. CBD/COP decision VI/24–Access and benefit-sharing as related to genetic resources, Bonn guidelines on Access to Genetic Resources and fair and Equitable Sharing of the benefits arising out of their Utilization, see http://www.biodiv.org/decisions/VI/24.
6. Farnsworth NR: The role of Ethnopharmacology in drug development. *In:* "Bioactive compounds from plants", Wiley Chichestor (Ciba Foundation Symposium) 1990, pp 2-21.

7. Govindarajan R, Vijayakumar M, Pushpangadan P: Review: Antioxident approach to disease management and the role of *Rasayana* herbs of Ayurveda. *J Ethnopharmacol* 2005, 99(2), 165-178.

8. Gupta VK: Traditional Knowledge Digital Library for protection, preservation and wealth creation, 2006.

9. Chaojin L: Management of Chinese Traditional Drugs. *In:* The Book of Traditional Medicine in Primary Health Care. 1987.

10. Posey D, Outfield G: Beyond Intellectual Property, Ottawa:IDRC, 1996.

11. Pushpangadan P: Ethnobiology in India–A Status Report. All India Coordinated Research Project on Ethnobiology (AICRPE). Ministry of Environment and Forests, Government of India, 1994

12. Pushpangadan P: Role of Traditional Medicine in primary health care. *In:* science for Health. (Ed. Iyengar PK), State Committee on Science Technology and Environment, Kerala, India, 1995.

13. Pushpangadan P: "Tropical Botanical Garden Research Institute: People Oriented Sustainable Development Programme", Paper presented at the UNEP/GEF Indigenous People's Consultation Meeting, Ganeva, 29-31 May,1996

14. Pushpangadan P: Biodiversity and Emerging Benefit Sharing Arrangements–Challenges and Opportunities for India. Proc. *Indian Natn Sci Acad* (PINSA) 2002, B68, 297-314

15. Pushpangadan P, Narayanan Nair K: "Access to Biological Resources and Associated Traditional Knowledge and Benefit-sharing" in The Group of Like Minded Megadiverse Countries–Realizing the Potential: Report of the Expert and Ministerial Level Meeting of Like Minded Megadiverse Countries, 17-21 January 2005, Ministry of Environment and Forests, Government of India, New Delhi, 2005, pp.10-13.

16. Pushpangadan P, Govindarajan R: Need for Developing Protocol for Collection/Cultivation and Quality parameters of Medicinal Plants for Effective Regulatory Quality Control of Herbal Drugs, Proceedings–International Conference on Botanicals, Kolkata, India, 2005, pp. 63-69.

17. Pushpangadan P, Govindarajan R: Need for scientific validation and standardization of TM to meet the Healthcare of the third world in 21st century. *In:* Herbal Medicine Phytopharmaceuticals and other Natural products: Trends and advances jointly published by centre for S&T of the Non-aligned and other Developing countries (NAM S&T Centre), India and Institute of Chemistry, Ceylon, Sri Lanka, 2006.

18. Pushpangadan P: Raw Material-Sustainable Availability and concern regarding Medicinal plants on Negative list in the proceedings of the International conclave on Traditional Medicine. 16-17 Nov 2006. Dept. of AYUSH&CSIR, N. Delhi, 2006, pp 144-152

19. Pushpangadan P: Important Indian Medicinal Plants of Global Interest in, 2006
20. TRIPS (Annex IC of 1994 Marrakesh Agreement Establishing the World Trade Organization; entered into force on 1 January 1995)
21. The WIPO Intergovernmental Committee on Intellectual Property and Genetic Resources, Traditional Knowledge and Folklore (IGC) was established by the WIPO General Assembly in October 2000 (see document WO / GA / 26 / 6 http://www.wipo.int/documents/en/document/govbody/wo_gb_ga/pdf/ga26_6.pdf
22. UNEP. Convention on Biological Diversity Decision VIII/5 BII on article 8 (j) and related positions-accessor on 27th June 2006. WW.Biod.org. 2006
23. WHO: Quality Control Methods for medicinal plant material WHO/PHARM/92.559, 1992.
24. WHO: Quality Control Methods for Medicinal plant material, WHO, Geneva, 1998.
25. WHO: http://www.who.int/mediacentre/factsheets/fs134/en, 2003.
26. WHO: National Policy on Traditional Medicine and Regulation of Herbal Medicines, Report of a Global Survey, World Health Organization, Geneva, 2005.
27. WIPO: Summary of Draft Policy and Core Principles, Annex I, http//www.wipo.int/edocs/mdcocs/tk/en wipo-grt/ftk-7 wipogrtkf-ic73.annex1.pdf, year
28. WIPO: Intellectual Property and Traditional Knowledge. Booklet No.2. WIPO Publication No. 920(E), World Intellectual Property Organization, Geneva, 2004.
29. WIPO: Intellectual Property and genetic resources, traditional knowledge and Cultural Expressions/ Folklores–WIPO/GRTKF/IC/a/4, 2006
30. WIPO: Intellectual Property and Genetic Resources, Traditional Knowledge and Traditional Cultural Expressions/Folklore. WIPO/GRTKF/INF/1, World Intellectual Property Organization, Geneva, 2006.
31. World Trade Organization (WTO), established on 1 January 1995 under the Uruguay Round negotiations 1986-1994, http//www.wto.org
32. WTO: Ninth session of Intergovernmental Committee on Intellectual Property and Genetic Resources, Traditional knowledge and Folklore. Protection of Traditional Knowledge revised objectives and principles, Geneva April 24-28, 2006.

Chapter 19

Antimitotic Polysaccharide from *Punica granatum*

T.T. Sreelekha[1]*, K.K. Vijayan[2], Prabha Balaram[1]**

[1]*Division of Cancer Research, Regional Cancer Centre, Thiruvananthapuram – 695 011, Kerala, India*

[2]*Department of Chemistry, University of Calicut, Thenjipalam, Kerala, India*

ABSTRACT

Drug development from natural products is an emerging area of medical research. Polysaccharides from plant products have attracted attention in the recent times. The advantage of these compounds is that they are generally non-toxic. The objective of this study was elucidation of anti cancer activity of polysaccharide from fruit rind of *Punica granatum*. Isolation and purification of the polysaccharide was carried out by standard procedures for water-soluble polysaccharides. Molecular weight was determined by gel filtration chromatography. For structural characterization, partial hydrolysis, periodate oxidation, methylation, hydrolysis, acetylation and trimethylsilylation were carried out and analysed by ^{1}HNMR, FABMS and GC-MS. Thin layer chromatographic analysis with hydrolysed polysaccharide and co-chromatography using standard sugars revealed the constituent monosaccharides to be glucose and mannose. The spectroscopic studies also revealed Pg polysaccharides to be a heteropolymer in which the constituent sugars are glucose and mannose. The results of the FABMS study of the native polysaccharide, the permethylated acetates and the trimethylsilylated samples support the above-mentioned observation. Biological activities were examined in cell cultures (peripheral lymphocytes and human leukemic cell line K_{562}) and in Swiss albino mice. *Pg polysaccharide* showed antiproliferative activities with mitotic abnormalities in malignant cell cultures suggesting that it possesses anti cancer properties. It was found to inhibit cell proliferation of cultured peripheral blood lymphocytes and the human leukaemic

* Phone: 0471-2522378, Email: lekhasree64@yahoo.co.in.

** Phone: 0471-2522203, Email: prabhabalaram@yahoo.co.in.

cell line, K_{562}. Animal studies revealed Pg polysaccharide to act at the early stages of M phase (prophase) and prevented most of the cells from further progression in division. This resulted in several morphological changes in prophase, stickiness of chromosomes at prophase, metaphase and anaphase leading to pycnotic irregular nuclei. These observations agree with the hypothesis that the goal of innovation of plant products with medicinal properties may serve as leads for the development of new drugs, which can be used as protective tools against diseases including cancer.

Introduction

Cancer, the second largest cause of death in people of various ages and racial background has led to much research efforts and clinical studies in the fight against the disease. Cancer cells originate from normal cells. A novel drug which is able to select and destroy only affected cells preventing carcinogenesis without injury to normal cells would be an ideal chemotherapeutic against cancer. This is a very difficult task facing cancer researchers. Recent investigations have been channeled towards the development of immunotherapy to target and remove cancer cells as well as on substances such as immunopotentiators, immunoinitiators and biological response modulators (BRM) that act to prevent carcinogenesis and induce carcinostasis (1).

The polysaccharides of higher plants occur mostly as glucans or glycans. Glycans are polysaccharides containing units other than glucose in their backbone. A wide range of antitumor or immunostimulating polysaccharides of different chemical structures have been investigated (2). Some correlation has been drawn between the chemical structure and antitumor activities of polysaccharides. A wide range of glycans extending from homopolymers to highly complex heteropolymers (3) exhibit antitumor activity. Differences in activity can be correlated with ability of the polysaccharide molecule to solubilize in water, size of the molecules, branching rate and form. Such structural features as β-(1→3) linkages in the backbone (main chain) of the glucan and additional β-(1→6)-branch points are needed for antitumor activity (2). β-glucans with only (1→6) glycosidic linkages have little or no activity. Higher molecular weight glucans have been reported by Mizuno *et al.* (4) and Mizuno (5) to be more effective than those of low molecular weight against tumors.

Three polysaccharide based carcinostatic (immunotherapeutic) agents, Krestin, Lentinan and Sonifilan, have already been developed from mushroom and are used currently in the treatment of cancer of the digestive organs, lung and breast, as well as cancers of the stomach and cervix.

In cancer chemotherapy, it is necessary to design an agent that suppresses or inhibits the targets that influence cell growth and apoptosis. Chemotherapeutic drugs are known to eliminate cancer cells by inducing apoptosis. The mechanism of action of various plant polysaccharides is through the induction of apoptosis in cancer cells.

Modern medical practice relies heavily on the use of highly purified pharmaceutical compounds because its purity can be easily assessed and the pharmaceutical activity and toxicity show clear structure-function relationships.

Traditional folk medicine and ethnopharmacology coupled to bioprospecting have been an important source of many anticancer agents as well as other medicines. Purified bioactive compounds derived from medicinal plants are a potentially important new source of anticancer agents. The structure and antitumor activity of a polysaccharide from the fruit rind of *Punica granatum* is presented here.

Materials and Methods

Isolation of Polysaccharides

The fruit rind of *Punica granatum* was shade dried and powdered. The powdered plant material (100 g) was extracted with petroleum ether (60°C–80°C) at room temperature for 72 h (3 x 300 ml) followed by methanol (2 x 300 ml), filtered and dried. This was then suspended in cold water (1000 ml) and kept overnight with occasional stirring. After filtration, the filtrate was concentrated (300 ml) under vacuum in a flash evaporator at 40°C. To this, 700 ml ethanol was added slowly with stirring for 6 h. It was then allowed to stand at 4°C for 24 h, and the precipitate collected by centrifugation at 20000 x g. The supernatant liquid was removed and the residue obtained was dissolved in a minimum quantity of distilled water (150 ml). This solution was again precipitated with ethanol (350 ml) and the precipitated polysaccharide collected by centrifugation at 20000 x g. The process was repeated 3 times and the residue was collected and dissolved in the minimum quantity of distilled water (50 ml) followed by dialysis against distilled water for 48 h with several changes of water. The contents of the dialysis bags were shaken with chloroform (50 ml) in a separating funnel to remove the denatured protein (6). This process was repeated until the water-chloroform interphase became clear. The aqueous layer was treated again with ethanol to precipitate the polysaccharide. This was then centrifuged at 20000 x g and the residue dissolved in water (100 ml), dialysed against distilled water and freeze dried.

Purification of Polysaccharides

The polysaccharide was purified by gel filtration Chromatography using Sephadex G-200 (Pharmacia Fine Chemicals) and Ultrogel AcA-44 (LKB), 0.001 M Phosphate Buffered saline (PBS) was used as the eluent. The lyophilized crude sample (500 mg) was suspended in the buffer and chromatographed through a column of Sephadex G-200 (3 cm x 75 cm) equilibrated with the buffer. 3 ml fractions were collected in test tubes and monitored by the absorbance of the eluent at 490 nm using phenol sulphuric acid and at 280 nm (7). For *Punica granatum* saccharide (Pgs) a single peak was obtained for both the columns. The fractions under the peak were pooled, lyophilized and stored at 4° C for further analysis.

Zone Electrophoresis

To test the homogeneity of the purified polysaccharide sodium dodecyl sulphate polyacrylamide gel (10 per cent) electrophoresis was performed (8). For this, sample was prepared in buffer containing 1 per cent (w/v) SDS and 5 per cent (v/v) 2-mercaptoethanol and kept at 100°C for 3 to 5 minutes. The prepared polysaccharide sample was then applied to the gel and electrophoresis was carried out at 3 mA current per gel until the bromophenol blue marker reached the other end of the gel. The gel was then treated with a solution of isopropanol, acetic acid and water (25: 10: 65) (2 times, 1 hour each) in borosilicate tubes to fix the polyacrylamide. This was then placed in a solution of thymol (0.2 per cent w/v) for 2 h, decanted and drained to remove the solution completely. A solution of concentrated sulphuric acid-absolute alcohol (80: 20 v/v, 10 ml) was added to the tube and shaken for about 2.5 h at 35°C until the opalescence disappeared. Zones containing polysaccharides stained red with yellow colour for the rest of the gel portion. Single band was obtained for the Pg polysaccharide.

Molecular Weight Estimation

Molecular weight of the purified polysaccharide sample was estimated from gel filtration chromatographic experiments using Sephadex G-200 column (2 cm x 75 cm). It was eluted with 0.001 M PBS at a flow rate of 20 ml per hour. A series of dextrans 10,20,40,70 and T-500 (Pharmacia Fine Chemicals) was used as reference standards. The molecular weight was estimated from a linear correlation between the logarithm of the molecular weights of the standards and the ratios of their elution volume to the void volume of the column (9).

Identification of Sugar Components (Complete Hydrolysis and Chromatography)

The polysaccharide sample (20 mg) was hydrolyzed with 1 N HCl (20 ml) at 100°C in sealed tubes for 24 h. After cooling, the excess acid was removed by passage over a small column (1 cm x 50 cm) of Dowex-1 (AcO^-) anion-exchange resin, and eluted with deionized water. The eluate was concentrated (10 ml) in a flash evaporator.

TLC

The hydrolysates (0.5 μl) were applied on a TLC plate coated with cellulose (1 mm thick 20 cm x 20 cm) and the chromatogram was developed using n-Butanol: Acetic acid: Water (3: 1: 2 v/v). For identification of the spots aniline diphenylamine–H_3PO_4 (10) spray reagent was used. Constituent saccharides were identified by comparison of Rf values with those of authentic samples and also by co-chromatography with authentic samples. Rf values of authentic samples were: D-glucose 0.25, D-mannose 0.30, D-galactose 0.21, D-fructose 0.29.

Reduction of the Hydrolysate, Peracetylation and Chromatographic Comparison

The polysaccharide hydrolysate (5 ml) was treated with sodium borohydride (10 mg) and kept at 50°C for 1 h. The excess of sodium borohydride was removed by treating with acetic acid (5 ml). The borohydride reduced samples were vacuum evaporated and extracted with pyridine/acetic anhydride mixture (10 ml; 1:1 v/v) and heated at 100°C for 1 h, cooled and passed through a column of Sephadex LH 20 (1 cm x 50 cm) and eluted with water. The eluate was evaporated in a flash evaporator. This concentrate was analyzed by paper chromatography (Whatman No.3 paper) with butanol/2-propanol/water (11:6:3 v/v) as solvent system. Samples were identified by their Rf values. The reduced and peracetylated samples were also analyzed by ^{1}HNMR.

Partial Acid Hydrolysis

The polysaccharide (50 mg) was hydrolysed with 0.05 M sulphuric acid (10 ml) in a sealed vial at 90°C for 14 h. The hydrolysate was then subjected to ion exchange chromatography on Dowex-1 (AcO^-) column (1 cm x 50 cm). Following elution with deionized water (100 ml), the eluate was lyophilized to powder form. One portion (5 mg) was used for FABMS studies. The rest of the lyophilized hydrolysate was subjected to preparative thin layer chromatography on cellulose plates (2 mm thick, 20 cm x 20 cm). The plates were developed using the solvent system ethylacetate: pyridine: water (2: 1: 2 v/v). TLC analysis showed the presence of the monosaccharides obtained from complete hydrolysis and also several other closely resolved components, which were then scraped out from the TLC plate, dissolved in distilled water and evaporated to dryness. Some of these could be identified from their melting points and further hydrolytic studies and reference to literature (11-14).

Methylation, Hydrolysis, Reduction and Acetylation

Pg polysaccharide (50 mg) in dimethyl sulfoxide (10 ml) in a small round bottomed flask was stirred using a magnetic stirrer under a nitrogen stream with an equal amount of methyl sulfinyl carbanion. Dissolving 20 mg of sodium hydride in dimethyl sulfoxide generated the carbanion. The mixture was stirred under the nitrogen stream for 6 h at room temperature. An excess of methyl iodide was then added and further stirred for overnight. Isolation of the product was done by dialysis in running water and lyophilization. One more repetition of the methylation gave completely permethylated products having no absorption band in the IR spectrum due to a hydroxyl group (15). The methylated polysaccharides were hydrolysed with 2 N H_2SO_4 at 90°C for 3 h. Hydrolysed samples (5 ml) were treated with sodium borohydride (10 mg) and kept at 50°C for 1 h. Excess of borohydride was removed, with acetic acid (5 ml) and was converted to the corresponding alditol acetate by reaction with pyridine-acetic anhydride (16). The borohydride-reduced samples were vacuum evaporated and extracted with 5 ml of pyridine: acetic anhydride (1: 1) mixture and was sealed in ampules. It was then heated at 100°C in a water bath for 1 h, cooled and passed through a column of Sephadex LH 20 (1 cm x 50 cm) and eluted with water. The eluate was evaporated in a flash evaporator. The concentrate was analysed by GC-MS.

Methylation, Hydrolysis and Acetylation

Methylation and hydrolysis were done as above. The hydrolysed sample was acetylated by reaction with pyridine–acetic anhydride mixture (16). This was subjected to ^{1}HNMR and FABMS studies.

Trimethyl Silylation

A mixture of anhydrous pyridine (reagent grade pyridine dried over KOH pellets) 5 ml, hexamethyl disilazane (1 ml) and trimethyl chlorosilane (0.5 ml) was used for the trimethylsilylation reaction (17). The polysaccharide (10 mg) was taken into a stoppered vial and 1 ml of the pyridine-silanes mixture was added. The mixture was shaken at intervals until the sugar had dissolved completely after which it was allowed to stand for 5 minutes at room temperature. The trimethyl silylated sample was analysed by FABMS.

Biological Assays

Sterile precautions were taken while carrying out these experiments. The Pg polysaccharide was studied for the following biological activities.

1. Leucocyte migration inhibition (LMI)
2. Phagocytosis
3. Toxicity profile
4. Cytogenetic studies

Leucocyte Migration Inhibition (LMI)

Leucocytes were collected from normal controls and prepared at a concentration of 1 x 10^8 cell/ml. LMI was carried out by the method of Roklin. The area of each migrated field was measured by planimetry (18).

$$\text{Calculation of migration index} = \frac{\text{Area of migration in test}}{\text{Area of migration in control}}$$

Tissue culture medium (TC 199) used alone, served as the control.

Phagocytosis

Ten ml of venous blood was collected for each test in heparinised tubes. The reaction mixture consisted of approximately 1.2 x 10^6 neutrophils in 1 ml of Hank's balanced salt solution and 5 per cent foetal calf serum and polysaccharide (5 µg in 50 µl). This mixture was preincubated in a water bath at 37°C for 7 minutes. A suspension of yeast particles was diluted with saline solution to 25 x 10^7 particles per millilitre and heated at 100°C for 30 minutes. To the preincubated reaction mixture, 0.1 ml of the suspension of yeast particles was added and incubation continued at 37°C for 60 minutes. The number of yeast particles phagocytosed by neutrophils was counted after staining with 5 per cent fuchsin in phenol solution (9).

$$\text{Phagocytosis index} = \frac{\text{No. of yeast phagocytosed by 100 neutrophils in test}}{\text{No. of yeast phagocytosed by 100 neutrophils in control}}$$

0.1 M phosphate buffered saline (PBS, pH 7.2) was used as the control.

Toxicity Profile

The toxicity studies for the polysaccharide in mice were carried out. The purified polysaccharide from Pg was administered intraperitonially at a dose of 100, 200, 500, 1000, 2000, or 5000 mg/kg body weight to a group of 6 animals. The animals were observed continuously for 2 h and then 4 h and finally overnight.

Cytogenetical Studies

The experiments were done in mice, in human leukemic cell line K_{562} and also in human peripheral blood lymphocytes.

Mice

Female Swiss inbred mice from our Laboratory were used. Selected mice were fed normally. Samples in saline at various concentrations such as 1 µg/ml, 10 µg/ml and 100 µg/ml were injected intraperitoneally (19). After 24 h the animals were sacrificed, femur separated and bone marrow collected in a fixative (3:1 methanol: acetic acid) and kept overnight. Slides were prepared by gentle vertical tapping and stained with acetocarmine.

Human Leukemic Cell Line K_{562}

Human leukemic cell line K_{562} was obtained from National Institute of Virology, Pune. RPMI 1640 (Sigma Fine Chemicals, UK) with 10 per cent Foetal Calf Serum was used for the culture. Three different sets of experiments were done.

1. Control: Cell line was cultured without any polysaccharide.
2. Polysaccharide was added at the time of initiation of the culture and incubated for 72 h.
3. Polysaccharide was added at the 70th hour of culture and incubation continued for further 2 h.

Polysaccharide in saline at various concentrations such as 1 µg/ml, 10 µg/ml and 100 µg/ml were used. After 72 h the cells were collected by centrifugation and treated with KCl (0.075 M) for 10 minutes. The supernatant was decanted and fixative (3:1 methanol: acetic acid) added. It was kept at 4°C for 30 minutes and washed with the fixative four or five times, smears were prepared and stained with Giemsa (20).

Peripheral Blood Lymphocytes

Peripheral blood lymphocytes from normal controls and from acute lymphoblastic leukemia (ALL) patients were collected and the experiment was done as above.

Results and Discussion

Chemical Studies

For the isolation and purification of the polysaccharide, standard procedures for water-soluble polysaccharides were followed. Final purification was carried out by gel permeation chromatography. The homogeneity of the purified compound was tested using sodium dodecylsulphate polyacrylamide gel electrophoresis. Molecular weights were determined by gel filtration chromatography using sephadex G-200 with a series of dextrans as standards. The molecular weights obtained for Pg polysaccharide was 1,10,000 Dalton.

For characterization, various chemical and spectroscopic analyses were carried out. Complete hydrolysis and thin layer chromatographic analysis and co-chromatography using standard sugars revealed that the constituent monosaccharides are glucose and mannose. Partial hydrolysis, periodate oxidation, methylation, hydrolysis, acetylation and trimethylsilylation were also carried out and analysed by various spectroscopic methods such as ^{1}HNMR, FABMS and GC-MS.

^{1}HNMR Spectroscopy

From the ^{1}HNMR spectrum of Pg polysaccharide, the characteristic proton absorption could be identified. The anomeric proton of the monosaccharides appeared in the region δ 4.58 to δ 5.19 indicating both α- and β-anomeric protons. Hydrolysis and chromatographic analysis of this polysaccharide gave glucose and mannose as constituent sugars. This also gave a complex NMR spectrum indicating a highly crosslinked structure. The anomeric proton signals are from δ 4.585 to δ 5.1911 indicating both α and β C-1 protons. Here also β-linkages are in preponderant amount. The peaks at δ 4.004, δ 4.097, δ 4.1757 etc may be assigned to H-2 of mannose[79] indicating that this polysaccharide contains a good percentage of mannose as the constituent co-monomer which is in conformity with chemical data. Methylation, hydrolysis and acetylation indicate that C-1 of the sugars is glycosidically linked because downfield shift upto δ 5.829 are observed. The nonanomeric protons are observed between δ 3.361 to δ 4.487 giving quite a number of peaks indicating the highly crosslinked nature of the Pg polysaccharides.

Similarly, in the ^{1}HNMR spectrum of the acetates of the methylated and hydrolysed polysaccharide, the methoxyl protons gave rise to a signal around δ 3.5 and the acetoxyl protons between δ 1.9–δ 2.4, as expected. The intensity of the methoxyl proton signal is almost equal to that of the acetoxyl signal strongly suggesting lower degree of cross linking in this polysaccharide suggesting that Pg polysaccharide is essentially linear. Linkages assigned from ^{1}HNMR spectra of Pg polysaccharide is given in Table 19.I.

Table 19.1

Linkage	*Fequency ppm (δ)*	*Reference*
α-glc-glycosidically linked	5.191	1. Goux WJ, Weber DS.
α-man or α-glc end group	5.179	Carbohydrate Research
α-man or α-glc	5.115	240: 57-69, 1993.
α-man–glycosidically	5.055	2. Frosberg LS, Dellg A,
linked 1→2 linkages		Walton DJ, Ballou CE.
α-gal	4.796	J Bio.Chem. 257 (7), 3555-3563, 1982.
β-glc	4.644	
β-D-man 1χ4 man	4.790	3. Vander Veer JM,
β-D-man 1→3	4.790	J.Org. Chem. 28, 564 1963.
β-D-glc 1→4	4.640	

FABMS

From the chemical studies it is revealed that Pg polysaccharide is a heteropolymer in which the constituent sugars are glucose and mannose. The results of the FABMS study of the polysaccharide, the permethylated acetate and the trimethylsilylated sample support the above-mentioned observation. The mass spectra of the polysaccharides from *Punica granatum* have several peaks in the low m/z region. The spectra of the partially hydrolysed samples of the polysaccharides also support the same observation. The peak at m/z 91 forms the base peak for this polysaccharide. The α and β anomers can be differentiated from the intensity of the peaks at m/z 145 and m/z 131. For α-anomer, the intensity of the peak at m/z 145 will be twice as intense as that of the peak at m/z 131, and for β–a reversed relationship being found. The peak at m/z 131 is more intense than that at m/z 145, but in the spectrum of the partially hydrolyzed and deionised samples, peak 131 is in much higher intensity. Hence it can be assumed that β-glycosidic linkages predominate.

The peak at m/z 342 and m/z 504 represents disaccharide and trisaccharide fragments. These di and tri saccharide units show the presence of (1→2), (1→4), (1→3) and (1→6) linkages by specific fragmentation pathways. The peaks at m/z 282 (+2), m/z 235 (±1,2) and m/z 119 seen in the spectrum of the Pg polysaccharide and in the spectrum of its partially hydrolysed samples are diagnostic of 1→2 and 1→4 glycosidic linkage. 1→4 linkage will give rise to peaks at m/z 282, 235 and 119 where as m/z 282 and 235 only are possible with 1→2 linkages. This observation is based on the studies of permethylated di and oligosaccharide acetates. Similarly peaks at m/z 269 and m/z 222 are diagnostic of 1→6 linkages. The peaks at m/z 311, m/z 293 and m/z 225 are also present very prominently in all the spectra indicating the glycosidic linkage at C-1. The occurrence of high quantity of pentaacetyl derivative of the monosaccharides may be rationalized to the highly crosslinked nature of the polysaccharides of *P. granatum*. Highly cross-linked structure inhibits methylation of free-OH group and in turn gets acetylated on hydrolysis and acetylation.

The mass spectrum of trimethyl silylated polysaccharides also gives a degradation pathway similar to those of the native samples and the permethylated acetates. Pg polysaccharide carries characteristic peaks of 1→2, 1→4 and 1→6 glycosidic linkages.

GC-MS

The GCMS experiments with the permethylated, hydrolysed, reduced and acetylated samples also largely supported the above-mentioned observations. For *P. granatum* compounds GC-MS gave 9 chromatographic fractions (Table 19.2).

The fragmentation patterns of each of the scans were analysed based on possible fragmentation in comparison with published data of partially methylated alditol acetates. In the case of the alditol acetates, the fragmentation is much more simpler than the pyranose forms of the saccharides because of the open chain structure of the alditol acetates. In this part, all the scans are not explained because the pathways for the primary fragmentation and also for the secondary fragments are same. One drawback in this study is that a GC plot is not available to calculate the relative areas of each fraction in the chromatogram in order to ascertain the molar ratios of the differently substituted alditol acetates. Further, the fragmentations of these derivatives do not give clear idea about the different stereoisomers of monosaccharides. However, the results of various fragments gave the glycosidic linkage positions in the monosaccharide units in the polysaccharides, as:

Table 19.2

Scan No	*Retention Time*	*M/z value (per cent intensity)*
1	8.5	233 (30), 205 (100), 189 (20), 173, 161 (40), 159 (55), 131 (60), 73
2	9	314 (18), 233 (40), 173 (25), 161 (30), 131 (45), 129 (60), 73 (100)
3	10.3	291 (15), 233 (35), 159 (30), 207 (100), 233 (20), 189 (30), 173
4	11.15	131 (45), 129 (100), 87 (30), 73 (80)
5	11.9	261 (40), 201 (100), 189 (25), 159 (30), 129 (35), 99 (40), 73 (40)
6	12.15	273 (30), 261 (45), 207 (100), 201 (20), 161 (35), 159 (35), 127 (30), 99, 73, 60, 43
7	12.45	261 (35), 207 (100), 201 (25), 189 (45), 159 (60), 98, 73, 45
8	12.75	405 (18), 389 (25), 247 (30), 215 (100), 201 (18), 174 (70), 161 (30), 98 (40), 73 (60), 45
9	16.4	433 (24), 417 (18), 373 (60), 247 (20), 215 (100), 174 (12), 159 (45), 99 (10), 73 (65)

C-1, 4, 6; C-1, 3; C-1, 4; C-1, 2, 3; C-3, 6; C-1, 2, 4; C-1, 6 substituted hexopyranoses.

From the above data the proposed structure of the Pg polysaccharide is as follows:

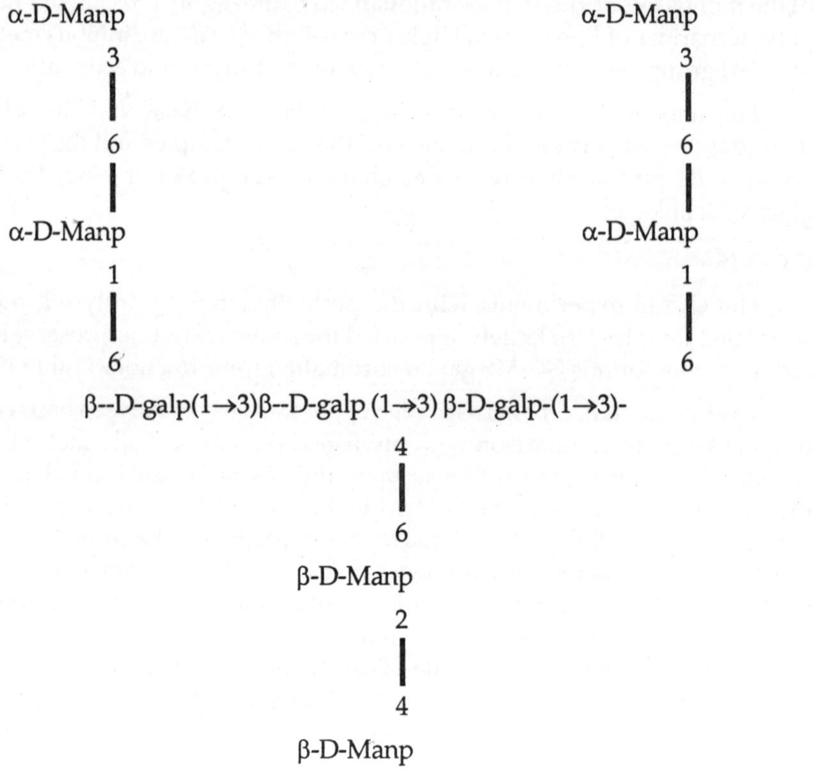

Biological Studies

Toxicity studies revealed that the Pg polysaccharide is non-toxic. The polysaccharide was found to inhibit cell proliferation of cultured peripheral blood lymphocytes and the human leukaemic cell line, K_{562}. It acted at the early stages of M phase (prophase) and prevented most of the cells from further progression in division. This resulted in several morphological changes in prophase.

The mode of action of the polysaccharide on cell proliferation could be better understood from cytological investigations on the bone marrow preparations of Swiss inbred mice which were given intraperitoneal injection with three different concentrations of the polysaccharide. The Pg polysaccharide caused cell division arrest mostly at prophase. Mitotic index, percentage of aberrations and percentage of aberrations in cells undergoing mitosis in the mouse bone marrow are given in Table 19.4.

Table 19.4

Drug Concentration	*Mitotic Index*	*Per cent of Aberrations*	*Per cent of Aberrations in Cells Undergoing Mitosis*
Normal controls	79	1	–
1 µg/ml	73	82	69
10 µg/ml	67.5	88	70
100 µg/ml	67	89	70.5

Per cent of aberrations in the control was taken as 1.

The effects of this polysaccharide at various concentrations on mouse bone marrow in different mitotic phases are shown in Table 19.5.

Table 19.5

Drug Concent-ration	*Nor-mal Inter-phase*	*Abnor-mal Inter-phase*	*Normal Pro-phase*	*Abno-rmal Pro-phase*	*Nor-mal Meta-phase*	*Abno-rmal Meta-phase*	*Nor-mal Ana-phase*	*Abno-rmal Ana-phase*	*Nor-mal Telo-phase*	*Abno-rmal Telo-phase*
Normal controls	200	10	300	-	80	-	20	-	390	-
1 µg/ml	140	130	40	650	-	30	-	10	-	-
10 µg/ml	120	185	-	690	-	10	-	-	-	-
100µg/ml	110	185	-	705	-	-	-	-	-	-

The polysaccharide from *Punica granatum* lowered the mitotic index in treated bone marrow. There was also a high incidence of mitotic aberrations. Stickiness of chromosomes at prophase, metaphase and anaphase leading pycnotic irregular nuclei was also observed (Figure 19.1).

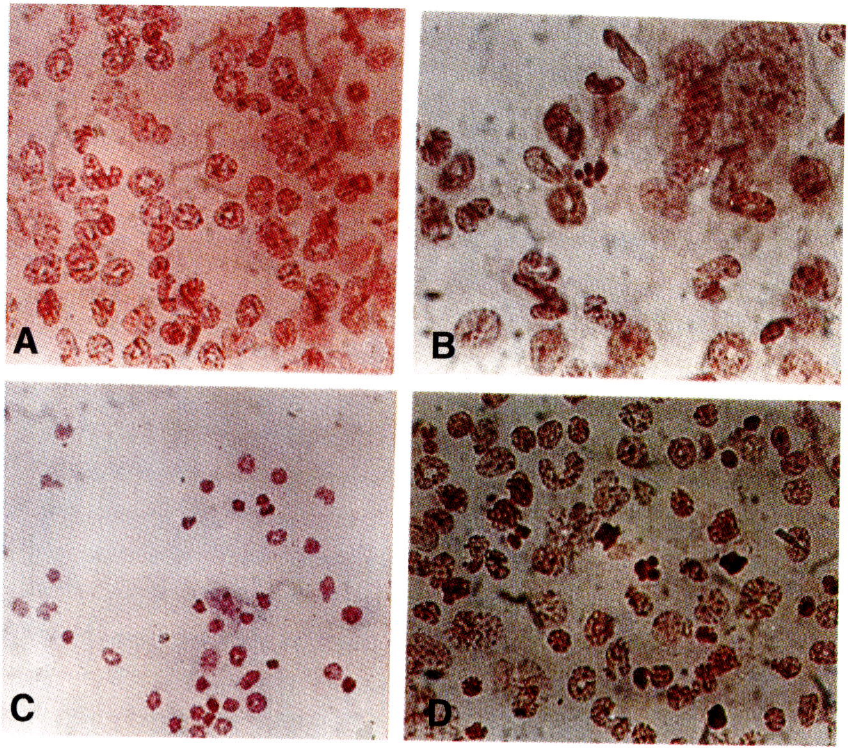

Figure 19.1: (A) Normal mouse bone marrow; (B) Mouse bonemarrow after 24 h treatment with 10 µg/ml Pg polysaccharide; (C) Mitotic arrest and stickiness at the metaphase resulting picnotic nuclei (10 µg/ml); (D) Mitotic arrest and stickiness at the prophase resulting picnotic nuclei (100 µg/ml).

The percentage of mitotic arrest and mitotic abnormalities increased with increasing concentrations. As in the case of cultured normal leucocytes and leukaemic cell line K_{562} the polysaccharide from *Punica granatum* blocked cell division at prophase. Clumping and stickiness of chromosome at prophase and metaphase was a salient feature of treated bone marrow cells. Structural aberrations of chromosomes and micronuclei were observed only rarely.

These effects qualify the polysaccharide to be in the group of antimitotic substances described by several authors (21,22). Nagl 1970 has expressed the view that endoreduplication, endomitosis and c-mitosis occur as a result of blockage to the cell cycle at G_2, early prophase and metaphase respectively (23). Blockage of the cell cycle at G_2 phase results in the lengthening of the synthetic phase (S-Phase) giving better chance for extra replication of chromatin, which results in endoreduplication. According to Nagl (1970) blockage of mitosis at early prophase results in endomitosis which is characterised by the visual replication of the chromosome inside intact nuclear membrane. Blockage of mitosis at metaphase results in C-mitosis, which can happen in the absence of colchicine either spontaneously or induced by antimitotic substances.

It has also been observed that the polysaccharide is capable of causing stickiness of chromosome, spindle abnormalities and arrest of cell cycle at interphase, prophase and early metaphase stages. Deysson 1968 stated that several antimitotic substances share these properties (22). The mechanism of action of mitotic inhibition of this polysaccharide may be attributed to apoptosis, which is being evaluated. In the light of the present results it is essential to evaluate further the mechanism of action of this polysaccharide as a mitotic inhibitor, a potential anticancer agent, by identification of the target proteins.

Structure Activity Relationship

Earlier reports suggest that there is a strong relationship between the structure and antitumor activities of polysaccharides.

Although common polysaccharides such as starch [an α-(1→4) glucan], dextran [an α-(1→6) glucan], and inulin (a fructan), do not have antitumor activity (10), →there is abundant evidence that mannans and selected glucans are potent anti-cancer agents (11). The factors that determine whether a polysaccharide will have antitumor activity are unclear. However, there appears to be a direct relationship between the antitumor activity of polysaccharides and their ability to interact with serum albumin (12). This may simply reflect the ability of these molecules to bind to proteins. The soluble D–glucans have antitumor activity if they are mainly linear, without excessively long branches, and are relatively resistant to degradation by glucanases. Thus, glycogen, starch, and dextrans are inactive. Compounds with long stretches of β-(l→3) linkages are effective (12). Loss of tertiary structure by denaturation also causes loss of activity. Dextrans may be activated if attached to diethylaminoethyl groups. Studies on synthetic β-(l→6) linked celluloses suggest that antitumor activity against sarcoma–l80 is greatest in molecules with a high degree of polymerization and a homogeneous distribution of side chains (13). The structure and antitumor activity of Smith-type degradation products (OL-2-I, OL-2-II and OL-2-III) of an alkali-soluble glucan, OL-2, isolated from a crude fungal drug "Leiwan" (*Omphalia lapidescens*) were investigated by Saito *et al.* (24) and the results indicated that the degree of beta-linked branching at position 6 was remarkably related to the antitumor activity. In the present study also a β-(1→3) linkages in the backbone (main chain) and additional β-(1→6)-branch points are observed which are reported for antitumor activity earlier (2).

Conclusion

Effective chemoprevention and therapy of cancer require the identification of specific molecular targets. Modulation of the chromatin status may enable us to develop rational chemopreventive/therapeutic strategies for human cancer. Many antimitotic natural compounds alter the polymerization dynamics of microtubules, blocking mitosis, and consequently, inducing cell death by apoptosis. eg. *Vinca* alkaloids, cryptophycins, halichondrins, estramustine, and colchicines.

Today drugs those are specific to defined cell cycle processes are available but are not adequate enough, which demands new chemotherapeutic drug development from natural sources. The biological activities of plant polysaccharides have attracted more attention recently in the biochemical and medical areas because of their antitumor effects. The present study unveils that the polysaccharide isolated from *Punica granatum*, a heteropolymer with mannose and galactose as monomer units, is a potent inhibitor of mitosis and inducer of apoptosis. The molecular mechanism of action is, however, not clear. Since mitosis forms the most important phase of cell cycle, inhibitors of this phase are found to be effective as antitumor agents. Hence, further studies on the mechanism of action of this polysaccharide as a mitotic inhibitor may be promising in its development as an antitumor drug.

References

1. Wasser SP, Weis AL: Medicinal properties of substances occurring in higher basidiomycete mushrooms: current perspectives (review). *Int J Med Mushrooms* 1999, 1, 31-62.
2. Wasser SP: Medicinal mushrooms as a source of antitumor and immunomodulating polysaccharides. *Appl Microbiol Biotechnol* 2002, 60, 258-274.
3. Ooi VE, Liu F: A review of pharmacological activities of Mushroom polysaccharides. *Int J Med Mushrooms* 1999, 1, 195-206.
4. Mizuno T, Yeohli P, Kinoshita T, Zhuang C, Ito H, Mayuzumi Y: Antitumor activity of chemical modification of polysaccharides from Nioshimeji mushroom *Tricholoma giganteum*. *Biosci Biotechnol Biochem* 1996, 60, 30-33.
5. Mizuno T: The extraction and development of antitumour-active polysaccharides from medicinal mushrooms in Japan. *Int J Med Mushrooms* 1999, 1, 9-29.
6. Alam N, Gupta PC: Structure of a water-soluble polysaccharide from the seeds of *Cassia angustifolia*. *Planta Med* 1986, 50, 308-310.
7. Dubois M, Gilles KA, Hamilton JK, Rebers PA, Smith F: Colorimetric method for determination of sugar and related substances. *Analytical Chemistry*, 1956, 28, 350-356.
8. Mathews MB, Decker L: *Biochim Biophys Acta*, 1971, 244, 30.
9. Yagi A, Nishimura H, Shida T, Nishioka I: Structure determination of polysaccharides in *Aloe arborescens* var. natalensis. *Planta Med* 1986, 50, 213-218.
10. Brantigam M, Franz G: Structural features of *Plantago lanceolata* mucilage. *Planta Med* 1985, 48, 293-97.
11. Bailey RW: Oligosaccharides, Pergamon Press Oxford. 1965, *V*, pp 97-101.
12. Chauhan AG, De Courters JE, Dizet PL: *Bull Soc Chem Biol* 1960, 42, 227-230.
13. Aspinall GO, Rashbrook RB, Kerster GK: *J Chem Soc* 1958, 215-221.
14. Tyminski A, Timell TE: *J Am Chem Soc* 1960, 82, 2823-2827.
15. Hakomoris: A rapid permethylation of glycolipid, and polysaccharide catalyzed by methylsulfinyl carbanion in dimethyl sulfoxide. *The J Biochem* 1964, 55, 205-208.

16. Sawardeker JS, Sloneker JH, Jeaner A: *Anal Chem* 1965, 37, 1602.
17. Sweeky CC, Wells WW, Bentley: Methods in Enzymology (Ed). Elizabeth F, Neufeld and Victor Ginsburg: Academic Press. 1966, 8, 96-97.
18. Roklin RE: Mediators of Cellular Immunity. *In:* Basic and clinical immunology. Los Altos CA: Lange Medical Publications 1976, 102-113.
19. Biesele JJ: Mitotic poisons and the cancer problem. Elsevier, Houston, 1958.
20. Morrehead PS, Nowell PC, Mellman WJ *et al.*: *Expt Cell Res* 1960, 20, 613-616.
21. Larramendry ML, Bulout FN, Bianchi NO, Olivero OA: *Mutation Research* 1980, 79,133-140.
22. Deysson G: Antimitotic substances. *Int Rev Cytol* 1968, 24, 99-148.
23. Nagl W: The mitotic and endomitotic nuclear cycle in *Allium cariantum*. II. Relations between DNA replication and chromatin structure. Caryologia 1970, 23, 71-78.
24. Saito H, Yoshioka Y, Uchara N, Aketagawa J, Tanaka S and Shibata Y: Relationship between conformation and biological response for (1→3)–β</ span>-D-glucans in the activation of coagulation Factor G from limulus amebocyte lysate and host-mediated antitumour activity. Demonstraiton of single-helix conformation as a stimulant. *Carbohydrate Research* 1991, 217, 181-190.

Chapter 20

Documentation of Traditional Knowledge and IPR Protection Related to Plants Used for Food and Medicine

S. Rajasekharan[1*], P.G. Latha[1] and P. Pushpangadan[2]

[1]*Division of Ethnomedicine and Ethnopharmacology, Tropical Botanic Garden and Research Institute, Palode, Thiruvananthapuram – 695 562*
E-mail: ethmed_tbgri@yahoo.co.in
**E-mail: drrajsek@yahoo.com*

[2]*Amity Institute for Herbal and Biotech Products Development, TC 10/910(1), VRA-173, Mannamoola, Peroorkada, Thiruvananthapuram – 695 005*
E-mail: palpuprakulam@yahoo.co.in

Introduction

The World Intellectual Property Organization (WIPO) uses the term "Traditional Knowledge" to refer the tradition based literary, artistic or scientific works; performances; inventions; scientific discoveries; designs; marks, names and symbols; undisclosed information; and all other tradition based innovations and creations resulting from intellectual activity in the industrial, scientific, literary or artistic fields. "Tradition based" refers to knowledge systems, creations, innovations and cultural expressions which have generally been transmitted from generation to generation and are generally regarded as pertaining to a particular people or its territory; they are constantly evolving in response to changing environment.

Categories of Traditional Knowledge

World Intellectual Property Organization (WIPO) has categorized Traditional Knowledge into different sectors like Agricultural knowledge, Scientific knowledge, Technical knowledge, Ecological knowledge, Ethnomedical knowledge etc.

Significance of Traditional Knowledge (TK)

Significance of TK is exclusively linked with culture and society, well connected with community practices, institutions, relationships, customs, beliefs, religions and rituals. Traditional Knowledge acts as a source for decision making of various developmental activities. This is also considered as a valuable asset of the community, helping them to shape and control their own development.

TK in development helps to increase efficiency and is cost effective and helpful for developing appropriate technology. Effectiveness of TK improves chances of adoption and is an integral part of local communities. Sustainability of TK facilitates mutual adoption and learning, and empowers local communities.

In the current IPR regime, documentation of TK with appropriate protection will prevent misappropriation and wrong patenting. Documentation of ethnomedical wisdom would further help the identification of promising plants/other materials to be selected for detailed scientific investigation and validation. It may also help in establishing linkages with the plan process, especially in the formulation of innovative programmes and projects that can be implemented at grass root level. Value addition of selected plants/other materials may help to enhance the socio-economic status of the knowledge providers/ custodians as well as the community as a whole.

Documentation of TK in India

Documentation of Traditional Knowledge (TK), especially ethnobiological aspects were carried out in India under the 'Man and Biosphere Programme'. This programme was originally conceived by Dr. M.S. Swaminathan and later it was formulated as a project namely 'All India Co-ordinated Research Project on Ethnobiology (AICRPE)' by Dr. T.N. Khoshoo in 1980 the then Director of NBRI, Lucknow. It was originally launched by DST, Govt. of India in 1982 and later it was brought under the newly created Ministry of Environment and Forest, Govt. of India for the documentation and scientific validation of TK related to plants, animals and micro-organisms in India. They set up a Co-ordination Unit at Regional Research Laboratory (CSIR) Jammu, with Dr. P. Pushpangadan, as the Chief Co-ordinator of the project.

AICRPE was a multi-institutional, multidisciplinary action oriented research programme aimed at documenting the multidimensional perspectives of the life, culture, tradition and knowledge of the tribal communities of India. The duration of the project was over a period of 16 years and it generated a vast wealth of database on Ethnobiological information.

The study revealed that over 10,000 wild plant species are used by tribal communities of India in meeting various requirements. About 8000 species are used for medicinal purposes, 3500 species for edible purposes, 550 species for fibre, 425 for gum, resin and dyes, 325 for pesticides and 1000 for other purposes.

An intensive survey conducted by Dr. S. Rajasekharan and his team in this sector in Kerala and Lakshadweep during the period from 1987 to 1992 has provided rich and varied ethnobiological data collected from the different tribal communities and local healers. It includes documentation on 500 single remedies and more than 200 simple formulations. Apart from this, the materials used for housing, fish poisoning, pesticides, food, fibre, dyes etc. were also collected and documented in the form of database.

The senior author and his team also carried out documentation of TK of the Kani and Malapandaram tribes of Kerala during 2001 and 2002 and have recorded the ethnomedical uses of 82 single drugs and 15 combinations.

The senior author and his team have conducted (2003-2004) another random survey on documentation of TK related to medicinal plants from 15 selected Grama Panchayats of 3 southern districts of Kerala under the project "Promotion of Traditional Technical Knowledge" sponsored by the Kerala State Planning Board. The study revealed that 200 to 225 medicinal plants are used as single drugs in each Panchayat, for treating various disorders like diabetes, jaundice, sinusitis, hypertension, cancer, diarrhoea, etc. and 250 polyherbal combinations are used by the local healers.

TK related to traditional medicine in India

Classical Health Tradition (CHT)

- Vedic / classical texts and treatises like Rig Veda, Atharva Veda, Charaka Samhita
- (Text on ancient Indian Medicine)
- Susrutha Samhita (Text on ancient Indian Surgery), Ashtangahridaya (Text on ancient Indian medicine and surgery) and numerous other related text books in both sanskrit and regional languages

Oral Health Tradition (OHT)

- Traditionally trained folk healers/ village physicians
- Not traditionally trained but experienced in certain health practices (*e.g.* Dai, bonesetters, specialists in treating poisons, jaundice, mental disorders).
- Aged people of different ethnic communities including women treating the patients based on the knowledge acquired from their predecessors.
- Individuals who acquired (educated group) certain knowledge from their predecessors.
- Tribal communities/ physicians/ aged individuals.

Methodology

Documentation of TK from individuals / communities / traditional / local / tribal healers of the selected Panchayats was one of the most difficult tasks, because

METHODOLOGY

↓

TRAINING / AWARENESS ON DOCUMENTATION OF IK/TK (INSTITUTE LEVEL)

↓

TRAINING/ AWARENESS ON IK DOCUMENTATION (PANCHAYATH LEVEL)

↓

TEAM BUILDING AND VISION DEVELOPMENT

↓

ENTRY TO PANCHAYATH

↓

INTERVIEW / MEETING WITH INDIVIDUALS/IK/TK HOLDERS

↓

DATA POOLING AND ANALYSIS

↓

PREPARATION OF DATABASE WITH ADEQUATE PROTECTION

↓

IK/TK DOCUMENTATION

↓

DIGITALISATION OF TK

↓

DEVELOPING VIABLE MODELS FOR THE PROTECTION OF IK/TK WITH LEGAL FRAME WORK

↓

RAPPORT ESTABLISHMENT WITH LOCAL BODY MEMBERS AND OWNERS OF IK/TK

↓

AWARENESS ON PRIOR INFORMED CONSENT

↓

ESTABLISHMENT OF DATA BANK

of the secretive nature of the information and the reluctance of the custodians to disclose, for fear of losing their source of income as well as occupation. Through seminars / discussions and contact programmes concerted efforts were made to win their faith and to persuade them to take a decision on the subject. They were also educated about the purpose and necessity of documenting this information in the larger interests of protection of IPR. They were assured that the information collected from them would not be exploited for monetary gain and in the event of development of a commercially useful product as a result of R&D efforts, they would receive the just and equitable share of the benefit accrued. Data were classified under three categories - Undisclosed, Partially Disclosed and Disclosed. Methodology adopted for the present study is given below in the flow chart. The informations were thus collected after obtaining a written Prior Informed Consent (PIC).

Intellectual Property Rights (IPR) and Benefit Sharing

The term 'intellectual property' is loosely defined as a 'Product of the mind'. According to World Intellectual Property Organisation, one of the specialized agencies of the U.N system, 'Intellectual Property', shall include rights related to:

1. Literary, artistic and scientific work.
2. Performance of performing artists, phonograms and broadcasts.
3. Invention in all fields of human endeavour.
4. Scientific discoveries.
5. Industrial design.
6. Trade marks, service marks and commercial names and designations.
7. Protection against unfair competition and all other rights resulting from intellectual activities in the industrial, scientific, literary or artistic fields.

Intellectual Property is a category of public law that generally includes Patents, Copyrights, Trademarks, Geographical Indications, Industrial Designs, Utility Models, Plant Breeders Rights, Integrated Circuits Rights and Trade Secrets. A *sui generis* regime for databases has also been established in some countries.

Patent

Patent is an exclusive right granted by a country to the owner of an invention, to make, use, manufacture and market the invention, provided the invention satisfies certain conditions stipulated in law. The conditions are: (*i*) Novelty , (*ii*) Inventiveness (Non-obviousness) , (*iii*) Usefulness.

Novelty

An invention will be considered novel if it does not form a part of the global state of art. Information appearing in magazines, technical journals, books, newspapers etc. constitutes the state of the art. Oral description of the invention in a seminar / conference can also spoil the novelty.

Inventiveness (Non-obviousness)

A patent application involves an inventive step if the proposed invention is not obvious to a person skilled in the art ie, skilled in the subject matter of the patent application.

Usefulness

An invention must possess utility for the grant of patent. No valid patent can be granted for an invention devoid of utility.

How to Protect TK Related Knowledge

The Convention of Biological Diversity (CBD) which has entered into force since 1993 is a unique international legal instrument to protect the sovereign rights of the countries and people over their biological resources including traditional knowledge.

CBD explicitly recognizes the sovereign rights of the state over their biological resources, [Article 15(1)], and the need to respect, preserve and maintain the knowledge, innovations and practices of indigenous and local communities and share with them the benefits arising from their use [Article (8)]. CBD also recognizes under Articles 15(1), the sovereign rights of state over their natural resources and the authority to determine access to genetic resources subject to national legislation. Article 15(4) and Article 15(5) subject this access to other contracting parties on 'mutually agreed terms' and 'prior informed consent'. The Convention thus establishes a new international legal frame work to assist the sovereignty of states over their genetic resources and authority of states to determine access to resources requiring prior informed consent on mutually agreed terms and confirming that countries providing genetic resources are entitled to fair and equitable share of benefits that arise from their commercialization. If we examine the Article 8 and 15 together we will get the implicit impression that the National Governments have to play the key role in the implementation of these Articles by due process of legislation and formulation of appropriate rules and regulations. Also fair equitable sharing of benefits from their knowledge will only be possible if the local communities are empowered to seek fair access and benefit sharing arrangements.

The benefit sharing provision envisaged in CBD under Article 8(j) and 15(1) was implemented in letter and spirit by Tropical Botanic Garden and Research Institute, Trivandrum, Kerala. The model relates to the development of the scientifically validated herbal drug named **'Jeevani'** based on a tribal lead. While obtaining the specific information about the medicinal value of wild plants from the tribal community, the researchers assured them, that the benefits will be shared with them in an equitable manner. TBGRI was successful in developing a scientifically validated herbal drug and while transferring the technology for the production of the drug to a pharmaceutical firm, it agreed to share the license fee and royalty with the tribal community on a 1:1 basis. The major players involved in the transaction are TBGRI and the Kani tribe. By this action, for the first time in India and perhaps in the world, the tribal intellectual property rights were recognized by TBGRI in a dignified manner. TBGRI also demonstrated to the world that Indigenous Knowledge system is a viable source and the owners of the Indigenous Knowledge should be rewarded whenever it is utilised for a commercially viable product and process.

Benefit Sharing (Mechanism Worked Out)

Kani tribe registered a Trust called 'Kerala Kani Samudaya Kshema Trust' with the guidance of TBGRI and the benefits received by the technology transfer and royalty has been remitted to the Trust's account.

Benefit Sharing (Mechanism Implemented)

Later, in consultation with TBGRI the Executive Committee of the Trust decided to felicitate the three Kani tribesmen who divulged the information about Arogyapacha. Accordingly, they were felicitated by the trust and two of them were given Rs. 20,000/- each (Sri. Mallan Kani and Sri Kuttimathan Kani) and Rs. 10,000/- was given to Eachan Kani (grand total Rs. 50,000/-) as prize / compensation. This amount has been taken from the first year interest of the 5 lakh rupees remitted to the trust's account. They also decided to maintain Rs. 5 lakh as the permanent asset of the trust in the bank and only the interest of that money would be utilised for the welfare activities of Kani tribe. Rs. 2500 is maintained as fixed deposit in the name of two Kani girls aged 8 and 10 whose mother was killed by a wild elephant in 2002. Recently they have constructed a community hall-cum-office of the Trust at Chonampara tribal settlement and they also purchased a Jeep for transportation of people, marketing goods and NWFP. Kerala Kani Samudaya Kshema Trust has given employment to two Kani tribesmen as Driver of the Jeep and Helper and both of them are drawing salary every month. Telephone facility has been installed in the office of the Trust. Construction of a small building is now in progress for providing computer facilities to the school children.

Negotiation is in progress to renew the manufacturing license of Jeevani to suitable pharmaceutical agencies for another 7 year-period. This will provide more financial benefit to the Kani Tribe. They are planning to do large scale cultivation of Arogyapacha involving 450 Kani families residing near the Agastiar Hills of Kerala.

Recognition to TBGRI Model of Benefit Sharing–UN Equator Initiative Award

TBGRI model of Benefit Sharing was acclaimed the world over and in the World Summit on Sustainable Development held at Johannesburg, in 2002 Dr. P. Pushpangadan received the UN Equator Initiative Award under individual category. The secretary of the trust, Sri. Kuttimathan Kani attended the World Summit as an invitee and received the Certificate of Excellence on behalf of the Kerala Kani Samudaya Kshema Trust.

For biodiversity rich nations documentation of traditional knowledge associated with biodiversity is of paramount importance especially with regard to the protection of IPR related to traditional knowledge. In recent years there has been a growing interest in aquiring traditional knowledge associated with plants especially by the pharmaceutical firms engaged in developing novel natural product based drugs. In this context in order to safeguard the interest of the knowledge providers it is necessary that such knowledge should be documented to establish the ownership rights of individuals, communities as well as nations.

Index